Antiviral Agents

Agents

Advances and Problems

Special Topic

Progress in Drug Research

Edited by Ernst Jucker, Basel

Board of Advisors
Joseph M. Colacino
Pushkar N. Kaul
Vera M. Kolb
J. Mark Treherne
Q. May Wang

Authors
Shijun Ren and Eric J. Lien
Noel A. Roberts
Q. May Wang and Beverly A. Heinz
Kirk A. Staschke and Joseph M. Colacino
Elcira C. Villarreal
Q. May Wang

Springer Basel AG

Editor

Dr. E. Jucker
Steinweg 28
CH-4107 Ettingen
Switzerland
e-mail: jucker.pdr@bluewin.ch

The reviews collected in this monograph are updated and revised versions of the articles published in PDR 50 (1998), PDR 51 (1998) and PDR 52 (1999), except for the unchanged reviews by Q. May Wang and Beverly A. Heinz (PDR 55, 2000), Elcira C. Villarreal (PDR 56, 2001) and Noel A. Roberts (PDR 56, 2001).

Deutsche Bibliothek Cataloging-in-Publication Data
Antiviral agents : advances and problems / ed. Ernst Jucker. Board of advisors Joseph M. Colacino ... Authors Shijun Ren ....
  (Progress in drug research ; Special topic)
  ISBN 978-3-7643-6547-9   ISBN 978-3-0348-7784-8 (eBook)
  DOI 10.1007/978-3-0348-7784-8

ISBN 978-3-7643-6547-9

Printed on acid-free paper produced from chlorine-free pulp. TCF ∞
Cover design and layout: Gröflin Graphic Design, Basel

ISBN 978-3-7643-6547-9
9 8 7 6 5 4 3 2 1

Contents

Contents

Foreword by the Editor

The unfortunate appearance of AIDS, the manyfold problems with herpesviruses and other viruses attacking humans have lead to an enormous dynamism of worldwide research and to an immense increase in the corresponding literature. With this first Special Volume of the monograph series *Progress in Drug Research*, the Editor and the Publishers undertake an effort to supply concise reviews on virus research and especially on efforts to develop new antiviral agents in a few selected classes of important and widespread viral diseases. Latest *Progress in Drug Research* articles dealing with new chemotherapeutics for the treatment of the most threatening viral diseases are presented here. These articles found a wide echo and were upgraded and supplemented with most topical chapters to form this actual overview of the achievements in the respective fields of virus research.

This Special-Topic Volume contains six review articles covering the latest studies on the HIV and hepatitis C and B virus as well as herpes- and influenzaviruses. Other worldwide diseases, like polio, hepatitis A and the common cold, are dealt with in context with the broad family of picornoviruses.

Despite certain advances in the treatment of the HIV virus infection, there is still a strong need for novel chemotherapeutics. A particularly interesting field of research is found in the HIV protease inhibitors. In "Development of HIV protease inhibitors: a survey", the structure-activity relationship of a number of HIV chemotherapeutics is discussed and a glance thrown at future drugs.

"Anti-influenza drugs and neuraminidase inhibitors" describes in great detail rationally designed neuroaminidase inhibitors that block the viral life cycle and appear to be well tolerated and effective against all types of influenza. It seems that the victory over influenza infections has become a realistic prospect within reach.

The still unsolved problems of chronic hepatitis in humans caused by the hepatitis C virus is today met with prophylactic vaccines on one hand, and the discovery of novel molecules to inhibit proteins essential for viral functions, on the other. "Recent advances in prevention and treatment of hepatitis C virus infections" summarizes the latest findings and will serve as a "buoy" to those who need fixed points in this rapidly changing field.

Innumerable humans suffering from chronic hepatitis throughout the world are victims of the hepatitis B virus. Despite the existence of a safe and effective vaccine, the prevalence of hepatitis B has not yet declined significantly. The resulting call for more selective antiviral agents is met with in "Drug discovery and development of antiviral agents for the treatment of chronic hepatitis B infection". This recently updated review presents novel approaches, including antisense and gene therapy. The authors also offer new perspectives on the challenging identification and development of anti-HBV agents.

Most up-to-date information on herpesvirus diseases as well as viral replication strategies are presented in a final article. So far, all approved treatments are uniquely based on the DNA-polymerase approach. Thus, the discussion of viral targets other than DNA polymerase are of utmost interest. Such new antiviral agents are discussed in "Current and potential therapies for the treatment of herpesvirus infections".

Another important virus family accounts for human pathogens including rhino- and hepatitis A virus. "Protease inhibitors as potential antiviral agents for the treatment of picornaviral infections" completes this special volume by documenting the essential role played by two viral proteases (2Apro and 3Cpro) in viral replication and summarizing recent approaches in the design of novel 2A and 3C protease inhibitors as potential antiviral agents.

The Editor is grateful to the authors for their profound research and comprehensively written articles. I would also like to thank the members of the Birkhäuser Publishing Inc. staff, and in particular Daniela Brunner from the Editorial Office: She was a great help in selecting the topics and putting emphasis on vital spots. I am also indebted to Ruedi Jappert, Bernd Luchner, Eduard Mazenauer and Gregor Messmer for having contributed their help, vast knowledge and experience. It is a great privilege to have such a harmonious and rewarding relationship with these persons.

My very special thanks go to Hans-Peter Thür, Birkhäuser Publishing's CEO. For decades Mr. Thür has put great personal interest and perseverance into the *Progress in Drug Research* series. Not surprisingly, this first and particular Special Volume of PDR owes its existence to Mr. Thür's initiative and support.

Basel, May 2001   Dr. E. Jucker

Antiviral Agents – Advances and Problems (E. Jucker, Ed.)
©2001 Birkhäuser Verlag, Basel (Switzerland)

Development of HIV protease inhibitors: A survey

By Shijun Ren and Eric J. Lien

Department of Pharmaceutical Sciences, School of Pharmacy, University of Southern California, Los Angeles, CA 90089-9121, USA

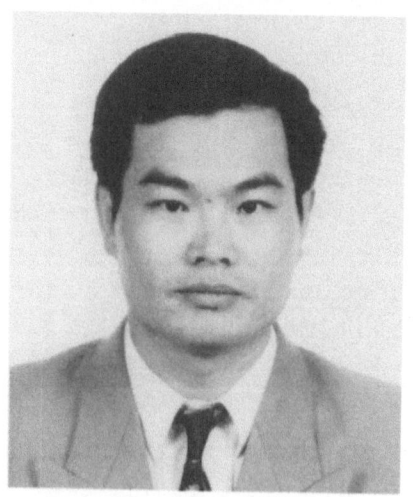

Shijun Ren

received his B. S. in pharmacy from Shandong Medical University, China, in 1987. In the same year, he joined the Institute of Pharmaceutical Research, Shandong Academy of Medical Sciences as a research assistant. From 1995 to 1997, he was a visiting research scholar in the School of Pharmacy, University of Southern California under the guidance of Dr. Eric J. Lien. In 1997, Mr. Ren was admitted to the School of Pharmacy, University of Southern California as a Ph.D. student. His research interests include structure-activity/permeability relationship, molecular modeling, cancer chemopreventive natural products, antioxidant phytophenolics, and anticancer and antiviral drug design and synthesis.

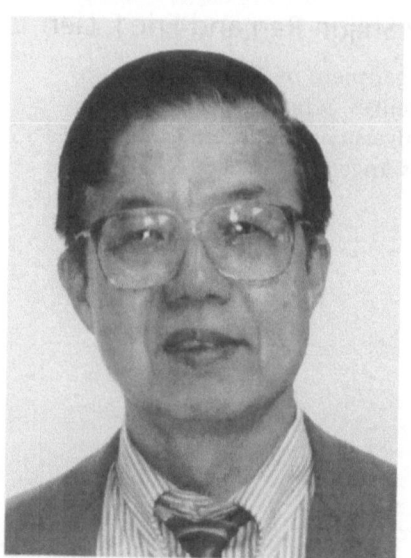

Eric J. Lien

received his Ph.D. from the University of California San Francisco Medical Center in 1966. In 1968, he joined the University of Southern California as a faculty member. Professor Lien's research interests include structure-activity relationship and drug design, physical organic chemistry and natural products. Ongoing research projects include design, synthesis, and testing of antiviral and anticancer agents; refinement of quantitative structure-activity relationship models for application in vivo and in vitro gastrointestinal and percutaneous absorption of drugs and isolation of bioactive natural products like immunostimulating polysaccharides from Chinese herbs. He has served as a consultant to various government agencies, universities and private cooperations. His most recent work deals with the evolution of biomacromolecules, from thermoneutrons to living organisms.

Summary

In the treatment of infections caused by rapidly mutating viruses like human immunodeficiency virus (HIV), combination therapy with multiple drugs acting by different mechanisms offers several advantages over monotherapy. It may provide: synergistic effect, possible reduction of dosages and side-effects, and reduction of the chance of drug resistance. In the past few years, hundreds of HIV protease inhibitors have been synthesized and tested in order to overcome the limitations of reverse transcriptase inhibitors like zidovudine and others. In this review, emphasis is placed on the development of HIV protease inhibitors as antiviral agents against HIV, and structure-activity relationship analysis of saquinavir and related compounds. Limitations of some protease inhibitors and ways to overcome the shortcomings are presented. Among these many protease inhibitors five have been marketed during 1995–1999. They are saquinavir, ritonavir, indinavir, nelfinavir and amprenavir. Their different structural features, important physicochemical, pharmacokinetic and clinical profiles are presented in a table form for easy comparison. It is hoped that in the future new drugs based on additional mechanisms can be developed for the treatment of AIDS.

Contents

Shijun Ren and Eric J. Lien

Keywords

AIDS; amprenavir; antiviral agents; chemotherapy; HIV protease inhibitors; indinavir; nelfinavir; ritonavir; saquinavir; structure-activity relationship (SAR).

Glossary of abbreviations

AHPBA: 3-amino-2-hydroxy-4-phenylbutanoic acid; AHPPA: 4-amino-3-hydroxy-5-phenylpentanoic acid; AIDS: acquired immunodeficiency syndrome; AZT: zidovudine; BN: β-naphthoyl; Boc: tert-butyloxycarbonyl; Clog P: calculated log P; CNA: β-cyanoalanyl; CYP3A4: cytochrome P450 3A4; C2: two-fold rotational symmetry; ddC: zalcitabine; ddI: didanosine; DIC: (4aS,8aS)-decahydro-3(S)-isoquinolinecarbonyl; d4T: stavudine; GT: glucuronosyl transferase; HIV: human immunodeficiency virus; Log P: partition coefficient in octanol/water; ; Mlog P: measured log P; MW: molecular weight; NRTI: nucleoside reverse transcriptase inhibitors; PIC: piperidine-2(S)-carbonyl; QC: quinoline-2-carbonyl; RT: reverse transcriptase; SAR: structure-activity relationship; SMC: S-methyl-cysteinyl; 3TC: lamivudine; tBu: tert-butyl; Z: benzyloxycarbonyl.

1 Introduction

Human immunodeficiency virus (HIV) has been identified as the determining agent of acquired immunodeficiency syndrome (AIDS). Many approaches such as HIV reverse transcriptase inhibitors have been used to prevent replication of this virus [1]. Unfortunately, the most widely used HIV reverse transcriptase inhibitors like zidovudine (Retrovir, AZT), didanosine (Videx, ddI), zalcitabine (Hivid, ddC), stavudine (Zerit, d4T) and lamivudine (Epivir, 3TC) have significant toxicity, and mutations in the viral target can lead to drug resistance [2]. Although reverse transcriptase inhibitors block viral replication in newly-infected cells by preventing an early step in the HIV replication cycle, such antiretroviral drugs have no effect on virus production by cells in which reverse transcription and integration have already occurred [3].

Recently, protease inhibitors, a newly developed drug class targeted at HIV protease, have shown considerable promise in prevention of HIV replication, especially in combination therapy. Five protease inhibitors are currently on the market: saquinavir mesylate (Invirase (hard gelatin capsule), Fortovase (soft gelatin capsule)), ritonavir (Norvir), indinavir sulfate (Crixivan), nelfinavir mesylate (Viracept), and amprenavir (Agenerase) [4a, 4b]. In this review, we shall focus on the development of HIV protease

4

inhibitors, SAR analysis of saquinavir and related compounds, comparison of five marketed HIV protease inhibitors and future prospect in new drug development.

2 HIV protease as a target for chemotherapy

HIV protease was first suggested as a potential target for AIDS therapy by Kramer et al. in 1986 [5]. HIV protease is a proteolytic enzyme responsible for cleaving large numbers of amino acid sequences. This enzyme regulates conversion of these large amino acid sequences into biologically active structural and functional protein products. Specifically, HIV protease is responsible for the enzymatic processing of the *gag* and *gag-pol* genes of HIV, which encode for functional core proteins and viral enzymes (reverse transcriptase, ribonuclease H, integrase, and HIV protease). The polyproteins encoded by the *gag* and *gag-pol* genes undergo post-translational processing by HIV protease to form functional protein products as the viral particles budding out from infected cells. Therefore, inhibition of HIV protease by a protease inhibitor results in the release of immature, noninfectious viral particles [4].

HIV protease inhibitors act at a late stage in the viral replication cycle, whereas the reverse transcriptase inhibitors inhibit reverse transcriptase, which is responsible for producing double-stranded DNA from viral RNA at an early stage. By targeting another site in the process of HIV replication, protease inhibitors have a greater impact on HIV replication, especially when combined with the nucleoside analogues [6].

3 Design of protease inhibitors

3.1 Basis of rational design of HIV protease inhibitors

On the basis of the primary amino acid sequence, inhibition by pepstatin and the crystal structure of HIV- 1 protease, this enzyme has been classified as an aspartic protease [7]. Further studies have shown that the HIV-1 protease is a C_2 symmetric homodimer in which each of the identical 99 amino acid subunits contributes a single aspartyl residue to the catalytic site. The two acid residues are juxtaposed about the C_2 axis of the diad [8, 9]. The native HIV-

5

1 protease comprises four interdigitated strands of β-sheet, a projecting loop from each monomer enclosing the catalytic cleft. The active site triad Asp[25]-Thr[26]-Gly[27] is located within a loop whose structure is stabilized by hydrogen bonds. The loops of each monomer are also interlinked by four hydrogen bonds. The structures of several enzyme-inhibitor complexes are similar to that of the native dimer, only with differences in the "flap" region [6]. In the early 1970s, Cohen, Lee and Lien have noted that molecular symmetry is an important property of a molecule regarding its activity and toxicity [10]. These axiomatic spatial relationships have served as a foundation for the design of protease inhibitors.

Catalysis by aspartic protease is generally considered to proceed via a high-energy tetrahedral transition state formed by addition of water to the scissile amide bond of the substrate. Since the transition state binds to the enzyme more tightly than either the substrate or the products, a stable transition-state mimetic has been used to design aspartic protease inhibitors [6]. So far, most of the HIV protease inhibitors are stable transition state analogues whose peptide-like structures mimic amide bonds (e.g. Phe-Pro or Tyr-Pro which are cleaved by HIV protease), but only very rarely recognized by other mammalian aspartic proteases. This results in the selective inhibition of HIV protease with no or limited effect on the activity of other structurally related human aspartic proteases such as renin and pepsin.

3.2   New development of HIV protease inhibitors

Three different kinds of approaches have been used in the design of protease inhibitors. One is the transition-state mimetic which includes hydroxyethylene dipeptide isostere, statine, phosphinic acid, difluoromethylketone, reduced amide, hydroxyethylamine, and hydroxyethylcarbonyl mimetics, while the second approach is based on the two-fold rotational (C2) symmetry of the native enzyme and interaction of protease/inhibitor via specific hydrogen bonds and hydrophobic interactions. In order to improve the pharmacokinetic profile of HIV protease inhibitors, the third approach uses non-peptidal strategy based on the first two approaches. Tables 1–3 summarize the structures, biological activities (Ki or IC_{50}) and physicochemical properties of novel protease inhibitors synthesized during 1992–1997 [11–43]. For the data before 1992, the readers should consult a good review by Kinchington et al. [6].

Table 1.
Substrate-based peptidomimetic HIV protease inhibitors

No.	Structure	Transition state	IC$_{50}$ (nM)	Ki (nM)	Properties	Ref.
1 KNI-174		hydroxymethyl-carbonyl analog	ATH8 cell: 399 PHA-PBM cells: 199		T$_{1/2}$: 3.97 h Bioavailability 5.37% in rats.	11
2 KNI-227		allophenylnorstatine	2.3 HIV-1 LAI: 100 HIV-1 RF: 20 HIV-1 MN: 30 HIV-1 ROD: 100		Log P: 3.79	6 12
3 KNI-272		allophenylnorstatine	6.5 HIV-1 LAI: 100 HIV-1 RF: 20 HIV-1 MN: 40 HIV-1 ROD: 100		Log P: 3.56 Bioavailability: 42% in rats	6 12
4 PD134922		renin inhibitor	15			13

8

Table 1 (continued)

No.	Structure	Transition state mimetic	IC$_{50}$ (nM)	K$_i$ (nM)	Properties	Refs
5 PD135390		renin inhibitor	2			13
6		AHPPA-containing	HIV-1 IIIB in MT4 cells: 250	9.5	Good bioavailability	14
7		hydroxyethylene dipeptide isostere, glycopeptide-containing	0.43			15
8		hydroxyethylene dipeptide isostere, glycopeptide-containing	0.17			15

Table 1 (continued)

No.	Structure	Transition state mimetic	IC$_{50}$ (nM)	Ki (nM)	Properties	Ref.
9		dihydroxyethylene isostere		5		16
10		dihydroxyethylene isostere		5		16
11		dihydroxyethylene isostere		4		16
12		cyclic sulfolanes	5.4			17

Table 1 (continued)

No.	Structure	Transition state mimetic	IC$_{50}$ (nM)	Ki (nM)	Properties	Ref.
13		cyclic sulfolanes	3.0			17
14		hydroxyethylene dipeptide isostere, phosphate prodrugs	HIV-1$_{IIIB}$ HPBM cells: 9.6 IC$_{90}$: 46.7			18
15		hydroxyethylene dipeptide isostere, phosphate prodrugs	HIV-1$_{IIIB}$ HPBM cells: 8.3 IC$_{90}$: 21.7			18
16		derived from saquinavir, tetrahydrofuranyl-glycine-containing	0.054 ClC$_{95}$: 8 (HIV-1$_{IIIB}$ in MT4 cells)			19

Table 1 (continued)

No.	Structure	Transition state mimetic	IC$_{50}$ (nM)	Ki (nM)	Properties	Ref.
17		derived from saquinavir, tetrahydrofuranyl-glycine-containing	0.071 CIC$_{95}$: 12 (HIV-1 IIIB in MT4 cells)			19
18		derived from saquinavir, tetrahydrofuranyl-glycine-containing	0.16 CIC$_{95}$: 3 (HIV-1 IIIB in MT4 cells)			19
19		reduced amide, β-turn-containing		430		20
20 SC-52151		hydroxyethyl urea	6 EC$_{50}$: 21		No antiviral activity in phase I/II study	21

Table 1 (continued)

No.	Structure	Transition state mimetic	IC_{50} (nM)	Ki (nM)	Properties	Ref.
21		hydroxyethyl urea isostere	3 EC_{50}: 10			22
22		hydroxyethyl urea isostere	3 EC_{50}: 21			22
23		hydroxyethylene dipeptide isostere, 3-tetrahydrofuran urethane-containing	<0.03 CIC_{95}: 3			23
24		hydroxyethylene dipeptide isostere, pyran urethane-containing	<0.03 CIC_{95}: 25			23

Table 1 (continued)

No.	Structure	Transition state mimetic	IC$_{50}$ (nM)	Ki (nM)	Properties	Ref.
25		hydroxyethylene dipeptide isostere, imidazole-derived	570	18	Bioavailability: 30% in rats 14% in monkeys	24
26 R-87366		AHPBA-containing	CEM/HIV-1$_{IIIB}$: 300 IC$_{90}$: 500 IC$_{90}$: 30–250	11	Water solubility: 4.2 mg/ml	25
27 SB206343		hydroxyethylene dipeptide isostere, imidazole-containing		0.6		26

Abbreviations: AHPPA, 4-amino-3-hydroxy-5-phenylpentanoic acid; AHPBA, 3-amino-2-hydroxy-4-phenylbutanoic acid; Boc: tertbutyloxycarbonyl

13

Table 2.
Symmetrical and pseudo-symmetrical HIV protease inhibitors

No.	Structure	Structural features	IC$_{50}$ (nM)	Ki (nM)	Properties	Ref.
28 XM323		cyclic urea non-peptide	IC$_{90}$: 63 (HIV-1 RF) IC$_{90}$: 160 (AZT-resistant isolates)			27
29 A77003		hindered peptide	<1 EC$_{50}$: 120–260		Solubility: 197 μg/ml in water. Under clinical investigation	6 28
30 SB204144		phosphinate	2.8			29
31		pseudo-symmetrical difluoroketones	0.1			30

14

Table 2 (continued)

No.	Structure	Structural features	IC$_{50}$ (nM)	Ki (nM)	Properties	Ref.
32		pseudo-symmetrical difluoroketones	0.02			30
33		pseudo-symmetrical difluoroketones	0.05			30
34		penicillin-derived C2 symmetric	3.0			31

15

16

Table 2 (continued)

No.	Structure	Structural features	IC_{50} (nM)	K_i (nM)	Properties	Ref.
35		penicillin-derived C2 symmetric	0.9 EC$_{50}$: 60 (C8166 cells) EC$_{50}$: 290 (MT4 cells)			32
36		cyclic urea C2 symmetric	IC$_{90}$: 4.2	0.04		33
37		cyclic urea C2 symmetric	IC$_{90}$: 8.7	0.14		33

Table 3.
Non-peptidal HIV protease inhibitors

No.	Structure	Structural features	IC$_{50}$ (nM)	Ki (nM)	Properties	Ref.
38 Evans blue		disulfonate-containing	480			34
39 Gardenin A		flavone	11000			35
40 Curcumin		polyphenol from *Curcuma Longa*	100000			36
41 α-MAPI		produced by *Streptomyces chromofuscus*	1300			37

Table 3 (continued)

No.	Structure	Structural features	IC$_{50}$ (nM)	Ki (nM)	Properties	Ref.
42		penicillin-derived	4.6 EC$_{50}$: 4700	0.25		38
43 Carnosic acid		diterpene isolated from rosemary (Rosmarinus officinalis L.)	IC$_{90}$: 0.08 mg/ml			39
44 MDL73669		difluorostatone		HIV-1 PR: 5		40
45 MDL 104168		macrocyclic inhibitor		HIV-1 PR: 20		40

Table 3 (continued)

No.	Structure	Structural features	IC_{50} (nM)	K_i (nM)	Properties	Ref.
46		cyclooctylpyranone	33400	4.0		41
47		cyclooctylpyranone	45300	3.0		41
48		derived from saquinavir, tetrahydrofuran-containing	1.8 CIC_{95}: 46			42
49		derived from saquinavir, tetrahydrofuran-containing	1.2 CIC_{95}: 50			42
50		sulfonamide, pyrone-containing	600 IC_{90}: 4500	0.52		43

Table 4.
Structures and activities of HIV protease inhibitors [7, 8]

No.	Stereo-chemistry at –CHOH–	Structure	IC$_{50}$ (nM)	
			HIV-1	HIV-2
51	R	Z-Asn-Pheψ[CH(OH)CH$_2$N]Pro-O-tBu	140	330
52	S	Z-Asn-Pheψ[CH(OH)CH$_2$N]Pro-O-tBu	300	
53	R	Z-Leu-Asn-Pheψ[CH(OH)CH$_2$N]Pro-O-tBu	600	
54	R	Z-Asn-Pheψ[CH(OH)CH$_2$N]Pro-Ile-NH-iBu	130	
55	R	Z-Leu-Asn-Pheψ[CH(OH)CH$_2$N]Pro-Ile-NH-iBu	750	
56	R	Z-Asn-Pheψ[CH(OH)CH$_2$N]Pro-NH-tBu	210	
57	R	BN-Asn-Pheψ[CH(OH)CH$_2$N]Pro-O-tBu	52	50
58	R	QC-Asn-Pheψ[CH(OH)CH$_2$N]Pro-O-tBu	23	
59	R	Z-Asn-Pheψ[CH(OH)CH$_2$N]PIC-NH-tBu	18	
60	R	Z-CNA-Pheψ[CH(OH)CH$_2$N]PIC-NH-tBu	23	
61	R	QC-Asn-Pheψ[CH(OH)CH$_2$N]PIC-NH-tBu	2	9.5
62 ,	S	QC-Asn-Pheψ[CH(OH)CH$_2$N]PIC-NH-tBu	470	
63	R	QC-SMC-Pheψ[CH(OH)CH$_2$N]PIC-NH-tBu	12	15
64	R	QC-Asn-Pheψ[CH(OH)CH$_2$N]DIC-NH-tBu	< 0.4	< 0.8

Abbreviations:
Z = benzyloxycarbonyl; tBu = tert-butyl; BN = β-naphthoyl; QC = quinoline-2-carbonyl; PIC = piperi-dine-2(S)-carbonyl; CNA = β-cyanoalanyl; SMC = S-methyl-cysteinyl; DIC = (4aS, 8aS)-decahydro-3(S)-isoquinolinecarbonyl; Pheψ [CH(OH)CH$_2$N]Pro indicates replacement of the imide group (CON<) in the Phe-Pro peptide bond by the hydroxyethylamine moiety –CH(OH)ĊHNH– (threo form), the hydroxy function has the configuration indicated in the table.

4   HIV protease inhibitors on the market

4.1   SAR of saquinavir and related compounds

Early attempts to design irreversible inactivator of the HIV protease have yielded only weak inhibitors [44]. Far greater success has been realized with competitive inhibitors designed to mimic the transition states [45]. Incorporation of the Phe-Pro hydroxyethylamine isostere Ψ[CH(OH)CH$_2$N] (threo form) into the pl7/p24 cleavage sequence provided the potent inhibitors **51** (see Tab. 4).

Based on the structure of potent compound **51**, the structural requirements for optimal binding at each subsite were systematically explored. More

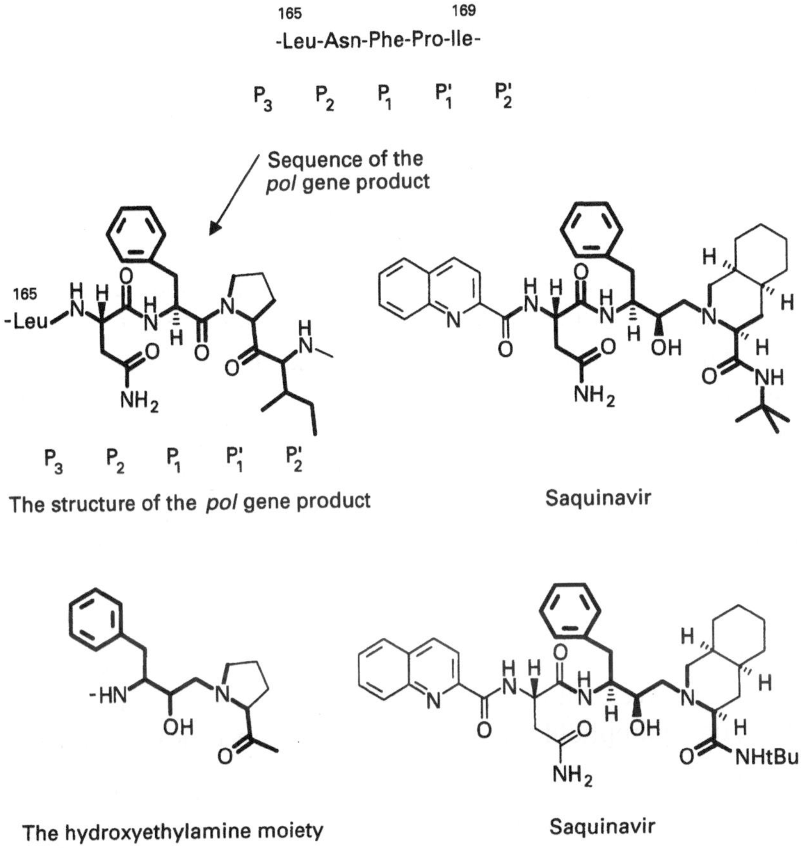

Fig. 1
Comparison of the structure of the *pol* gene product and the structure of saquinavir. Note that the common backbones in these structures are presented in boldface for easier comparison.

than 100 compounds were synthesized in which the steric and electronic properties of each side chain and terminal substituent were individually modified [7]. The most important findings were that (a) extension at the amino terminus or carboxyl terminus or both did not result in further improvement in potency (compounds 53 and 54); (b) a preference for R stereochemistry at the hydroxyl-bearing carbon atom was initially indicated by compounds 51 and 52. This effect was more dramatically confirmed with compounds 61 and 62; (c) a large hydrophobic pocket at P_3 was inferred from the high potency shown by compounds 57 and 58; (d) at the P_2 subsite no improvement over asparaginyl was found, although the β-cyanoalanyl (CNA) and S-methylcysteinyl (SMC) analogues (compounds 60 and 63, respectively) displayed comparable potencies. Similarly, at P_1 no improvement was found over the benzyl side chain of Phe; (e) the most marked improvements in potency were achieved by varying the amino acid at P_1', highly effective replacements for prolyl being piperidine-2-(S)-carbonyl (PIC) (compound 59) and (S, S, S)-decahydro-isoquinoline-3-carbonyl (DIC) (compound 64, saquinavir, see Tab. 4 and Fig. 1 for the structure); (f) at the carboxyl terminus tert-butyl ester could be replaced by a tert-butylamide group without significant change in potency (compounds 51 and 56), but no better replacement was identified.

The hydroxyethylamine moiety of saquinavir mimics the *pol* product sequence of HIV protease (see Fig. 1). Lipophilic benzyl and DIC, as well as the linkage between the benzyl and DIC are favored in the symmetry-related P_1 and P_1' subsite while there is a clear preference for Asn at the P_2 site, t-Bu group mimics Ile at P_2' site. Planar, aromatic end pieces may mimic the peptide backbone rather than the P_3 and P_3' side chains. The studies of HIV protease/inhibitor complexes revealed that the molecular forces involved in the interactions between inhibitor and HIV protease were mainly hydrogen-bonding and hydrophobic interactions in addition to a water molecular bridge [8].

4.2 Advantages and disadvantages of saquinavir

Saquinavir, the first HIV protease inhibitor marketed in 1995, is an extremely potent *in vitro* inhibitor of both HIV-1 and HIV-2 proteases. The inhibition constant Ki at pH 5.5 is 0.12 nM against HIV-1 protease, and binding to HIV-2 protease is even stronger (Ki < 0.1 nM) [7]. Saquinavir has an IC_{50} of 2 nM against HIV-1 (strain RF) in C8166 cells [7], and an IC_{90} of 16.1 nM in HIV-infected JM cells [3]. Moreover, this compound is highly selective, causing less than 50% inhibition of the human aspartic proteases like renin, pepsin, gastricsin, cathepsin D, and cathepsin E at a concentration of 10 μM [7]. Cytotoxicity studies with saquinavir in C8166 and JM cells have given TD_{50} (toxic dose) values in the range from 5 to 100 μM which is at least 2000-fold greater than the concentration required for antiviral activity [7].

Phase II clinical studies have shown that saquinavir therapy, given either alone or in combination with nucleoside analogues, increased CD4 lymphocyte cell counts and decreased viral burden. The combination of saquinavir with zidovudine, or zidovudine and zalcitabine, resulted in greater improvement in laboratory markers of disease than saquinavir monotherapy, with the combination delaying the onset of resistance to either drug alone [1, 3, 46a]. Like other therapies, the durability of the surrogate marker responses was limited, but longer with combination therapy than with monotherapy. The emergence of HIV-1 resistance to saquinavir has been reported in laboratory strains and in clinical isolates from saquinavir-treated patients with HIV infection [46b–46e]. Saquinavir is well tolerated alone and in combination with nucleoside analogues [3, 47].

Saquinavir has a high molecular weight (670.86 for the free base), a low aqueous solubility (2.22 mg/mL) [47], high lipophilicity (calculated partition coefficient ClogP = 4.66 for the free base, calculated using the CQSAR program [48]), and significant peptide character. Historically, peptide based leads have presented significant obstacles to drug development. Saquinavir has a low oral bioavailability (4%) due to a combination of incomplete absorption and extensive first-pass metabolism [47]. Moreover, systemic clearance of saquinavir is rapid. The mean residence time of saquinavir is 7 h [47].

4.3 Possible methods to overcome the disadvantages of saquinavir

To overcome these disadvantages, further investigations have been carried out on saquinavir. Improvement of the oral bioavailability is being met through the development of a new soft gelatin capsule formulation (Fortovase, marketed by Roche in 1998) [46f]. Available data indicate that the oral bioavailability of saquinavir soft gelatin capsule is 3 to 4 times higher than that of the hard gelatin capsule formulation. Although the mean absolute bioavailability of saquinavir soft gelatin capsule has not been determined, a single 600 mg dose of this formulation was estimated to have a relative bioavailability of 331% compared with a single 600 mg dose of saquinavir hard gelatin capsule. Recent studies indicate that saquinavir is mainly metabolized by human intestinal cytochrome P450 3A4 (CYP3A4), this metabolism may contribute to its poor oral bioavailability, and that combination therapy with indinavir, ritonavir, ketoconazole, and troleandomycin (selective inhibitors of CYP3A4) may attenuate its relatively low bioavailability [49, 50]. Recent work in the renin area has shown that systematic structural modifications can lead to compounds with acceptable pharmacokinetic properties [51]. Structural modifications may improve the oral bioavailability through lowering the log P to a value closer to ideal log P_0 of around 2–3 for maximum gastrointestinal absorption [52]. Efforts to design inhibitors based on enzyme protein structure rather than substrate sequence may offer another source of new drug candidates. The availability of x-ray crystallographic structures of HIV protease/inhibitor complexes will undoubtedly provide another view for *de novo* design of non-peptide inhibitors which take advantage of specific hydrogen bonding and hydrophobic interactions with the active site. Random screening with high throughput assays might also yield useful, non-peptide leads. The delivery of protease inhibitors via non-oral routes, such as nasal spray, intravenous or subcutaneous injection, may a have a role in antiviral therapy.

4.4 Comparison of saquinavir, ritonavir, indinavir, nelfinavir and amprenavir

Five HIV protease inhibitors, saquinavir, ritonavir, indinavir, nelfinavir and amprenavir (see Table 5 for the structures), have been marketed by different pharmaceutical companies during 1995–1999 [4a, 4b, 47, 53–64]. Their different structural features, physicochemical, pharmacokinetic and other properties are summarized in Table 5.

5 HIV protease inhibitors undergoing clinical studies

The worldwide AIDS epidemic has stimulated a large research effort directed toward identifying therapeutic agents effective for control of the disease and its causative agent HIV. Of hundreds of HIV protease inhibitors synthesized and tested over the past few years, highly potent transition-state peptidomimetic, symmetrical/pseudo-symmetrical, and non-peptidic protease inhibitors have been described in the literature [6, 66]. Recent advances have

Table 5.
Differential features of protease inhibitors currently on the market [4a, 4b, 47, 53–64].

Generic name	Saquinavir	Ritonavir	Indinavir	Nelfinavir	Amprenavir
Trade name and company No.	Invirase Ro318959	Norvir ABT-538	Crixivan MK-639 L-735524	Viracept AG 1343	Agenerase 141W94 VX-478
Company and year marketed	Roche 1995	Abbott 1996	Merck 1996	Agouron 1997	Glaxo Wellcome 1999
Structure					
Physico-chemical properties	Clog P: 4.66a (free base) MW: 670.86 (free base) 766.96 (salt)	Clog P: 3.77a MW: 720.95	Clog P: 2.79a (free base) Log P: 2.92a MW: 613.79 (free base) 711.88 (salt)	Clog P: 5.52a (free base) Log P: 4.1b MW: 567.78 (free base) 663.90 (salt)	Clog P: 3.29 MW: 505.64
Licensed indication	Late-stage infection, Combination therapy-NRTI (ddC)	Late-stage infection, Combination therapy-NRTI (AZT, ddI)	Late-stage infection, Combination therapy-NRTI (AZT, ddI, 3TC)	For the treatment of HIV infection when antiretro-viral therapy is warranted. The first protease inhibitor to be approved simul-taneously in adult and pediatric formulations.	HIV infected adults and children at least four years old

Table 5 (continued)

Generic name	Saquinavir	Ritonavir	Indinavir	Nelfinavir	Amprenavir
Dose forms	200 mg hard gelatin capsules	100 mg capsules 80 mg/ml solution	200 and 400 mg capsules	250 mg tablets 50 mg/g oral powder	50 mg and 150 mg capsule, 15 mg/ml solution
Dose	600 mg tid	600 mg bid	800 mg every 8 hours	750 mg tid or 1250 mg bid.. Pediatric dosing: 20–30 mg/kg/dose tid	1200 mg bid. Pediatric dosing: (1) capsule: 20 mg/kg bid or 15 mg/kg tid; (2) solution: 22.5 mg/kg bid or 17 mg/kg tid
Dosage consideration	Take with food up to 2 h after meals. No fluid requirement. Avoid taking oral solution (contains alcohol) with metronidazole to prevent disulfiram-like reaction.	Take with food. No fluid requirement.	Take on empty stomach 1 h before or 2 h after meal with water at exact 8-h intervals. May be taken with light meal or skim milk, juice, coffee, or tea. Hydrate with 1.5 l/day (48 oz.) of fluids. Space dose from didanosine.	Take with meal or light snack. May mix oral powder with water, milk, formula or soy milk. Avoid concomitant administration of acidic food or juice (may result in bitter taste). Space dose from didanosine.	Take with or without food. Avoid high-fat meal. Patients taking antacids or didanosine should take amprenavir at least 1 h before or afterward.
Pregnancy category	B	B	C	B	C
Approximate wholesale price	$580/month	$670/month	$460/month	$580/month	$600/month
Adverse effects	Headache, rash, peripheral neuropathy, gastrointestinal disturbances. Laboratory abnormalities – increased serum calcium, serum transaminases and	Gastrointestinal intolerance – diarrhea, nausea, vomiting, abdominal pain, taste perversion. Circumoral paraesthesia, rash, asthenia, vasodilatation,	Nephrolithiasis, asymptomatic hyperbilirubinaemia. Dry skin, rash, taste perversion, gastrointestinal disturbances.	Diarrhea, abdominal pain, asthenia, nausea, , flatulence, rash.	Rash, diarrhea, or loose stools, headache, nausea, vomiting, oral and peri-oral paresthesias. Rashes can be severe or life-threatening.

Table 5 (continued)

Generic name	Saquinavir	Ritonavir	Indinavir	Nelfinavir	Amprenavir
	creatinine phosphokinase, reduced neutrophil counts and glucose levels.	peripheral neuropathy. Increased lipid levels and hyperuricaemia.			
Interactions	*Inadvisable combinations:* Rifampicin, riftabutin, phenobarbital, phenytoin, dexamethasone, carbamazepine, terfenadine, astemizole, cisapride. *Careful monitoring advised:* Ketoconazole, fluconazole, itraconazol, miconazole, calcium antagonists, clindamycin, dapsone, quinidine, triazolam or midazolam.	*Contraindicated in combination with:* Amiodarone, astemizole, bepridil, bupropion, cisapride, clozapine, dextropropoxyphene, encainide, flecainide, meperidine, pimozide, piroxicam, propafenone, quinidine, terfenadine, alprazolam, clorazepate, diazepam, flurazepam, midazolam, triazolam, zolpidem and riftabutin. *Careful monitoring recommended with:* Immunosuppressants, macrolide antibiotics, various steroids, non-sedating antihistamines, calcium channel antagonists, antidepressants, neuroleptics, antifungals, co-trimoxazole, theophylline, morphinomimetics, carbamazepine, warfarin and tolbutamide.	Rifabutin, ketoconazole, itraconazole, phenobarbital, phenytoin, carbamazepine, dexamethasone, terfenadine, astemizole, cisapride, triazolam, alprazolam, midazolam and tiazolam. Co-administration of indinavir with ritonavir is likely to result in significant increases in plasma concentrations of indinavir.	*Contraindicated in combination with:* Amiodarone, quinidine, ergot derivatives, midazolam terfenadine, astemizole, cisapride, rifampin. *Careful monitoring advised:* rifabutin, carbamazepine, phenobarbital, phenytoin, indinavir, ritonavir and oral contraceptives (ethinyl estradiol and norethindrone).	Co-administration of amprenavir with ritonavir and ketoconazole increases the plasma concentration and/or AUC of amprenavir. Co-administration of amprenavir with ribafutin or rifampin or efavirenz, or DMP-266 decreases the plasma concentration and AUC of amprenavir. *Inadvisable combinations:* midazolam, triazolam, bepridil, ergotamine, di-hydroergotamine, and cisapride. *Combinations that might cause serious toxicity:* amiodarone, systemic lidocaine, quinidine, -warfarin, tricyclic anti-depressants, ribafutin, and sildenafil

27

Table 5 (continued)

Generic name	Saquinavir	Ritonavir	Indinavir	Nelfinavir	Amprenavir
Pharmaco-kinetics	Absolute bioavailability: 4% $T_{1/2}$: 1.5–2.0 h Plasma protein binding: >98% Urinary elimination: 1% Fecal excretion: 88% Metabolism: CYP3A4	Absolute bioavailability: 60–70% $T_{1/2}$: 3.0–5.0 h Plasma protein binding: 98–99% Urinary elimination: 11% Fecal excretion: 86% Metabolism: CYP3A4 & CYP2D6	Absolute bioavailability: >>30% $T_{1/2}$: 1.5–2.0 h Plasma protein binding: >>60% Urinary elimination: 19% Fecal excretion: 83% Metabolism: CYP3A4 & GT	Absolute bioavailability: 20–80% $T_{1/2}$: 3.5–5.0 h Plasma protein binding: >>98% Urinary elimination: 1–2% Fecal excretion: 87% Metabolism: CYP3A4 CYP2C, CYP2D6 & GT	Absolute bioavailability: 35–90% $T_{1/2}$: 7.1–9.5 h Plasma protein binding: 90% Urinary elimination: <2% Fecal exretion: most Metabolism: CYP3A4
Storage	15–30°C	Refrigerator, protect from light.	Sensitive to moisture.	15–30°C	Room temperature, shold not be refrigerated.
Resistance	Does not appear to lead to cross-resistance with ritonavir and indinavir In vivo primary mutations: positions 48, 90	Does not appear to lead to cross-resistance with saquinavir. May lead to reduced susceptibility to indinavir. In vivo primary mutation: position 82	Appears to confer cross-resistance to all protease inhibitors. In vivo primary mutation: position 82	In vivo primary mutation: position 30	Limited cross-resistance to saquinavir or indinavir in vitro. No evidence of resistance in clinical isolates from 42 patients treated with amprenavir for 4 weeks. In vivo primary mutation: position 50

a Calculated using CQSAR program [48].
b From ref. [65].

28

led to protease inhibitors with reduced peptidic nature which generally exhibited improved pharmacokinetic properties. Several new protease inhibitors such as ABT-378, PNU-140690, DMP-450, DMP-851, KNI-272 and palinavir are in clinical trials [64, 66–75]. Their characteristics are briefly summarized in Table 6.

6   Conclusion

The protease inhibitors offer a novel and promising approach to the treatment of HIV infection. Among available anti-HIV drugs, protease inhibitors produce the greatest suppression of viral replication. In spite of their potency, currently available HIV protease inhibitors are limited by their gastrointestinal intolerance, drug-drug interactions, moderate bioavailability, and cross-resistance. The cost of protease inhibitors may present an economic burden. Protease inhibitors must be taken compliantly, without interruption, or else resistance may develop. There are limited guideline available as to when and which protease inhibitor to add to a specific regimen. A new generation of protease inhibitors with higher potency, improved pharmacokinetic profile, fewer drug interactions, better tolerability and convenient dosing schedule will be highly desirable. Development of new classes of agents aimed at other targets such as HIV integrase, zinc-finger [76] and ribonucleotide reductase [77] is also warranted, and may produce additional armament in the fight against AIDS.

Combination therapy of viral infection with multiple drugs acting by different mechanisms may offer several advantages over monotherapy: (1) potential synergistic effect; (2) possible reduction of dosages and side-effects; (3) reduction of the chance of drug resistance, for example, if a single drug has a 1% chance of producing resistance viral particles, the combination of three different drugs will reduce the chance to $1/10^6$ during the same period of time. This may be of the greatest advantage in treating infections caused by rapidly changing viruses like HIV.

Acknowledgement

The authors wish to express their sincere thanks to the Hong-yen Hsu & Lin-run Charitable Foundation for generous support of this work.

Table 6.
HIV prote inhibitors undergoing clinical studies [64, 66-75].

Name/Company no./Company	Chemical structures	Physico-chemical properties	In vitro activities	Pharmacokinetic & phase I clinical studies	Refs.
ABT-378 Abbott	Peptidomemitic	Clog P = 6.10	Ki = 1.3-3.6 pM for wide-type and for V82A/F mutant HIV protease. EC$_{50}$ = 100 nM in the presence of 50% human serum. EC$_{50}$ = 6.5 nM for HIV patient isolates.	Bioavailability: 25% in rats.	64, 67
Tipranavir PNU-140690 Pharmacia Upjohn	Non-peptide	Clog P = 7.76	Ki = 8 pM IC$_{50}$ = 0.03 μM IC$_{90}$ = 0.10 μM Ki < 1 nM for HIV-2 protease. Ki = 3.0 nM for V82A mutant HIV-2 protease. Ki = 0.25 nM for V82F/I84V mutant HIV-2 protease.	Bioavailability: 30% in rats. T$_{1/2}$ = 5.4 h iv dosing in rats.	64, 68–70
DMP-450 Triangle	Symmetric cyclic urea, non-peptide (C2 symmetry)	Clog P = 4.78	Ki = 0.28 nM. EC$_{50}$ = 10~20 nM against different HIV strains	Bioavailability: 24% in chimpanzees, 79% in dogs. Cross-resistance to ritonavir and indinavir.	64, 71

Table 6. (continued)

Name/Company no./Company	Chemical structures	Physico-chemical properties	In vitro activities	Pharmacokinetic & phase I clinical studies	Refs.
DMP-851 DuPont Merck	Asymmetric cyclic urea, non-peptide	Clog P = 6.25	Ki = 21 pM. IC_{90} = 56 nM for HIV RF virus. IC_{90} = 114 nM for clinical isolate. EC_{50} = 0.8 µM for wild-type HIV-1 protease. EC_{50} = 3.8 µM for the I84V mutant HIV-1 protease	Bioavailability: 63% in dogs. Less cross-resistance with other HIV protease inhibitors.	64, 72
KNI-272	Peptidomimetic	Mlog P = 3.56 Clog P = 4.73	IC_{50} = 6.5 nM for HIV-1 protease.	Bioavailability: 22–55% in patients, 40–60% in dogs, 42% in rats. $T_{1/2}$ = 0.39–0.52 h in patients. Dose limiting toxicity: hepatic transaminase elevation.	66, 73–74
Palinavir	Peptidomimetic	Clog P = 4.64	IC_{50} = 4 nM for HIV-1. IC_{50} = 10 nM for HIV-2. EC_{50} = 0.5–30 nM for clinical isolates.	Bioavailability: 26.1% in rats. $T_{1/2}$ = 0.7 h.	75

References

1   S.M. Hammer: AIDS 10 (suppl. 3), S1–S11 (1996).
2   C.A.B. Boucher, M. Tersmette, J.M.A. Lange, P. Kellam, R.E.Y. De Goede, J.W. Mulder, G. Darby, J. Goudsmit and B.A. Larder: Lancet 336, 585–590 (1990).
3   K. Bragmann: Adv. Exp. Med. Biol. 394, 305–317 (1996).
4a A. Pakyz and D. Israel: J. Am. Pharm. Asso. NS 37, 543–551 (1997).
4b Anonymous: Med. Letter 41 (1057), 64–66 (1999).
5   R.A. Kramer, M.D. Schaber, A.M. Skalka, K. Ganguly, F. Wong-Staal and E.P. Reddy: Science 231, 1580–1584 (1986).
6   D. Kinchington and S. Redshaw, in: D.J. Jeffries and E. De Clercq (eds.): Antiviral chemotherapy. John Wiley & Sons, Chichester 1995, pp. 3–40.
7   N.A. Roberts, J.A. Martin, D. Kinchington, A.V. Broadhurst, J.C. Craig and I.B. Duncan: Science 248, 358–361 (1990).
8   D.W. Norbeck and D.J. Kempf: Ann. Rep. Med. Chem. 26, 141–150 (1991).
9   A.L. Swain, M.M. Miller, J. Green, D.H. Rich, J. Schneider, S.B.H. Kent and A. Wlodawer: Proc. Natl. Acad. Sci. USA 87, 8805–8809 (1990).
10 J.L. Cohen, W. Lee and E.J. Lien: J. Pharm. Sci. 63, 1068–1072 (1974).
11 A. Kiriyama, T. Mimoto, Y. Kiso and K. Takada: Biopharm. Drug Dispo. 14, 199–207 (1993).
12 S. Kayeyama, T. Minoto, Y. Murakawa, M. Nomizu, H. Jr. Ford, T. Shirasaka, S. Gulnik, J. Erickson, K. Takada and H. Hayashi: Antimicrob. Agents Chemother. 37, 810–817 (1993).
13 C.C. Humblet, E.A. Lunney, R.W. Jr. Buckheit, C. Doggett, R. Wong and T.K. Antonucci: Antiviral Res. 21, 73–84 (1993).
14 M. Sakurai, M. Sugano, H. Handa, T. Komai, R. Yagi, T. Nishigaki and Y. Yabe: Chem. Pharm. Bull. 41, 1369–1377 (1993).
15 A.K. Ghosh, S.P. McKee, W.M. Sanders, P.L. Darke, J.A. Zugay, E.A. Emini, W.A. Schleif, J.C. Quintero and J.R. Huff: Drug Design Disco. 10, 77–88 (1993).
16 S. Thaisrivongs, S.R. Turner, J.W. Strohbach, R.E. TenBrink, W.G. Tarpley, T.J. McQuade, R.L. Heinrikson, A.G. Tomaselli, J.O. Hui and W.J. Howe: J. Med. Chem. 36, 941–952 (1993).
17 A.K. Ghosh, W.J. Thompson, H.Y. Lee, S.P. McKee, P.M. Munson, T.T. Duong, P.L. Darge, J.A. Zugay, E.A. Emini, W.A. Schleif: J. Med. Chem. 36, 924–927 (1993).
18 K.T. Chong, M.J. Ruwart, R.R. Hinshaw, K.F. Wilkinson, B.D. Rush, M.F. Yancey, J.W. Strohbach and S. Thairsrivongs; J. Med. Chem. 36, 2575–2577 (1993).
19 A.K.Ghosh, W.J. Thompson, M.K. Holloway, S.P. McKee, T.T. Duong, H.Y. Lee, P.M. Munson, A.M. Smith, J.M. Wai and P.L. Darke: J. Med. Chem. 36, 2300–2310 (1993).
20 K.A. Newlander, J.F. Callahan, M.L. Moore, T.A. Jr. Tomaszek and W.F. Huffman: J. Med. Chem. 36, 2321–2331 (1993).
21 M. Bryant, D. Getman, M. Smidt, J. Marr, M. Clare, R. Dillard, D. Lansky, G. DeCrescenzo, R. Heintz and K. Houseman: Antimicrob. Agents Chemother. 39, 2229–2234 (1995).
22 D.P. Getman, G.A. DeCrescenzo, R.M. Heintz, K.L. Reed, J.J. Talley, M.L. Bryant, M. Clare, K.A. Houseman, J.J. Marr and R.A. Muller: J. Med. Chem. 36, 288–291 (1993).
23 A.K. Ghosh, W.J. Thompson, S.P. McKee, T. T. Duong, T.A. Lyle, J.C. Chen, P.L. Darke, J. A. Zugay, E.A. Emini and W.A. Schleif: J. Med. Chem. 36, 292–294 (1993).
24 M.S.S. Abdel, B.W. Metcalf, T.J. Carr, P. Demarsh, R.L. DesJarlais, S. Fisher, D.W. Green, L. Ivanoff, D.M. Lambert and K.H. Murthy: Biochem. 33, 11671–11677 (1994).

25   K. Tomoaki, Y. Ryuichi, S. Hisayo and S. Mitsuya: Biol. Pharm. Bull. *20*, 175–180 (1997).

26   S.K. Thompson, K.H. Multhy, B. Zhao and E. Winborne: J. Med. Chem. *37*, 3100–3107 (1994).

27   M.J. Otto, C.D. Reid, S. Garber, P.Y. Lam, H. Scarnati, L.T. Bacheler, M.M. Rayner and D.L. Winslow: Antimicrob. Agents Chemother. *37*, 2606–2611 (1993).

28   J.J. Kort, J.A. Bilello, G. Bauer and G.L. Drusano: Antimicrob. Agents Chemother. *37*, 115–119 (1993).

29   M.S.S. Abdel, B. Zhao, K.H. Murthy, E. Winborne, J.K. Choi and R.L. DesJarlais: Biochem. *32*, 7972–7980 (1993).

30   H.L. Sham, D.A. Betebenner, N. Wideburg, A.C. Saldivar and W.E. Kohlbrenner: Febs Lett. *329*, 144–146 (1993).

31   A. Wonacott, R. Cooke, F.R. Hayes, M.M. Hann, H. Jhoti, P. McMeekin, A. Mistry, R.P. Murray, O.M: Singh and M.P. Weir: J. Med. Chem. *36*, 3113–3119 (1993).

32   D.C. Humber, M.J. Bamford, R.C. Bethell and N. Cammack: J. Med. Chem. *36*, 3120–3128 (1993).

33   D.A. Nugiel, K. Jacobs, L. Cornelius, C.H. Chang and P. K. Jadhav: J. Med. Chem. *40*, 1465–1474 (1997).

34   R.I. Brinkworth and D.P. Fairlie: Biochem. Biophy. Res. Communi. *188*, 624–630 (1992).

35   R.I. Brinkworth, M.J. Stoermer and D.P. Fairlie: Biochem. Biophy. Res. Communi. *188*, 631–637 (1992).

36   Z. Sui, R. Salto, J. Li, C. Craik and P.R. Ortiz de Montellano: Bioorgan. Med. Chem. *1*, 415–422 (1993).

37   R. Kaneto, H. Chiba, K. Dobashi, I. Kojima and K. Sakai: J. Antibio. *46*, 1622–1624 (1993).

38   D.S. Holmes, R.C. Bethell, N. Cammack and I.R. Clemens: J. Med. Chem. *36*, 3129–3136 (1993).

39   A. Paris, B. Strukelj, M. Renko, V. Turk, M. Pukl, A. Umek and B.D. Korant: J. Nat. Prod. *56*, 1426–1430 (1993).

40   B.L. Podlogar, R.A. Farr, D. Friedrich, C. Tarnus, E.W. Huber, R.J. Cregge and D. Schirlin: J. Med. Chem. *37*, 3684–3692 (1994).

41   K.R. Romines, K.D. Watenpaugh, W.J. Howe, P.K. Tomich, K.D. Lovasz and J.K. Morris: J. Med. Chem. *38*, 4463–4473 (1995).

42   A.K. Ghosh, J.F. Kincaid, D.E. Walters, Y. Chen and N.C. Chaudhuri: J. Med. Chem. *39* 3278–3290 (1996).

43   S. Thaisrivongs, M.N. Janakiraman, K.T. Chong, P.K. Tomich, L.A. Dolak and S.R. Turner: J. Med. Chem. *39*, 2400–2410 (1996).

44   J.J. Blumenstein, T.D. Copeland, S. Oroszlan and C.J. Michejda: Biochem. Biophys. Res. Commun. *163*, 980–987 (1989).

45   D.H. Rich: J. Med. Chem. *28*, 263–273 (1985).

46a   J.C. Craig, I.B. Duncan, D. Hockley, C. Grief, N.A. Roberts and J.S. Mills: Antiviral Res. *16*, 295–305 (1991).

46b   D.D. Richman: Antimicrob. Agents Chemother. *37*, 1207–1213 (1993).

46c   S. Vella: AIDS Clin. Care *9* (6), 47–52 (1997).

46d   C. Boucher: AIDS *10* (suppl. 1), S15–19 (1996).

46e   N.A. Roberts: AIDS *9* (suppl. 2), S27–32 (1995).

46f   C.M. Perry and S. Noble: Drugs *55*, 461–486 (1998).

47   Physicians' Desk Reference, 51st ed., Medical Economics Co., Inc., Montvale, NJ, USA, pp. 2291–2294 (1997).

48   CQSAR database, BioByte Corp., 201 W, 4th St. Clarement, CA, USA (1999).

49   C. Merry, M.G. Rarry, F. Mulcahy, M. Ryan, J. Heavey, ,T.F. Tjia, S.E. Gibbons, A.M. Breck-enridge and D.J. Back: AIDS *11*, F29–33 (1997).

50   M.E. Fitzsimmons and J.M. Collins: Drug Met. Disp. *25*, 256–266 (1997).

51   S.H. Rosenberg, H.D. Kleinert, H.H. Stein, D.L. Martin, M.A. Chekal, J. Cohen, D.A. Egan, K.A. Tricarico and W.R. Baker: J. Med. Chem. *34*, 469–471 (1991).

52   E.J. Lien: Ann. Rev. Pharmcol. Toxicol. *21*, 31–61 (1981).

53   Physicians' Desk Reference, 51st ed., Medical Economics Co., Inc., Montvale, NJ, USA, pp. 447–451 (1997).

54   Physicians' Desk Reference, 51st ed., Medical Economics Co., Inc., Montvale, NJ, USA, 1670–1673 (1997).

55   P. Galatsis: Ann. Rep. Med. Chem. *32*, 310 (1997).

56   P. Galatsis: Ann. Rep. Med. Chem. *32*, 317 (1997).

57   X. M. Cheng: Ann. Rep. Med. Chem. *31*, 349 (1996).

58   J. Misson, W. Clark and M.J. Kendall: J. Clin. Pharm. Ther. *22*, 109–117 (1997).

59   Anonymous: US Pharmacist, October: 148–154 (1997).

60   Physicians' Desk Reference, 52nd ed., Medical Economics Co., Inc., Montvale, NJ, USA, 476–480 (1998).

61   J.C. Adkins and D. Faulds: Drugs *55*, 837–842 (1998).

62   B.M. Sadler, C.D. Hanson, G.E. Chittick, W.T. Symonds and N.S. Roskell: Antimicrob. Agents Chemother. *43*, 1686–1692 (1999).

63   Anonymous: Am. J. Health-Syst. Pharm. *56*, 1057–1058 (1999).

64   A. Molla, G.R. Granneman, E. Sun. D J. Kempf: Antiviral Res. *39*, 1–23 (1998).

65   M. Longer, B. Shetty, I. Zamansky and P. Tyle: J. Pharm. Sci. *84*, 1090–1093 (1995).

66   S.J. Ren and E.J. Lien: Prog. Drug Res. *51*, 1–31 (1998).

67   H.L. Sham, D.J. Kempf, A. Molla, K.C. Marsh, G.N. Kumar, C. Chen, W. Kati, K. Stewart, R. Lal, A. Hsu et al.: Antimicrob. Agents Chemother. *42*, 3218–3224 (1998).

68   S.M. Poppe, D.E. Slade, K.-T. Chong, R.R. Hinshaw, P.J. Pagano, M. Markowitz, D.D. Ho, H. Mo, R.R. Gorman III, T.J. Dueweke et al.: Antimicrob. Agents Chemother. *41*, 1058–1063 (1997).

69   S. Thaisrivongs, H.I. Skulnick, S.R. Turner, J.W. Strohbach, R.A. Tommasi, P.D. Johnson, P.A. Aristoff, T.M. Judge, R.B. Gammill, J.K. Morris et al.: J. Med. Chem. *39*, 4349–4353 (1996).

70   S.R. Turner, J.W. Strohbach, R.A. Tommasi, P.A. Aristoff, P.D. Johnson, H.I. Skulnick, L.A. Dolak, E.P. Seest, P.K. Tomich, M.J. Bohanon et al.: J. Med. Chem. *41*, 3467–3476 (1998).

71   G.V. De Lucca, U.T. Kim, J. Liang, B. Cordova, R.M. Klabe, S. Garber, L.T. Bacheler, G.N. Lam, M.R. Wright, K.A. Logue: J. Med. Chem. *41*, 2411–2423 (1998).

72   J.D. Rodgers, P.Y. Lam, B.L. Johnson, H. Wang, R. Li, Y. Ru, S.S. Ko, S.P. Seitz, G.L. Trainor, P.S. Anderson et al.: Chem. Biol. *5*, 597–608 (1998).

73   R.W. Humphrey, K.M. Wyvill, B. Nguyen, L.E. Shay, D.R. Kohler, S.M. Steinberg, T. Ueno, T. Fukasawa, M. Shintani, H. Hayashi et al.: Antiviral Res. *41*, 21–33 (1999).

74   B.U. Mueller, B.D. Anderson, M.Q. Farley, R. Murphy, J. Zuckerman, P. Jarosinski, K. Godwin, C.L. McCully, H. Mitsuya, P.A. Pizzo and F.M. Balis: Antimicrob. Agents Chemother. *42*, 1815–1818 (1998).

75   F. Liard, J. Jaramillo, W.L. Paris and C. Yoakim: J. Pharm. Sci. *87*, 782–785 (1998).

76   M.B.V. Hui, E.J. Lien and M.D. Tronsdale: Antiviral Res. *24*, 261–273 (1994).

77   E.J. Lien: Prog. Drug Res. *31*, 1–26 (1987).

Antiviral Agents – Advances and Problems (E. Jucker, Ed.)
© 2001 Birkhäuser Verlag, Basel (Switzerland)

Anti-influenza drugs and neuraminidase inhibitors

By Noel A. Roberts

Roche Discovery Welwyn
Broadwater Road
Welwyn Garden City
Hertfordshire AL7 3AY, UK
<noel.roberts@roche.com>

Noel A. Roberts

studied at University of Hull (UK) and gained a B.Sc. (Chemistry) in 1965, followed by his Ph.D. (Chemical Microbiology) in 1968. He became Team Leader in the Biochemical Development Department of BDH Chemicals Ltd, then joined Roche in the UK in 1973 to study the biochemistry and inhibition of proteinases, initially in the field of inflammation and then for HIV. Dr. Roberts led the biology team responsible for the discovery and development of saquinavir (Invirase/Fortovase). This drug has been awarded 4 Prix Galien awards, and several other prizes. Dr. Roberts is a recipient of The Roche International Research Award 1995, The Royal Society for Medicines Research Award for Drug Discovery 1997 and The Pharmaceutical Manufacturers of America Drug Discoverers Award 1999. Dr. Roberts is head of Product Support in the area of viral diseases at Roche and is responsible for clinical resistance studies. He is also preclinical manager for integrated health care in viral diseases.

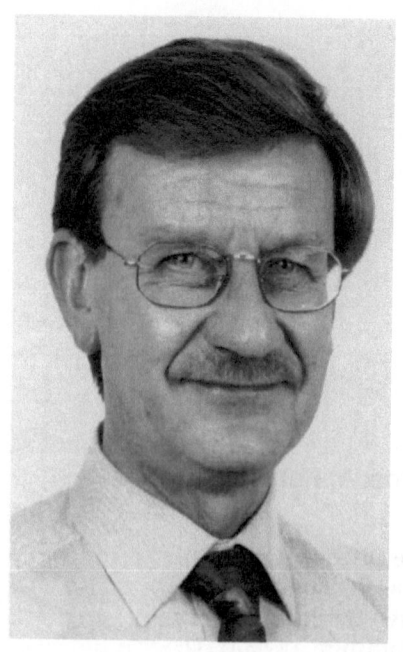

Summary

Each year, influenza viruses are responsible for considerable illness, complications and mortality. An effective treatment will have a major impact on the severe personal and economic burden that this disease incurs. There are several points in the influenza life cycle that may be potentially inhibited. One critical point is the release of newly synthesized virions from the host cell surface. Viral neuraminidase (NA) cleaves the virus from host cell sialic acid residues allowing infection of other host cells. Rationally designed NA inhibitors that block the viral life cycle are now in the clinic and these molecules are effective and safe for the treatment of influenza. Compared with other anti-influenza agents the NA inhibitors are well tolerated, effective against all influenza types and there has been little evidence of the emergence of viral resistance. NA inhibitors provide an important new therapeutic weapon for the management of influenza infection.

Contents

Noel A. Roberts

Key words

Antivirals, clinical efficacy, haemagglutinin, influenza, inhibitor design, neuraminidase, neuraminidase inhibitors, prophylaxis, treatment, viral replication.

Glossary of abbreviations

CYP, cytochrome P450; HA, haemagglutinin; IC_{50}, concentration for 50% enzyme inhibition; NA, neuraminidase; NP, nucleoprotein; RNP, ribonucleoprotein.

1 Influenza viruses

Influenza viruses are negative-strand RNA viruses with a segmented genome. There are eight RNA segments in influenza A and B viruses and seven segments in influenza C virus. The viruses are classified as types A, B and C according to the antigenic determinants of two of the major structural proteins, the nucleoprotein (NP) and the matrix (M1) protein. The spherical lipid envelope of the influenza virus is roughly (80–120 nm) in diameter with projecting glycoprotein spikes of haemagglutinin (HA) and neuraminidase (NA) (Fig. 1). Within the lipid envelope is a matrix protein that in turn encloses the viral RNA associated with NP. Type A influenza virus is further subtyped according to variations in the surface glycoproteins that project from the surface of the virus, HA and NA (Fig. 1). Also embedded in the surface is the tetrameric M2 ion channel protein that allows acidification of the interior of the virus during the uncoating process.

To date there have been 15 HAs (H1–H15) and nine NAs (N1–N9) described, and influenza A viruses are named according to the combination of molecules that are displayed e.g. H1N1, H2N2, H3N2 etc. [1]. Type A influenza viruses infect pigs, horses, birds and humans, but only birds are affected by all HA and NA subtypes. Human influenza strains comprise combinations of H1, H2 and H3 and N1 and N2, although recently new strains, H5N1 and H9N2, emerged in a limited number of individuals in Hong Kong. Influenza B and C viruses show less variation in their HA molecules and were thought to generally infect only humans prior to a recent report of influenza B in seals [2]. Influenza A and B viruses are widespread and both cause clinical disease in humans. Influenza C infection is not widespread and it is not an important clinical pathogen.

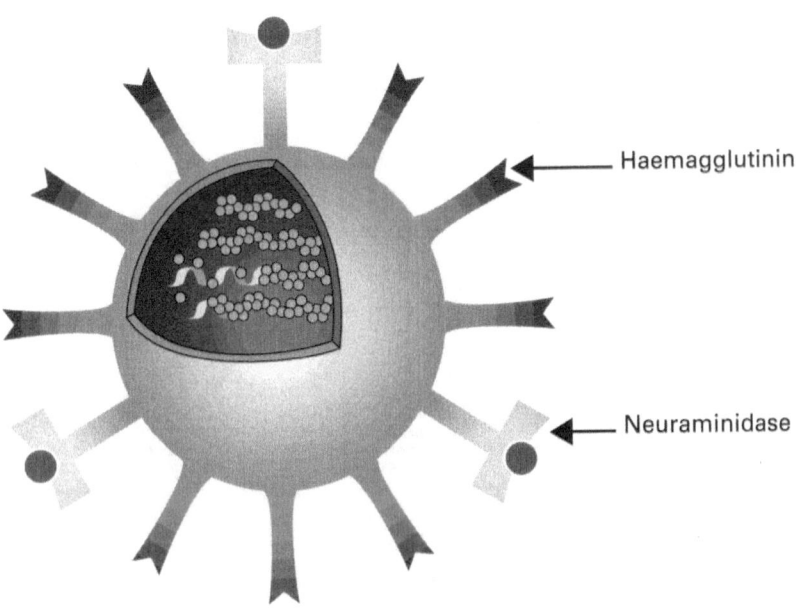

Haemagglutinin

Neuraminidase

Fig. 1
Structure of the influenza A virus.

1.1 Influenza virus replication

HA and NA are both essential to influenza virus replication (Fig. 2). The HA on an influenza virus particle binds to terminal sialic acid residues on glyco-conjugates on the surface of a host cell, inducing uptake of the infecting virus. The viral RNA and proteins are replicated within the host cell nucleus and assembled into new viral particles at the cell surface. When the new viruses bud off from the host cell, they too carry terminal sialic acid residues on glycoconjugates. Thus the progeny virus becomes attached by its HA to both the cell surface and also to other virus particles which form aggregates. The NA enzyme catalyses the hydrolysis of glycosidic linkages between a terminal sialic acid and its adjacent carbohydrate moiety, thus cleaving sialic acid from the cell and virus, and allowing release of the virus to infect new cells. Infection with influenza virus ultimately leads to host cell death.

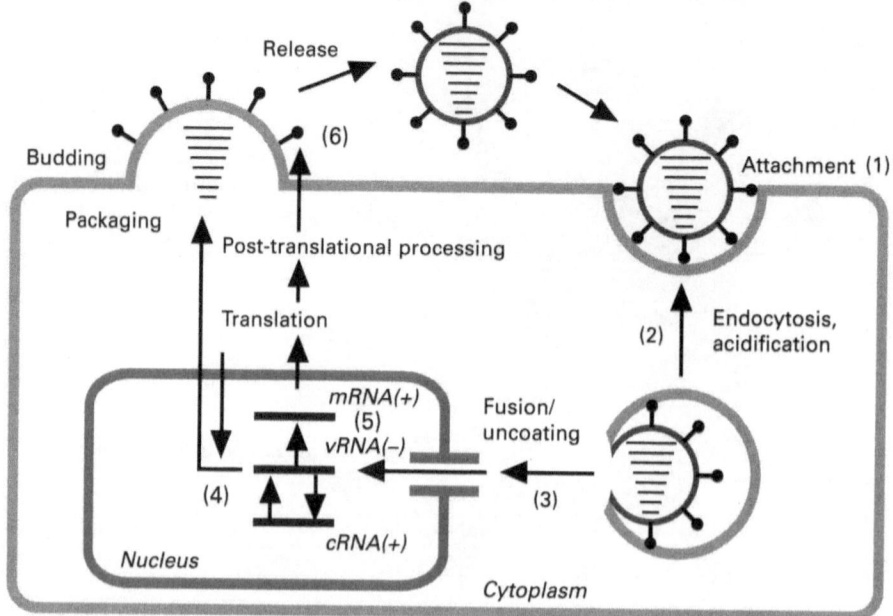

Fig. 2.
The life cycle of the influenza virus (adapted from source:
http://www-micro.msb.le.ac.uk/335/Orthomyxoviruses.html).
Life-cycle of the influenza virus: (1) The virus particle binds to the surface of the target cell by the HA molecule binding to sialic acid. (2) Entry into the cell is by fusion with the cell membrane and internalisation of the endosome. (3) Lowering of the intraendosomal pH through the M2 channel (influenza A) or NB channel (influenza B) dissociates the RNP from the protein coat, allowing the RNP to enter the cell nucleus. (4) Viral RNA is copied. 5. mRNA is formed using the host cell's transcription machinery. (6) Newly assembled viral particles bud from the cell and are liberated by the action of viral neuraminidase.

1.2 Antigenic drift and shift

The surface antigens on the virus are the dominant target for the host antibody response (and therefore also for influenza vaccines). However, minor mutations in the amino acid sequences of HA and NA occur frequently and this enables the viruses to evade the host immune system. The continual mutation process is known as antigenic drift and necessitates the yearly update and administration of influenza vaccines [3].

The segmented genome of the influenza virus gives the potential for a more dramatic alteration in the viral surface and other proteins. This process is called antigenic shift and involves the reassortment of two viral strains within one host. This mechanism produces a totally new virus strain giving the potential for, or threat of an influenza pandemic.

1.3   Influenza symptoms

Influenza is spread by virus-ladened respiratory secretions expelled during coughing and sneezing from an infected to a susceptible person [4]. The symptoms of influenza disease are both systemic and respiratory, and include fever, cough, headache, malaise and myalgia. The systemic symptoms usually disappear after 3–5 days but cough and malaise may last considerably longer (2–4 weeks). In some patients, influenza can exacerbate underlying conditions such as asthma or pulmonary or cardiac disease. It may also lead to secondary infections that require antibiotic therapy, e.g. bacterial pneumonia, bronchitis or otitis media.

2   Why treat influenza?

Outbreaks of influenza occur every winter resulting in about 10% of the global population contracting the disease and leading to considerable debilitating illness. The impact of the disease varies with age and is worse in people with chronic pulmonary diseases. Complications lead to the hospitalization of about 300 000 patients in each annual outbreak and up to 40 000 deaths in the USA alone [5]. Complications and deaths occur with greater frequency in the very young, elderly and other at-risk groups, but otherwise healthy individuals are also affected. The cumulative toll of morbidity and mortality during interpandemic years exceeds that of pandemics. It has been estimated that influenza epidemics accounted for 426 000 deaths during the interpandemic period from 1972 to 1992 in the USA [6]. This contrasts with 104 000 excess deaths during the pandemic outbreaks of 1957 and 1968 [7].

A substantial economic burden accrues as a result of the annual outbreaks of influenza, with considerable loss of productivity and earnings. In addition, healthcare resources become strained as hospitalization rates increase, primary care staff shortages occur (due to illness) and drug use (particularly antibiotics) rises [8, 9].

3   Symptomatic treatment and vaccination

The symptoms of fever, cough, headache and myalgia experienced with influenza illness naturally prompt the patient to seek relief. Medications that are usually taken for the symptom relief include analgesics, antipyretics, and cough remedies. However, these palliatives treat only the symptoms and not the cause of the disease, the influenza virus. Therefore, although there may be some modest symptomatic relief from using these agents, viral replication and cell damage will continue and the illness will run its course.

The mainstay of preventative measures against the impact of influenza is vaccination of groups of patients most at risk from the disease. However, the effectiveness of influenza vaccine depends on the level of similarity between the vaccine virus strains and those circulating in the community. Prediction of the composition of the annual vaccine helps determine its protective efficacy and when the match is close, the vaccine prevents illness in approximately 70–90% of healthy subjects under 65 years old [10]. However, long-lasting immunity is impossible because of the antigenic drift that continually occurs in influenza viruses. The age and immunocompetence of the vaccine recipient are also important variables in vaccine efficacy, even if the match is good. Elderly patients and those with chronic disease (i.e. those normally targeted for influenza vaccination) may develop lower post-vaccination antibody titres than younger, healthy recipients due to an impaired immune response [11]. A new influenza virus appearing unpredictably through antigenic shift would render current vaccines completely ineffective, leaving the global population unprotected against pandemic disease.

4   Antiviral agents

Antiviral therapy, used in conjunction with vaccination, is a logical approach to the management of influenza. By targeting viral replication, viral titres are reduced, thereby minimizing cell damage. There are a variety of points within the influenza virus life cycle at which virus replication may be inhibited (Fig. 2).

4.1   Inhibition of haemagglutinin binding

The first opportunity to inhibit influenza virus replication is at attachment of the virus to the host cell membrane (Fig. 2, inhibition point 1). The influenza virus HA attaches to oligosaccharides on the host cell membrane bearing sialic acid in the terminal position. One potential advantage for an inhibitor of HA binding is that it would not have to enter the cell in order to be active.

Early attempts to block the binding of HA to sialic acid were based on monovalent sialic acid derivatives. However, these were of low potency, typically with dissociation constants in the low mM range. The natural influenza inhibitor α_2-macroglobulin achieves high affinity-binding to HA by multivalent attachments [12]. This strategy has been used to incorporate sialic acid residues into a polymer, which enhances HA inhibition because hydrophobic constituents increase the affinity for the virus receptor binding site. Furthermore, spacing of the sialic acid residues 55 Å apart on the backbone (mimicking the natural gap found between these residues on the cell membrane) increase the binding potency of the compound by 100-fold. These polymers inhibited influenza A haemagglutination of erythrocytes with an IC_{50} of 0.6 nM [13]. *In vivo* efficacy of these compounds is yet to be established, but they would clearly require topical or systemic administration.

4.2   Fusion inhibitors

The influenza virus HA is synthesized as a single polypeptide precursor (HA_0) and is cleaved into HA_1 and HA_2 subunits by host proteases. Cleavage of HA at the virion surface is essential for the infectivity of all three influenza virus types (A, B and C) [14]. Therefore, the potential exists for protease inhibitors to prevent this essential cleavage. The protease inhibitor ε-aminocaproic acid (E-ACA) decreases virus replication in the lungs of influenza challenged mice [15]. The sodium salt of E-ACA, acemin, protects mice from a lethal influenza virus challenge when dosed subcutaneously [16]. Mechanistic studies with E-ACA on proteases in mice infected with influenza virus suggests that this compound may act at least in part by inhibition of HA cleavage [17].

Influenza virus is believed to enter mammalian cells by endocytosis in clathrin-coated pits. The virus fuses with the endosomal membrane through an irreversible conformational change in the HA molecule caused by a lowering of vesicle pH by the action of an ATP-dependent H^+ pump. A number of compounds inhibit viral fusion by stabilizing the HA structure, preventing the acid mediated alteration to the fusogenic state (Fig. 2, inhibition point 2). BMY–27709 (Fig. 3a) inhibits fusion of H1 and H2 influenza viruses by specifically binding in a hydrophobic pocket around the fusion peptide [18]. Other structurally similar compounds have also been found to be fusion inhibitors of influenza A virus, for example CL 61917, CL 385319 and CL 62554 (Wyeth-Ayerst) (Figs. 3b–d) [19]. These compounds were more effective against H1 (IC_{50}s 0.1–12 µg/ml) and H2 (IC_{50}s 0.4–1 µg/ml) than against H3 virus (IC_{50} 25 µg/ml).

Polyoxometalates are clusters of polyoxonic acid molecules that contain transition metal ions (e.g. tungsten, manganese, vanadium). These compounds inhibit the fusion between the influenza A viral envelope and the cell membrane. PM-523, a titanium containing polyoxotungstate is thought to inhibit HA conformational change by binding to the interface edges of the HA trimers. An aerosol of PM-523 4.8 mM, over 2 h, bid for 4 days protected 50% of mice from a lethal exposure of influenza A (H1N1) [20].

In contrast to stabilizing the HA at low pH, some compounds are able to destabilize it at neutral pH, causing inactivation by a conformational change before endosomal entry. A series of derivatives of podocarpic acid (Fig. 3e) interact with HA at neutral pH and prevent the low pH-induced change to the fusogenic conformation. These compounds are similarly effective against H1 and H2 influenza viruses but are less active against H3 or influenza B viruses. In mice infected with a lethal challenge of influenza A, two such compounds, LY314177 and LY311912 (Figs. 3f–g), gave survival rates of 90% and 80%, respectively, with intraperitoneal doses of up to 200 mg/kg bid for 8 days [21].

In general, all of the fusion inhibitors appear to have a narrow spectrum of activity against H1, H2 or H3 influenza A viruses.

4.3 Uncoating the virus

The M2 inhibitor amantadine, and the structurally related molecule rimantadine (Figs. 4a, b) are both clinically effective for the treatment of influenza A, but not influenza B virus infections. This is because their mechanism of

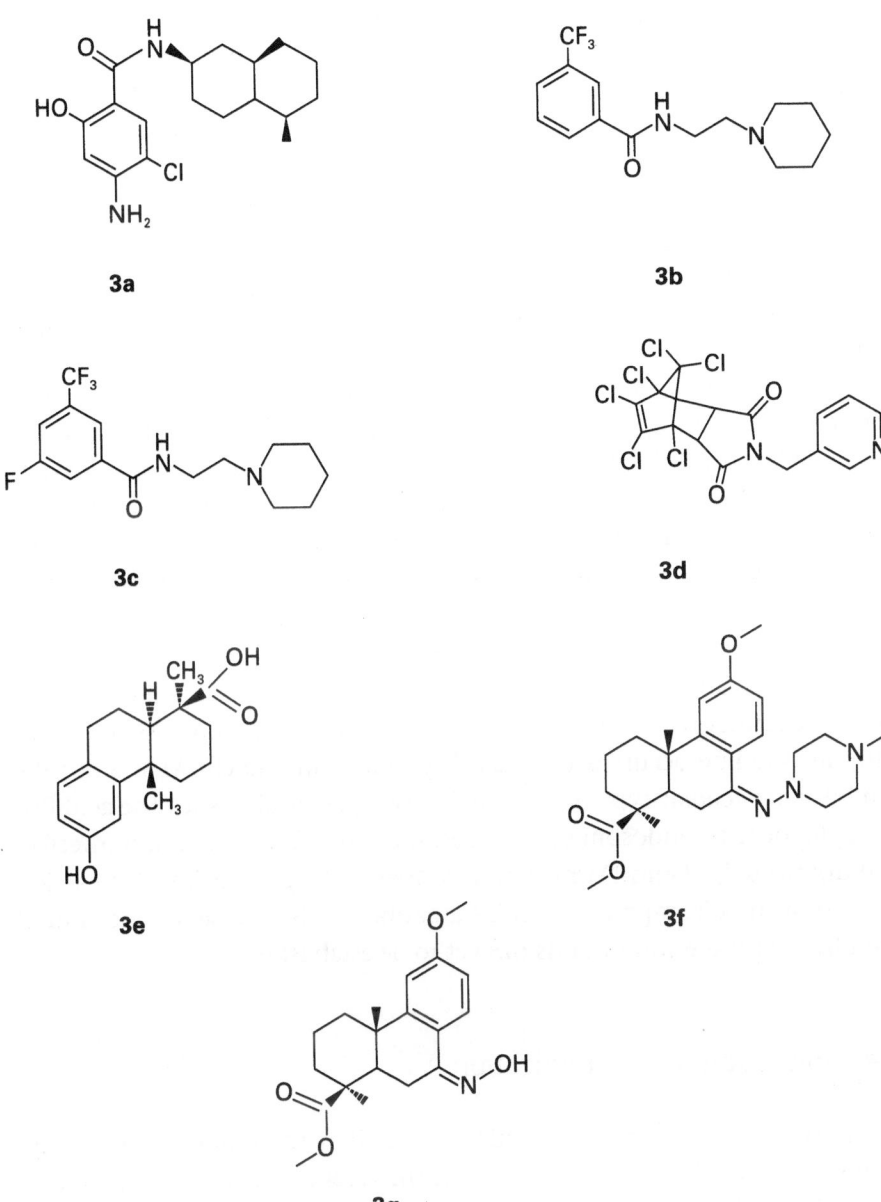

Fig. 3.
Structures of influenza virus fusion inhibitors. (a) BMY–27709, (b) CL 61917, (c) CL 385319, (d) CL 62554, (e) podocarpic acid, (f) LY314177, (g) LY311912.

action is through inhibition of the influenza virus M2 protein, an acid pH-activated ion channel, which is not present in influenza B viruses. Functioning of this channel normally results in acidification of the interior of the virion, which allows the M1 matrix protein to dissociate from the ribonucleoprotein (RNP) complex (Fig. 2, inhibition point 3). Transport of the RNP complex to the nucleus is required for genomic transcription, translation and viral assembly [22].

Although approved for treatment for influenza A infections for many years, the use of amantadine and rimantadine has been limited by the rapid emergence of drug-resistant virus, often occurring as rapidly as two days after start of therapy [22, 23]. Transmission of drug-resistant influenza A has been demonstrated during prevention programmes with rimantadine following treatment of infected patients in contact with persons receiving prophylaxis [24]. In addition, adverse events associated with these agents are commonly reported [25]. Central nervous system (CNS) side-effects include dizziness, anxiety, nervousness, insomnia, loss of concentration and insomnia. In general, rimantadine is better tolerated than amantadine [26].

Newer agents related to M2 function include a novel spiro compound, BL-1743 (Fig. 4c), and bafilomycin A1, a macrolide antibiotic. BL-1743 blocked the M2 channel when expressed in *Xenopus* oocytes [27]. Cross-resistance with amantadine occurs with this compound. Bafilomycin A1 is a specific inhibitor of vacuolar-type H$^+$ ATPase that completely abolished the acidified cell components (endosomes and lysosomes) in influenza A and B infected, and uninfected, Madin-Darby canine kidney (MDCK) cells [28]. The action of both of these compounds, unlike amantadine, is reversible. The clinical usefulness of these compounds has yet to be established.

4.4 Inhibition of viral replication

The host cell transcriptional machinery is used by the influenza virus polymerase complex during viral RNA transcription for capping, cap-methylation and splicing of viral mRNAs. The transcription complex of influenza viruses consists of a trimeric polymerase. This complex comprises PB1 (transcriptase), PB2 (cap-binding protein and possibly endonuclease) and PA (essential cofactor of unknown function). Association of the polymerase with the RNA template, which harbours essential and influenza virus specific sequence motifs,

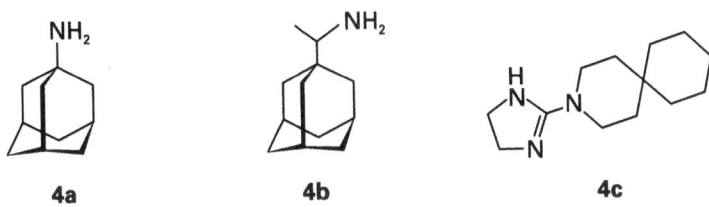

Fig. 4.
Structures of selected influenza M2 channel inhibitors. (a) amantadine, (b) rimantadine, (c) BL–1743.

and with the nucleoprotein (NP, RNA binding protein) is required for full transcriptase activity [29]. Known inhibitors of viral replication are targeted to several of these points (Fig. 2, inhibition points 4 and 5).

Influenza viruses have a unique mechanism for the cap formation of their mRNAs – hijacking that of the host cell. The polymerase contains an endonuclease activity that cuts the host cell mRNA at approximately 10–16 nucleotides from the cap structure. It then uses the capped oligonucleotides as primers for the generation of capped, viral mRNAs. The endonuclease is a unique and highly conserved target present in all influenza virus types, including influenza A and B viruses.

Divalent metal ions are required for enzymatic catalysis of the endonuclease reaction [30], and a number of potential metal ion chelating-compounds have been described for this target. Flutimide (Fig. 5a), isolated from the fungus *Delitschia confertaspora*, selectively inhibits the cap-dependent transcriptase of influenza A and B viruses. In MDCK cells, flutimide inhibited influenza virus replication with an IC_{50} of 5.9 µM and exhibited no cytotoxicity at concentrations up to 100 µM [31].

Structurally similar compounds include BMY-26270 (Fig. 5b) which was obtained from library screening. BMY-26270 also selectively inhibits the endonuclease activity of influenza A and B viruses [32].

L735,882 (Fig. 5c) is an example of a series of 4-substituted 2,4-dioxobutanoic acid endonuclease inhibitors. This compound showed antiviral activity in cell culture against influenza A and B viruses with IC_{50}s of 6 and 2 µM respectively, and had no apparent cytotoxic effects in MDCK cells at concentrations up to 100 µM [33]. Other members of this series showed antiviral activities with IC_{50}s of 0.18 µM and higher, and efficacy in a

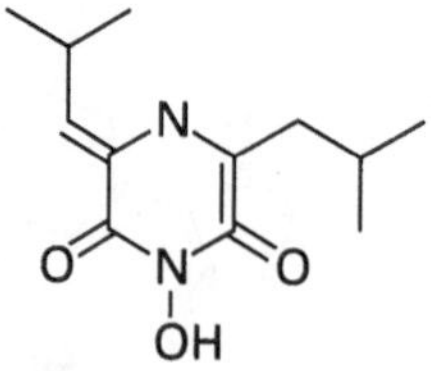

Fig. 5.
Structures if inhibitors of influenza virus replication. (a) flutimide, (b) BMY-26270, (c) L-735,882, (d) 2-FDG.

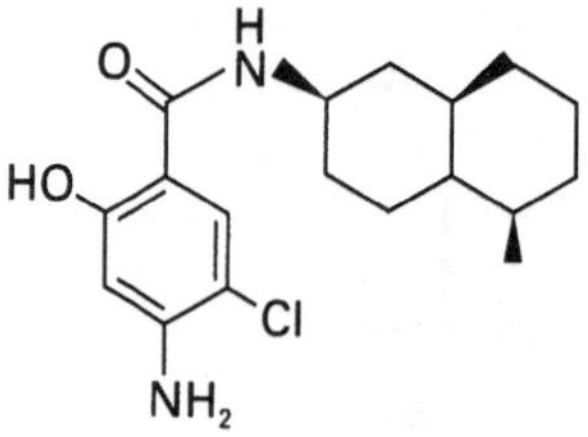

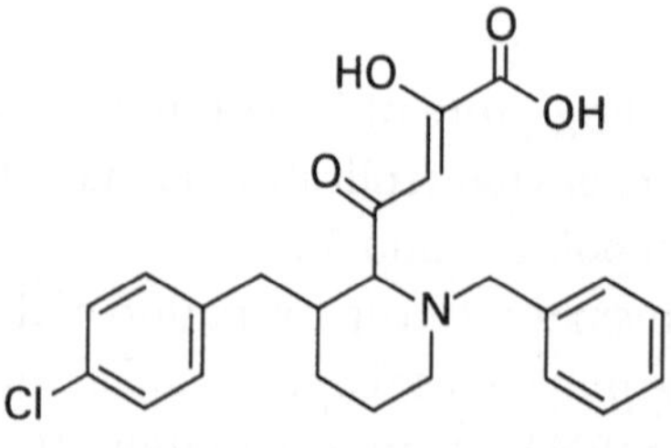

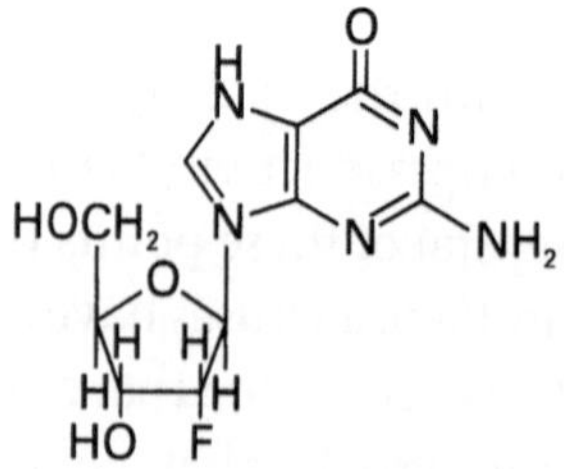

mouse model was demonstrated for a selected compound after intranasal administration [34].

The nucleoside analogue deoxyfluoroguanosine (2-FDG) (Fig. 5d) appears to be a specific inhibitor of influenza transcriptase activity that targets the active site of the polymerase subunit PB1. The triphosphate of 2-FDG showed competitive inhibition with GTP *in vitro*, and incorporation of this nucleoside analogue in place of GTP by the influenza virus polymerase leads to chain termination during transcription initiation [35]. Different strains of influenza A and B viruses were sensitive to 2-FDG with IC_{50}s ranging from 0.2–1 µM in chicken embryo fibroblast cells and from 2–22 µM in MDCK cells [36]. The mean pulmonary viral titre of influenza A and B in mice was significantly reduced after intraperitoneal treatment with 2-FDG (120 mg/kg up to 24 h postinfection) as compared with untreated controls. This compound also appeared to be more effective than amantidine (against influenza A) and ribavirin (against influenza B) [37]. Both 2-FDG and a prodrug (2,6-diamino-purine-2'-fluororiboside) have not progressed beyond preclinical development.

A synthetic, zinc binding peptide, peptide 6, derived from amino acids 148–166 of influenza virus strain A/PR/8/34 M1 protein has been reported to possess significant antiviral activity in cell culture when added up to 1 h after infection. On a molar basis, peptide 6 was about 1000-fold more active than amantidine or ribavirin in preventing MDCK cell death due to influenza virus infection, although the protective effect was quite variable among different virus strains [38]. Efficacy in preventing death was demonstrated in the mouse model after intranasal administration of 30 or 60 mg/kg/day, three times daily for 5 days with two influenza A virus strains. In contrast, there was only a rather small or insignificant effect on lung consolidation and lung virus titres [39]. The mechanism of action of this peptide remains unclear. As the whole M1 protein can inhibit influenza virus RNA synthesis *in vitro* at least partially, a possible effect of the M1-derived peptide on the transcription activity of the polymerase complex has been considered. However, others have not been able to detect significant inhibition of a similar peptide in the presence or absence of zinc in contrast to whole M1 protein [40], and the zinc binding residues of isolated peptide 6 do not form a zinc finger in the crystal structure of this protein [41].

Small nucleic acids have also shown potential to inhibit influenza virus replication. Capped RNA molecules too small to be endonuclease substrates can inhibit influenza virus transcription *in vitro* with IC_{50} values between 0.083 and 17 nM [42, 43]. In addition, RNA molecules containing the conserved influenza virus vRNA or cRNA ends can function as polymerase binding decoys to prevent replication in cell culture [44]. An antisense phosphorothioate oligonucleotide directed against the initiation codon of the influenza virus PB2 mRNA has been shown to inhibit virus replication in MDCK cells in a sequence specific manner, with an IC_{50} of 0.15 µM when encapsulated in cationic liposomes. Free oligonucleotides could interfere with virus attachment in a sequence independent manner, with IC_{50}s between 1 and 3 µM [45]. Protective efficacy of a liposomal preparation was also demonstrated in the mouse model after intravenous administration of 40 mg/kg twice daily for 5 days. The oligonucleotide treatment had a sequence specific effect on mouse survival, virus titre and lung consolidation, similar to treatment with 40 mg/kg ribavirin, although the levels of PB2 mRNA were only partially reduced. Interestingly, intranasal or intraperitoneal administration of encapsulated oligonucleotides were not protective, due to a lack of liposome mediated oligonucleotide transfer into the lung [46].

4.5 IMPDH inhibition

Inhibition of inosine monophosphate dehydrogenase (IMPDH; E.C. 1.1.1. 205) results in a decrease in the intracellular pool of GTP, required for the synthesis of nucleic acids (Fig. 2, inhibition point 5). This mechanism of action accounts for the anti-influenza activity of amitivir (LY 217896) (Fig. 6a). Amitivir is effective against several influenza A and B viruses in MDCK cells with IC_{50} values of 0.37–1.19 and 0.75–1.54 µg/ml respectively [47]. In addition, this compound protected against influenza A and B infection in mice when administered orally immediately, or several days after, experimental infection. However, development of amitivir has been discontinued because of a lack of clinical efficacy and increased patient serum uric acid levels [48].

Ribavirin (Virazole) (Fig. 6b), a synthetic guanosine derivative, is a broad spectrum antiviral that is active against several RNA virus families. Three possible mechanisms of action have been proposed for the anti-influenza virus action of ribavirin: IMPDH inhibition; inhibition of 5'-cap formation of mRNAs and inhibition of the function of virus-coded RNA polymerases that are necessary to initiate and elongate viral mRNAs [49]. Uncontrolled studies have shown that high doses of ribavirin reduce the duration of fever and respiratory symptoms resulting from influenza A and B infections by about one day [50]. Although oral and intravenous infusions are reported to be effective [51, 52], it is usually administered by a small particle aerosol (20 mg/ml) in hospitals and is consequently very costly. This and poor tolerance limits its use.

None of the above compounds are ideal for the antiviral treatment of influenza. Therefore there was a need for a new therapeutic class of anti-influenza treatment with wide specificity against influenza strains including pandemic strains and a good safety profile.

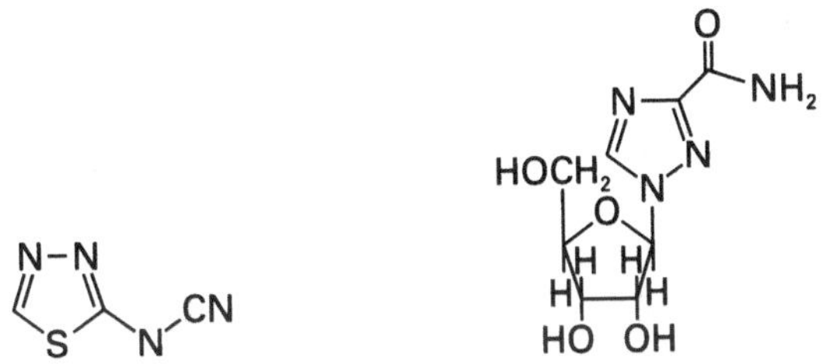

Fig. 6.
Structures of anti-influenza virus IMPDH inhibitors. (a) amitivir, (b) ribavirin.

4.6 Inhibiting neuraminidase

4.6.1 Role of neuraminidase in the virus life cycle

Neuraminidase (sialidase; acylneuraminyl hydrolase; E.C. 3.2.1.18) (Fig. 7) performs a vital function in the final stage of the viral life cycle. Without functional NA, newly-formed viral particles remain attached to the host cell membrane and form viral aggregates (Fig. 2, inhibition point 6). This binding is to sialyloligosaccharides *via* the viral HA and thus the essential function of HA at virus entry becomes a liability to virus release. Hence virus spread to infect naïve cells is limited when NA function is inhibited. The viral NA catalyses the hydrolysis of α-(2,3) or α-(2,6) glycosidic linkages between a terminal sialic acid and its adjacent carbohydrate moiety, thus cleaving sialic acid from cell surface oligosaccharides and from those on the virus. NA is also responsible for removing sialyl residues from mucins in the mucus of the respiratory tract similarly facilitating the movement of the virus towards its target epithelial cells [14]. HA can bind to the sialyl residues on mucin thus reducing propagation of the virus.

4.6.2 Predicted effect of neuraminidase inhibition

The role of viral NA was predicted when two mutant strains of influenza virus with defective NA (but not HA) were grown at a non-permissive temperature

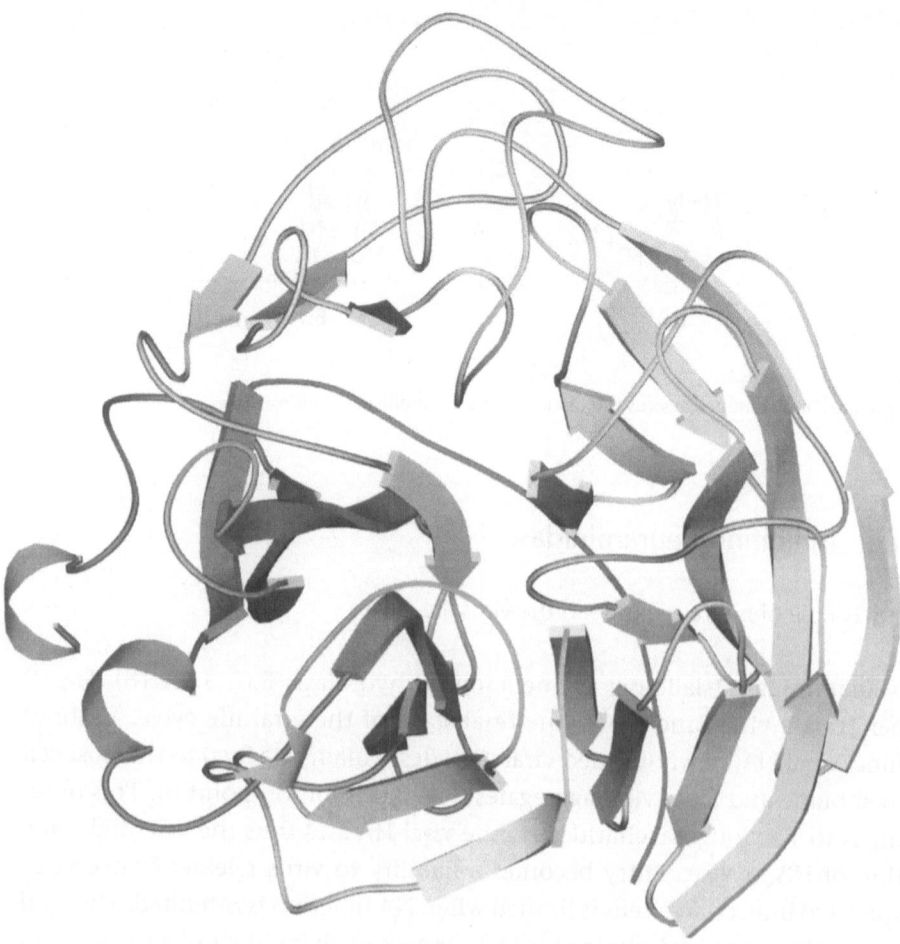

Fig. 7.
Neuraminidase subunit folding (Figure from Dr B. Graves).

(39.5°C) [53]. Electron microscopy revealed that viral particles formed aggregates near the cell surface, although the virus particles themselves were morphologically intact. Aggregates were not seen when NA was added to the culture. These findings demonstrated the requirement of normal NA activity for viral dispersal.

The active site of NA is highly conserved across all influenza A and B strains studied [54]. Despite 70% sequence variation in NAs, 24 amino acids

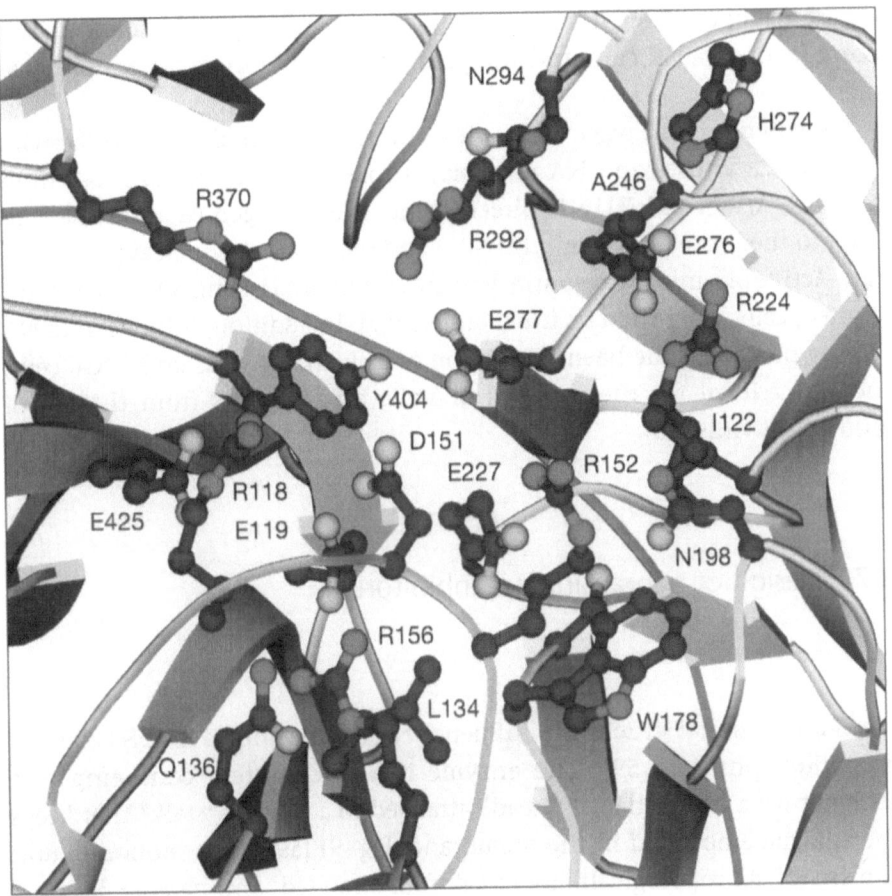

Fig. 8.
Minor mutations at the influenza virus neuraminidase active site compromise virus viability (Figure from Dr B. Graves).

at the active site are conserved, suggesting that even minor mutations at this site might compromise virus viability (Fig. 8). Laboratory-induced mutations at the active site on NA produce unstable or inactive viral strains [55]. Strains with mutations in HA have been produced that show resistance to NA inhibitors *in vitro* in MDCK cells [56], presumably because the HA is less adhesive and therefore NA is not required to cleave it from sialic acid. However, such strains are not resistant to inhibitors in the ferret *in vivo*. This may be an artefact of differential HA binding between the predominant α-(2,3) receptors on MDCK cells and the predominant α-(2,6) in ferret epithelial tract.

Proteolytic HA cleavage at the virus surface is essential for the infectivity of influenza viruses and NA may play a role in facilitating this. NA from influenza A/WSN/33 (H1N1) directly binds plasminogen (that can be activated to the protease plasmin by t-PA) and sequesters it for cleavage activation. Active plasmin cleaves and activates influenza HA and allows the virus to infect cells other than its usual targets [57]. In addition, inhibition of NA activity prevented the haemadsorbtion of influenza B virus on MDCK cells, and was critical for the removal of sialic acid residues from the HA of influenza B virus [58].

4.7   Design of neuraminidase inhibitors

4.7.1 Enzyme structure

The 3-dimensional structure of influenza NA was elucidated in 1983 by x-ray crystallography [54, 59]. The enzyme is a glycoprotein consisting of a tetramer with a box-shaped "head" attached to a slender "stalk" that keeps the enzyme embedded in the membrane (Fig. 9) [59]. Each monomer unit consists of six topologically identical, four-stranded, anti-parallel β-sheets, arranged in a "propeller" formation [59].

The active site is a deep cleft on the surface of the protein, lined by an unusually high proportion of charged amino acids (Fig. 9). The site has been identified and studied by means of its interactions with sialic acid [54, 59–61]. The three guanidinium groups of Arg118, 292 and 371 interact with the carboxylate of the sugar in sialic acid. The N–H group of the 5-N-acetyl side chain is held to the floor of the active site cleft *via* a bound water molecule. A hydrophobic pocket near Ile222 and Trp178 surrounds the methyl group and the oxygen of the 5-N-Acetyl side chain is hydrogen bonded with Arg152. On the 6-glycerol side chain, the last two hydroxyl groups are hydrogen bonded to Glu276, the 4-hyroxyl interacts with Glu119, and the glycosidic oxygen interacts with the carboxylate oxygen of Asp151.

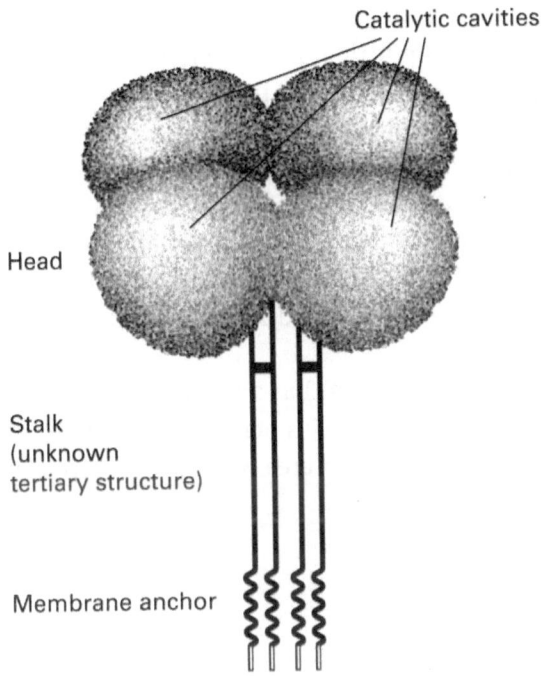

Catalytic cavities

Head

Stalk
(unknown
tertiary structure)

Membrane anchor

Fig. 9.
The active site on the surface of influenza virus neuraminidase.

4.7.2 Early substrate analogues

The first NA inhibitor to be described in 1969 was Neu5Acen (2-deoxy-2,3-dehydro-N-acetyl neuraminic acid; DANA) (Fig. 10a) [62]. It is an analogue of sialic acid. Neu5Acen inhibits influenza NA *in vitro* with a K_i in the micromolar range, has poor specificity for influenza NA, and has shown no beneficial effects in animal models of influenza [63].

2-deoxy-2,3-dehydro-N-trifluoroacetylneuraminic acid (FANA) (Fig. 10b) is a DANA derivative [64], with a K_i of 0.8 µM. Although FANA retards viral shedding in culture [53, 65], it is ineffective in animals with influenza infection [63].

4.7.3 Zanamivir

The characterization of the influenza NA active site by x-ray crystallography in 1983 [54] was a breakthrough for rational drug design. Computer modelling of the site [66] produced a derivative of Neu5Acen, zanamivir (4-guanidino-Neu5Acen; GG167; Relenza) (Fig. 10c), which is both potent and selective *in vitro*. Zanamivir inhibits the NA of all human influenza A and B virus strains tested *in vitro* [66] at low-nanomolar concentrations. However, the positively-charged guanidino group confers low oral bioavailability [67], and it must therefore be administered intranasally or by inhalation.

Zanamivir, derived from DANA, has a guanidino group on the 4-carbon position of DANA that interacts with acidic residues Glu119, Glu227 and Asp151 in a previously unoccupied area within the active cleft of influenza NA [66].

4.7.4 Oseltamivir

Rational medicinal chemistry at Gilead Sciences produced the NA inhibitor oseltamivir carboxylate (Ro 64–0802; GS 4071) (Fig. 10d) [68]. Although more lipophilic than zanamivir and not possessing a guanidino group, Ro 64-0802 also suffers from low oral bioavailability [69] due to a negatively charged carboxylate moiety. The goal to generate a convenient oral formulation was achieved by the development of its ethyl ester derivative, oseltamivir ((3R, 4R, 5S)-4-acetamido-5-amino-3-(1-ethylpropoxy)-1-cyclohexane-1-carboxylic acid; Ro 64-0796; GS 4104; Tamiflu) (Fig. 10e).

Oseltamivir is highly orally bioavailable and is metabolized by liver esterases to its active form (Fig. 11). Oseltamivir carboxylate is a very specific competitive inhibitor of NA from all influenza A and B strains tested, active at low nanomolar concentrations *in vitro* [70]. It is also active against avian influenza strains [71] and the H5N1 and H9N2 Hong Kong strains [72]. This inhibitor binds through an interaction between the lipophilic 3-pentyloxy side chain and a hydrophobic pocket in the region corresponding to the glycerol subsite of sialic acid [68].

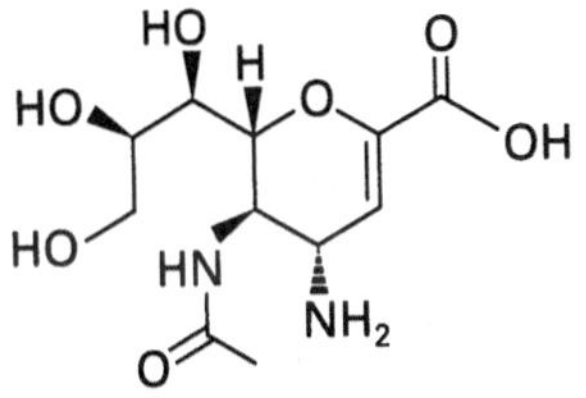

10a

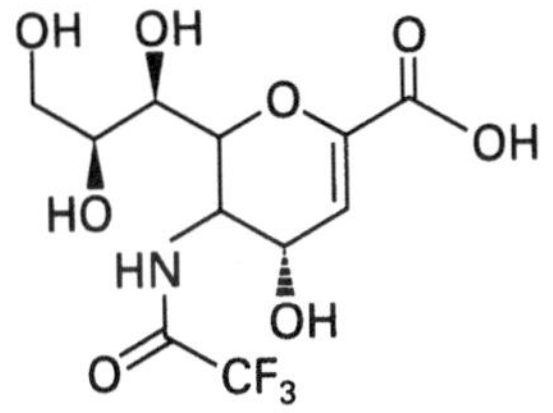

10b

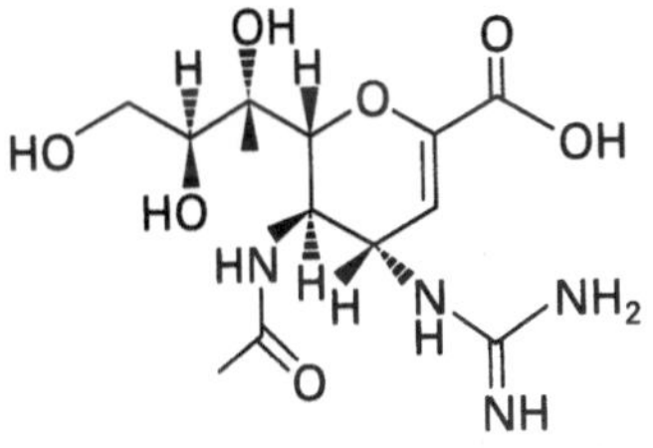

10c

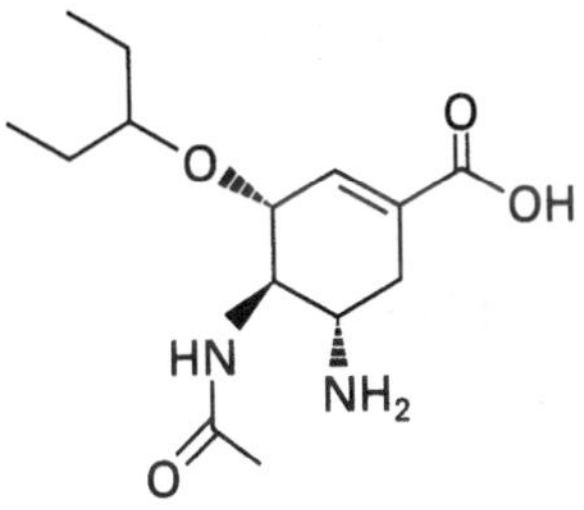

10d

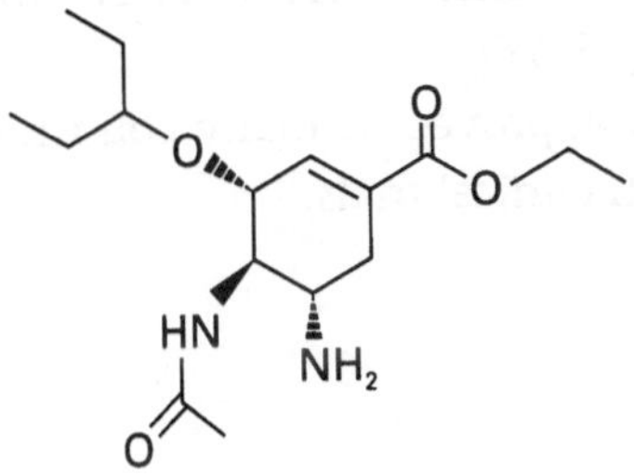

10e

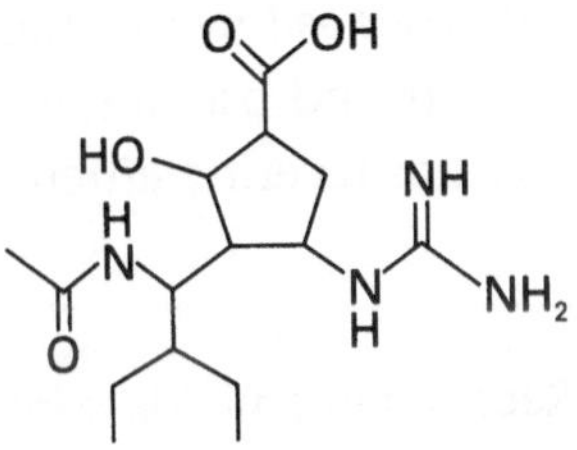

10f

Fig. 10.
Structures of the neuraminidase inhibitors. (a) DANA, (b) FANA, (c) GG167, (d) Ro 64-0802, (e) Ro 64-0796, (f) BCX-1812.

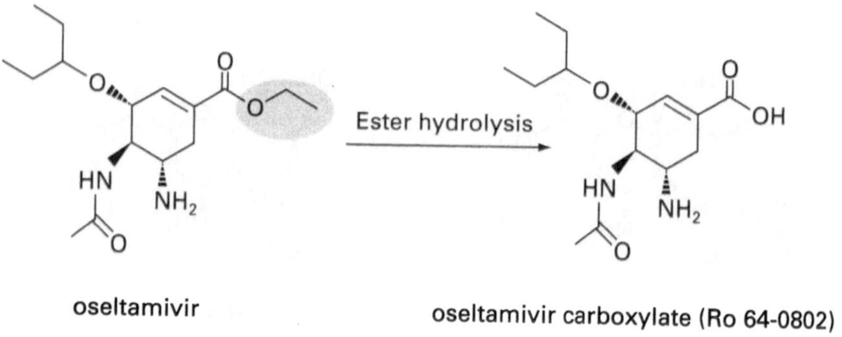

oseltamivir

oseltamivir carboxylate (Ro 64-0802)

Fig. 11.
Liver and gut esterases hydrolyse Ro 64-0796 to its active metabolite, Ro 64-0802.

4.7.5 BCX-1812

Another compound, BCX-1812 (4-(acetylamino)-3-guanidinobenzoic acid, RWJ-270201) (Fig. 10f), is a potent inhibitor of influenza A and B viral NA, with IC_{50} values ranging from 0.1 to 11 µM, and is active orally [73]. BCX-1812 inhibited the replication of most influenza A and B virus strains in MDCK cells (IC_{50} ranges from 0.037 to 7 µM) [74]. This agent prevented death in mice infected with lethal doses of influenza A (H1N1 or H3N2) and B viruses at doses as low as 1 mg/kg/day [75, 76].

Zanamivir and oseltamivir are now approved in many countries while BCX-1812 has recently entered phase III clinical trials.

4.7.6 Recent neuraminidase inhibitors

Since the discovery of zanamivir, GlaxoWellcome have sought to identify further NA inhibitors as possible clinical candidates. 4H-pyran 6-ether and ketone analogues of zanamivir were potent and selective inhibitors for influenza A NA [77]. Representative tetrasubstituted bicyclo[3.2.1]octenes were weak inhibitors of NA from influenza A and B, being 10- to 100-fold less active than DANA [78], but a bicyclo[2.2.2]octane was inactive against these same enzymes [79].

4.7.7 Specificity of neuraminidase inhibitors

As well as conferring high affinity for the influenza virus enzyme, substitutions in the C4 position of NA inhibitors lead to an increased specificity in enzyme inhibition. The 4-hydroxyl group of sialic acid points in the direction of (but does not directly interact with) two glutamic acid residues (Glu119 and Glu227) that sit in a small cleft in the active site and are unique to influenza virus NA [66]. Basic substitutions at C4 that are larger than the hydroxyl group of sialic acid yield high affinity, specific influenza NA inhibitors. NAs from other viral, bacterial or mammalian sources are therefore not significantly inhibited by zanamivir [66, 80] or oseltamivir carboxylate [70].

5 *In vitro* properties of neuraminidase inhibitors

The NA inhibitors zanamivir, oseltamivir carboxylate and BCX-1812 inhibit NA activity in the low nanomolar range from a wide variety of laboratory strains and clinical isolates of influenza A and B viruses (Tab. 1). In addition, these three compounds inhibit the NA activity of a variety of avian influenza strains [74, 81, 82]. Inhibition of NA activity across the spectrum of influenza viruses provides strong evidence that these agents will be active against potential new pandemic strains.

   NA inhibitors also effectively inhibit laboratory strains of influenza virus replication in cell culture. For example, zanamivir inhibits plaque formation by laboratory strains of influenza A and B viruses with IC_{50} values between 5 and 15 nM in MDCK cells [83]. The potency and antiviral activity of oseltamivir carboxylate is at least comparable to zanamivir for a variety of influenza A and B viruses in MDCK cells and a transformed human bronchial epithelial cell line (BEAS-2B) [71]. In contrast, drug inhibition of plaque formation by clinical isolates of influenza viruses is less effective, despite potent inhibition of NA activity. This phenomenon is likely due to a different sialic acid linkage present on MDCK cells (a combination of predominantly α-(2,3) and α-(2,6) compared with human respiratory epithelial cells (α-(2,6)). Clinical isolates will be adapted to α-(2,6) linkages while laboratory passaged virus will have adapted to the MDCK cell receptors favoured by viral HA [84, 85]. This mismatch in clinical isolates may reduce the affinity of HA for the MDCK

Table 1.
Inhibition of influenza virus A and B neuraminidase activity by neuraminidase inhibitors

Virus	IC_{50} (nM)[a]		
	Zanamivir[b]	Ro 64-0802[b]	BCX-1812[c]
Laboratory strains			
A/WS/33 (H1N1)	0.7	1.0	7.0
A/Victoria/3/75 (H3N2)	1.7	0.5	<0.1
B/Port Chalmers/1/73 (H3N2)	1.1	0.3	0.02
B/Mass/3/66	1.7	0.8	NR
B/Hong Kong/5/72	1.0	1.7	2.0
Clinical isolates			
A/Texas/36/91 (H1N1)	0.3	0.5	0.1
A/Texas/36/91-like (H1N1)	0.5	0.4	NR
A/Taiwan/1/86-like (H1N1)	0.5	1.3	NR
A/Johannesburg/33/94/ (H3N2)	4.6	0.8	0.015
A/Victoria/7/87-like (H3N2)	2.6	0.7	NR
A/Shangdong/09/93-like (H3N2)	0.7	0.2	<0.1
A/Virginia/305/95 (H3N2)	0.6	0.1	NR
B/Harbin/07/94	2.1	2.0	<0.1
B/Beijing/184/93-like	1.2	2.6	7.0
B/Victoria/2/87-like	1.4	2.6	NR

[a] IC_{50} = concentration required to inhibit the neuraminidase activity by 50%
[b] Oxford & Lambkin 1998 [81]
[c] Huffman et al 1999 [74]
NR, not reported

cellular receptor [86, 87] and hence the requirement for NA activity. Enzyme assay is therefore a more useful tool in evaluating NA inhibitors than antiviral assay MDCK culture.

Electron microscopy of *in vitro* NA inhibition confirms the predicted effect of NA in the influenza virus life cycle. Figure 12 clearly demonstrates clustering of virus particles on the host cell surface, preventing the release of newly synthesized virus and infection of other target cells.

5.1 Reduced sensitivity to neuraminidase inhibitors

In contrast to the M2 inhibitors amantadine and rimantadine, with which drug resistant viruses can be easily generated after one to two passages in cell culture [88], viruses with reduced sensitivity to NA inhibitors are generated

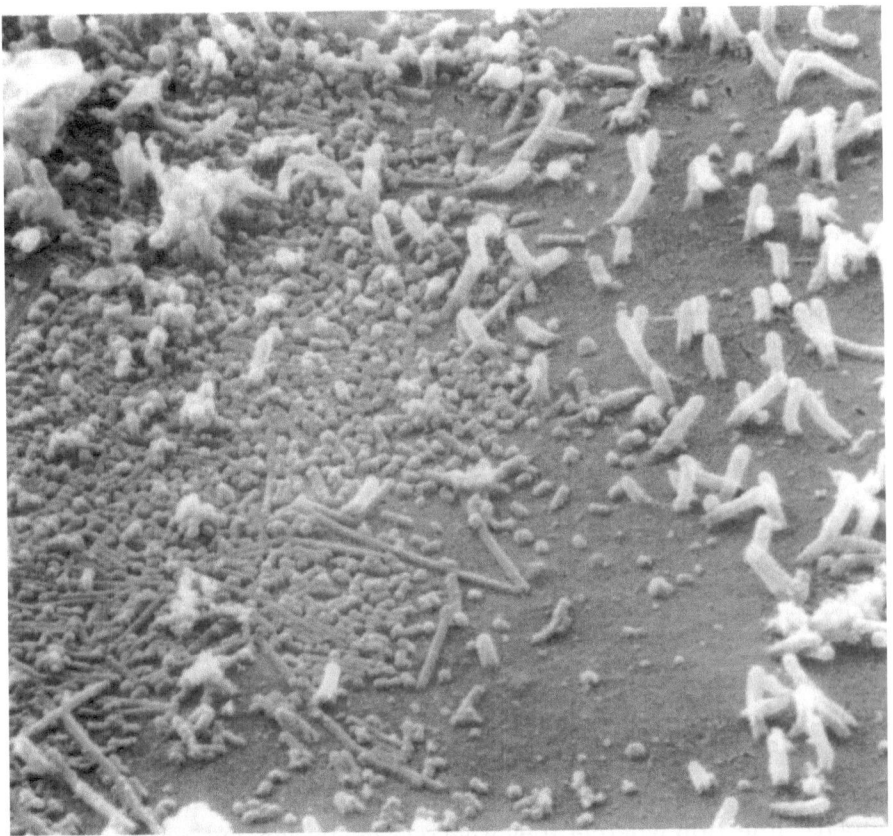

Fig. 12.
Electron micrograph of clusters of virus particles bound to the host cell as a result of the effect of neuraminidase inhibition (× 20 000 magnification).

less readily. Following isolation and sequencing, viruses resistant to the NA inhibitors *in vitro* have mutations within the HA and/or NA genes. HA mutations are generated within fewer passages.

Most HA mutations generated by passage with zanamivir result in marked (100- to 10 000-fold) decrease in virus sensitivity to drug [56, 87, 89–91]. The resistant virus strains bind less avidly to sialyl receptors which have a reduced requirement for NA function. Virus variants selected in the presence of oseltamivir carboxylate with combined mutations at Ala28 (in HA1) and Arg124 (in HA2) only have about an 8-fold decrease in sensitivity to drug [92].

It was not possible to determine which mutation contributed to the decrease in sensitivity. The 8-fold decrease was within the range (ten-fold) that other studies have shown can be generated by passage in MDCK cells alone in the absence of any drug [89]. The greater decrease in drug sensitivity in viruses with HA mutations selected with zanamivir suggest that they confer a greater advantage to the virus and therefore may be more likely to arise.

In general, mutations in the HA molecule lower the binding affinity for sialic acid and lessen the dependence on NA activity for cleavage of the attachment that facilitates viral spread, thereby reducing the sensitivity to NA inhibitors [87]. However, there is no guarantee that mutations that result in decreased binding to MDCK cells will predict a decrease in binding to human respiratory epithelial cells. In fact the evidence suggests that they do not [86].

Mutations within NA have been found at Arg292 following extensive virus passage in the presence of zanamivir [89], Ro 64-0802 [92] and BCX-1812 [93]. This residue is important for substrate binding and stabilization of the transition state. Following passage with zanamivir, other mutations have been isolated with substitutions at Glu119 [89, 94]. Because oseltamivir carboxylate contains an amino group in the position corresponding to the guanidino group of zanamivir, its activity is essentially unaffected by the mutations at Glu119 that confer resistance to zanamivir.

Influenza viruses containing Lys at residue 292 (Arg292Lys) in NA were found to be far less infectious than the wild type virus in a mouse model of influenza infection whether they were selected by zanamivir or oseltamivir [92, 95]. In contrast, the mutation Glu119Ala selected by zanamivir did not alter the infectivity of the virus compared with the wild-type [95]. This suggests that should these mutant viruses arise in humans, the likelihood of transmission of the Arg292Lys mutant will be less than either the Glu119Ala mutant or wild-type virus. However, viruses resistant to zanamivir have not been generated in animals using conditions equivalent to those that create viruses resistant to the M2 inhibitors [66]. Similarly, viruses recovered from mice protected from a lethal dose of influenza A virus by doses of oseltamivir were just as susceptible to Ro 64-0802 in vitro as those from infected vehicle-treated animals [55]. Under the same conditions, virus recovered following treatment with amantadine or rimantadine may be 1000-fold less sensitive to the M2 inhibitors [55].

The novel mutant of influenza A (H1N1), His274Tyr, selected in vivo by oseltamivir or in vitro by oseltamivir carboxylate is approximately 400-fold less sensitive to inhibition by Ro64-0802 [96, 97]. The growth of this variant is reduced by 100-fold in MDCK cells and by at least 1000-fold in animal models, indicating that impaired replication of this mutant means it is unlikely to be transmitted in man [96, 97]. This mutant shows only minor resistance to zanamivir [98] and studies have shown that the amino-acid side chain at position 274 can influence the interaction of influenza NA with zanamivir and oseltamivir [99].

Influenza B virus resistant to oseltamivir carboxylate has not yet been selected despite several attempts. Binding of this compound to influenza B NA does not result in the same reorientation of Glu276 as occurs with influenza A NA. It is this reorientation which is thought to be prevented by the Arg292Lys and His274Tyr mutations in H3N2 and H1N1 viruses respectively (B Graves, personal communication).

6   *In vivo* properties of neuraminidase inhibitors

6.1   Efficacy

Mice infected with influenza virus develop pneumonia with a high degree of mortality [100, 101]. Intranasally administered zanamivir (0.01 mg/kg) significantly reduced influenza mortality, viral titres in pulmonary homogenates and lung consolidation [102]. Oral oseltamivir dose-dependently protected mice infected with influenza A and B strains; 1 mg/kg dosed twice daily for 5 days beginning 4 h prior to influenza inoculation gave total protection against influenza A (H1N1) induced mortality. A higher dose, 10 mg/kg, was similarly effective against influenza A (H3N2), A (H1N1) and influenza B infections and lung viral titres were substantially reduced [55]. Delaying administration of oseltamivir by 60 h protected all mice challenged with an LD_{85} dose of influenza A (H1N1) compared with vehicle-treated controls (85% mortality). Oseltamivir 10 mg/kg/day, administered up to 36 h post inoculation of a 100-fold increase in the viral inoculum was 50% protective [103]. BCX-1812 at doses as low as 1 mg/kg/day for 5 days protected mice from the lethal effects of influenza A (H3N2) or influenza B, weight loss and reduced viral lung titres [75, 76]. As observed for oseltamivir, delaying the administration of BCX-1812 10 mg/kg as long as 60 h after inoculation prevented death following infection by influenza A (H1N1) [76].

The ferret is a useful experimental animal model of influenza infection as infection is characterized by a display of lethargy, fever and nasal symptoms, all signs seen in humans with this disease. In addition, the ferret can be infected with most human influenza virus isolates without adaptation. Intranasal zanamivir 50 µg/kg administered twice daily 1 day before and 6 days following infection with influenza A virus effectively abolished fever and reduced nasal virus titres in ferrets [66]. Oral oseltamivir is also effective in this animal model. When administered to ferrets twice daily for 3 days starting 2 h after inoculation with influenza A (H3N2), oral oseltamivir 5 mg/kg and 25 mg/kg dose-dependently lowered the febrile response to infection by 58% and 93%, respectively. In addition, oseltamivir treatment reduced nasal signs and lethargy, lowered the numbers of inflammatory cells in nasal lavages and reduced peak viral titres [70]. Similar effects were seen with influenza A (H1N1), A (H3N2) and influenza B induced infections (F. Hoffmann-La Roche, data on file).

Intranasal zanamivir (1 mg/kg) is effective prophylactically against lethal influenza A (H7N7) infection in chickens, but not against infection by other virulent viruses of the N1, N2 or N3 subtype [82]. However, oseltamivir carboxylate was effective against H5N1 and H9N2 avian influenza viruses *in vitro* (EC_{50} values from 7.5 to 12 µM in MDCK cells) and oral oseltamivir at 1 and 10 mg/kg/day prevented death, inhibited lung viral titres and prevented the spread of virus to the brains of mice infected with these viruses [72].

Neither zanamivir nor oseltamivir administration has been shown to adversely affect the primary immune response to influenza infection in animals [104–106].

6.2 Bioavailability

Zanamivir is readily bioavailable in mice by the intranasal, intraperitoneal and intravenous routes, but not after oral administration [102]. The highly polar, zwitterionic nature of zanamivir is responsible for its poor oral bioavailability. When administered intranasally to ferrets the bioavailability of zanamivir is 7.8% which contrasts with 43% in the mouse [104].

Administration of oral oseltamivir gave bioavailabilities of oseltamivir carboxylate of 30–73% in several species, including rodents, ferrets, dogs and marmosets [69, 107]. Most of the absorbed prodrug was hydrolysed to oseltamivir carboxylate in these species [107].

6.3 Biodistribution

Influenza viruses replicate throughout the respiratory tract and may cause complications in the middle ear and sinuses. It is therefore important that antiviral agents penetrate these sites at therapeutic concentrations. Whole-body autoradiography in ferrets after a single oral dose of 5 mg/kg [^{14}C]-oseltamivir demonstrated that levels of label in the lungs was over five times greater than in the blood. There was also good drug penetration to the middle ear and nasal mucosa [107]. In a similar study in rats using 30 mg/kg [^{14}C]-oseltamivir, drug concentrations in the lung were double those in the plasma at 6 h, and at 24 h the difference was 30-fold greater [107]. The drug moiety in the lungs of rats dosed with labelled oseltamivir was confirmed as Ro 64-0802 [108]. In addition, Ro 64-0802 was cleared from bronchoalveolar lavage fluid slower than from plasma [107]. There are no animal distribution data for inhaled zanamivir.

7 Clinical properties of neuraminidase inhibitors

7.1 Drug interactions

No clinically relevant drug interactions are expected with either zanamivir or oseltamivir [107, 109]. Zanamivir is not metabolized and is renally excreted [110]. It does not alter the metabolism of a number of cytochrome P450 (CYP) probe substrates by human liver microsomes and its plasma protein binding is low. These properties indicate that zanamivir has low potential for clinical interaction with co-administered drugs [109].

Oseltamivir has 43% plasma protein binding and the carboxylate (which represents over 95% of the total exposure following oral dosing in humans) is ~ 3% bound. Both of these values are below protein binding levels associated with interactions. Oseltamivir is eliminated *via* metabolism to the carboxylate which is excreted *via* the kidney through a combination of glomerular filtration and anionic renal tubular secretion. Oseltamivir carboxylate has weak affinity for the anionic tubular transporter and does not interact with other drugs excreted *via* this route, e.g. amoxicillin [107]. Neither oseltamivir nor oseltamivir carboxylate are substrates for human CYPs or glucuronosyl-transferases [107].

There is no effect on the immune response to vaccination when zanamivir is co-administered with influenza vaccine [111]. Similarly, the immune response to influenza infection is unaffected by treatment with oseltamivir in clinical trials [112].

7.2   Human pharmacokinetics

In human volunteer studies, a 16 mg dose of zanamivir was given by one of three routes: inhaled, intranasal or intravenous. Intravenous zanamivir gave the highest peak serum levels (C_{max} 1275 µg/mL) followed by the inhalation (C_{max} 136 µg/mL) and then the intranasal route (C_{max} 4.2 µg/mL) [113]. Topical administration gave a longer half-life (intranasal $t^1/_2$, 3.4 h; inhaled $t^1/_2$, 2.9 h; intravenous $t^1/_2$, 1.7 h). This reflects slow or complex adsorption rather than changes to the elimination phase.

In most clinical studies, zanamivir has been administered by inhalation using the currently approved dry-powder aerosol containing lactose. The deposition of drugs into the lung is a function of particle size and inspiratory flow rates (PIFR). PIFR is lower in young children and some elderly subjects compared to healthy adults [114, 115]. As lactose particles are large (> 40 µM), nearly 80% of the zanamivir dose deposits in the oropharynx of uninfected healthy adults. Only 13–15% of the zanamivir dose deposits in the trachea, bronchi and lungs [110, 116]. Inspiratory flow rate reductions may also adversely affect lung deposition.

About 80% of an oral dose of oseltamivir reaches the circulation as oseltamivir carboxylate. The active metabolite is detectable in plasma within 30 min of the dose and peak levels are attained after 2 to 3 h exceeding those of the prodrug (Fig. 13). Mean peak plasma concentrations of oseltamivir carboxylate ranged from 77.1 µg/mL (oseltamivir 20 mg) to 4490 µg/mL (oseltamivir 1000 mg). The steady-state volume of distribution of oseltamivir carboxylate is 23 to 26 L (after an intravenous dose), suggesting that the drug will penetrate systemic sites of viral infection at concentrations similar to those in plasma [107]. Recently, antiviral concentrations of

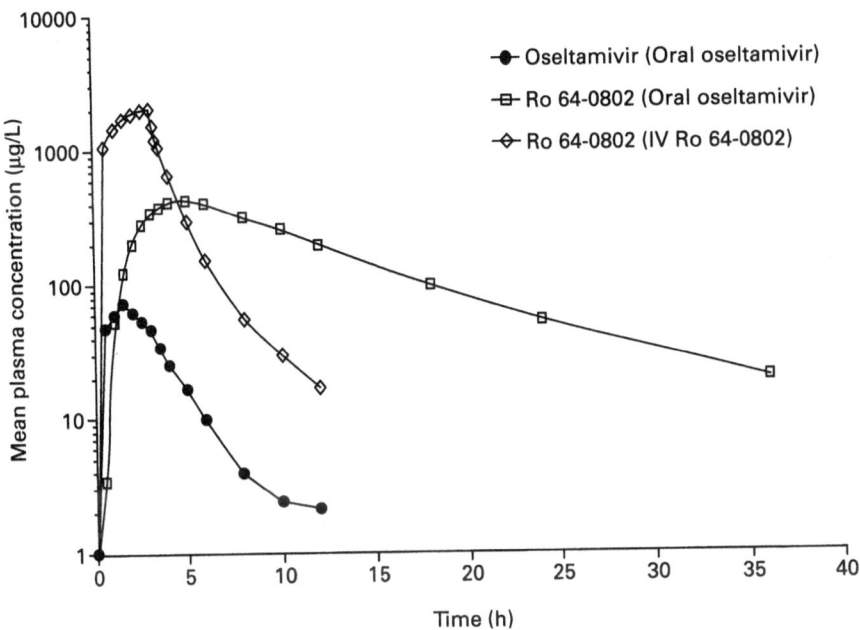

Fig. 13.
Mean plasma concentrations time profiles of oseltamivir and its active metabolite, Ro 64-0802 after oral oseltamivir 150 mg or intravenous Ro 64-0802 150 mg to healthy volunteers (n = 12) [107].

oseltamivir carboxylate have been detected in middle ear fluid and maxilliary sinuses from patients dosed with oseltamivir 75 mg and who required surgical drainage [117].

7.3 Experimental influenza

The NA inhibitors are effective in treating and preventing influenza A (H1N1) infection in volunteers experimentally infected with the virus [118, 119]. Viral shedding, symptom severity and symptom duration were reduced by treatment with both oseltamivir and zanamivir. Both drugs were also effective against influenza B infection [120, 121]. BCX-1812, is effective in experimental influenza A infection [122] and has recently entered phase III clinical trials.

Virological and clinical features of experimentally infected influenza A illness correlate well with proinflammatory cytokine levels in nasal lavage fluid [123]. Oseltamivir treatment abolished the increased levels of TNFα, IL-6 and IFNγ resulting from experimental influenza A infection [124].

7.4   Natural influenza

A number of randomized, placebo-controlled studies have demonstrated the efficacy of zanamivir and oseltamivir for both the treatment and prevention of naturally acquired influenza infections in healthy adults.

Inhaled zanamivir 10 mg twice-daily for 5 days reduced the median duration of symptoms in those patients with influenza by 1–2.5 days compared with placebo [125–127]. Oseltamivir 75 mg or 150 mg twice daily for 5 days reduced the duration of fever, the severity of symptoms and reduced the duration of illness by > 1 day (Fig. 14) [112, 128]. Because of differences in study endpoint definitions and outcome analyses, the efficacy of the two agents cannot be directly compared. However, results from phase III studies conducted during the influenza season of 1997–98 were very similar. Recent publications show that both agents are effective in the treatment of influenza in children. Zanamivir reduced the duration of acute influenza by 1.25 days in children aged 5–12 years of age [129]. Oseltamivir suspension was administered to children aged 1–12 years and reduced both the duration of influenza by 1.5 days and the incidence of acute otitis media by 44% [130].

Fewer secondary complications requiring antibiotic use resulting from influenza infection occur following treatment with the NA inhibitors compared with placebo treatment. For example, the collective incidence of pneumonia, bronchitis, sinusitis or otitis media in influenza patients was reduced by half in oseltamivir recipients compared with placebo treatment [112]. Similarly, patients thought to be at a high risk of developing complications (e.g. those with existing respiratory, cardiovascular disorders) developed a third fewer complications and had a lower antibiotic use than placebo recipients [125].

Significant benefits to the quality of life are also apparent following treatment of influenza illness with NA inhibitors. Patients treated with oseltamivir returned to normal activities 2 to 3 days sooner than those patients in the placebo group [112]. Zanamivir treatment also reduced the period taken for

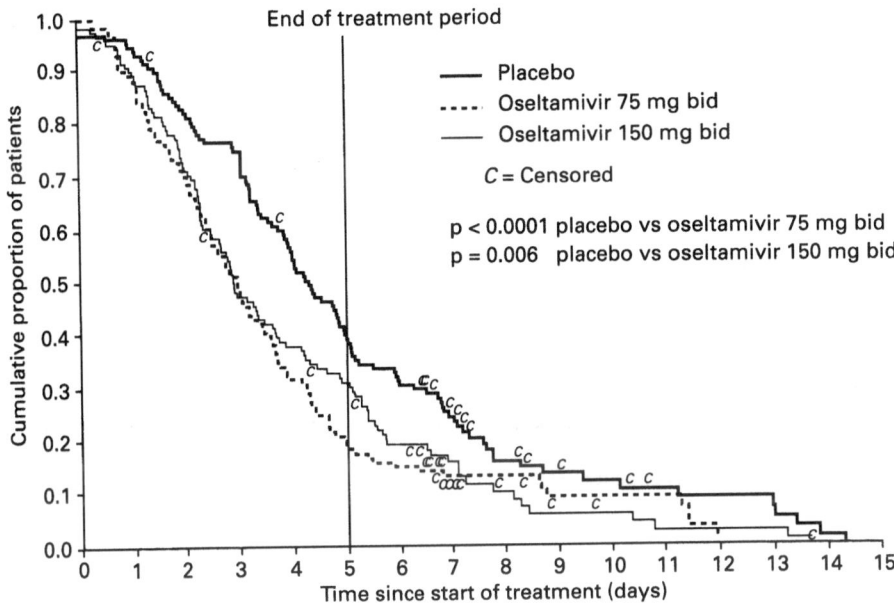

Fig. 14.
The effect of oral oseltamivir 75 or 150 mg twice daily on the time to alleviation of all symptoms in influenza infected patients. p < 0.001 for placebo vs oseltamivir 75 mg twice daily; p = 0.006 for placebo vs oseltamivir, 150 mg twice daily [112].

patients to return to normal activities (Fig. 15) and experienced a median of two fewer symptom-disturbed nights compared with the placebo group [125, 131].

The NA inhibitors are also effective in preventing influenza infection. Zanamivir 10 mg inhaled once daily over a 4-week period in adults was 67% protective against laboratory confirmed influenza [131]. Administration of oral oseltamivir 75 mg once or twice daily for 6 weeks gave a protective efficacy of 74% for laboratory confirmed influenza [124]. This dosing regime for oseltamivir was effective in frail elderly residential subjects (92% protective efficacy, p = 0.0015) [132]. In addition, oseltamivir 75 mg once daily for 7 days reduced the post-exposure spread of influenza in families (89% efficacy, p < 0.0001) [133].

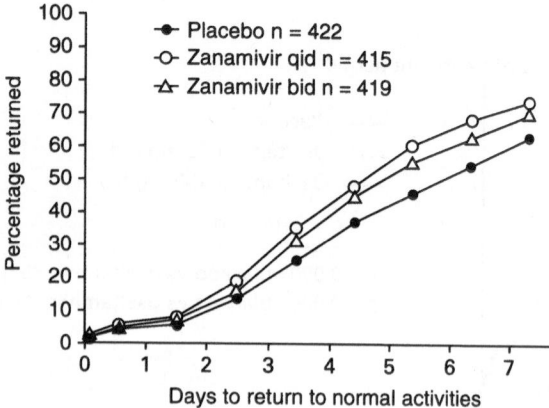

Fig. 15.
The effect of zanamivir 10 mg inhaled and 6.4 mg intranasally administered either twice (bid) or four times (qid) daily for 5 days on the time taken for patients to feel able to return to normal activities compared with placebo treatment [131].

7.5   Safety and tolerability

Both zanamivir and oseltamivir are well tolerated. During pharmacokinetic studies, single intravenous doses of zanamivir 600 mg, multiple intranasal doses of 16 mg, or multiple inhaled doses of 10 mg were well tolerated with no adverse event or laboratory changes reported [110]. Oseltamivir was well tolerated after single doses of up to 1000 mg. Both drugs have also been well tolerated in clinical studies. In patients with confirmed influenza infection, the adverse events reported for zanamivir were confined to the gastrointestinal and respiratory tracts and were indistinguishable from influenza symptoms [125, 134]. However, GlaxoWellcome advise caution in prescribing zanamivir to patients with underlying asthma or chronic obstructive pulmonary disease because of a risk of bronchospasm [135]. Mild gastrointestinal intolerance (mainly nausea and vomiting) occurred more frequently in oseltamivir recipients compared with placebo [112].

Elderly patients are at a high risk of developing complications following influenza infection [136]. Adequate delivery of an inhaled medication requires that the patient has been trained to competently use the inhaler device and frail elderly patients may find this difficult [137]. In contrast, oseltamivir is an oral preparation and is appropriate for use in all age groups.

7.6 Drug resistance in the clinic

So far there have been limited reports of the generation of resistant virus with the clinical use of NA inhibitors. The first event occurred with the use of zanamivir in an immunocompromized child (who subsequently died) with a prolonged influenza B virus infection that was unresponsive to ribavirin treatment [86]. The resistant virus emerged at day 12 of treatment and upon isolation was found to have mutations in NA (Arg152Lys) and HA (Thr198Ile). NA activity was 1000-fold less sensitive to zanamivir, and the virus was less virulent than wild type when inoculated into ferrets. However, the sensitivity to zanamivir was unaffected when tested in cell culture (MDCK cells) providing further evidence of the difference in receptor specificity between these cells and those in respiratory epithelia [86].

Data on the emergence of resistance to oseltamivir carboxylate following treatment of naturally acquired influenza with oseltamivir has yet to be published in detail. However, the study of virus from several hundred influenza-infected oseltamivir-treated patients has shown that resistant mutations observed *in vitro* are predictive of those found to be the predominant resistant genotypes in the clinical setting. No resistant virus has been found until late in the treatment period (day 4 or later) and only from small numbers of patients; (approximately 1% in oseltamivir treated adults). These data suggest that the frequency with which resistant virus is found may be affected by the timing of sampling relative to the onset of treatment and is an important consideration when assessing the frequency of emergence of resistance to neuraminidase inhibitors.

The patients carrying resistant virus show no clinical deterioration. The resistant virus genotypes are all compromised with respect to wild-type virus having low infectivity/replicative ability in mice and ferrets [96, 138, 139]. These data suggest a reduced capacity for transmission in man.

8 Conclusion

The NA inhibitors are an exciting new class of antiviral drugs for the management of influenza. They have been rationally designed from a detailed knowledge of the highly conserved active site of influenza virus NA and the interaction with the natural substrate, sialic acid. *In vitro* and *in vivo* studies

Noel A. Roberts

have established the NA inhibitors as effective and safe antiviral agents against influenza A and B viruses. Two of these compounds, orally active oseltamivir and inhaled zanamivir, have shown the value of this class of compound in the clinic, with safe and effective treatment and prevention of experimental or naturally acquired influenza infections. The NA inhibitors provide an important new therapeutic weapon in the management of influenza infection.

Acknowledgements

The author is grateful to Dr K. Klumpp and Dr P. Ward for critical reading of the manuscript. The help of Dr B. Graves and Dr A. Cann (Leicester University) in the preparation of selected figures is gratefully acknowledged.

References

1   N.J. Cox and C.A. Bender: Semin. Virol. *6*, 359–370 (1995).
2   A.D. Osterhaus, G.F. Rimmelzwann, B.E. Martina, T.M. Bestebroer and R.A. Fouchier: Science *288*, 1051–1053 (2000).
3   R.G. Webster, W.G. Laver, G.M. Air and G.C. Schild: Nature *296*, 115–121 (1982).
4   K.G. Nicholson, in: K.G. Nicholson, R.G. Webster and A.J. Hay (eds.): Textbook of influenza, Blackwell Science, Oxford 1998, 219–264.
5   Centers for Disease Control and Prevention: MMWR Morb. Mortal Wkly. Rep. *48* (RR-04), 1–28 (1999).
6   L. Simonsen, M.J. Clarke, G.D. Williamson, D.F. Stroup, N.H. Arden and L.B. Schonberger: Am. J. Public Health *87*, 1944–1950 (1997).
7   G. Noble, in: A.S. Beare (ed.): Basic and applied influenza research, CRC Press, Boca Raton, FL 1982, 11–50.
8   T.R. Cate: Am. J. Med. *82* (Suppl. 6A), 15–19 (1987).
9   M. Keech, A.J. Scott and P.J.J. Ryan: Occup. Med. *48*, 85–90 (1998).
10 A.M. Palache: Drugs *54*, 841–856 (1997).
11 R.G. Webster: Vaccine *18*, 1696–1689 (2000).
12 Pritchett TJ and Paulson JC: J. Biol. Chem. *264*, 9850–9858 (1989).
13 M. Mammen, G. Dahmann and G.M. Whitesides: J. Med. Chem. *38*, 4179–4190 (1995).
14 H.D. Klenk and R. Rott: Adv. Virus Res. *34*, 247–281 (1988).
15 V.P. Lozitsky, L.E. Puzis and R.Y. Polyar: Acta Virol. *32*, 117–122 (1988).
16 V.P. Lozitsky, A.S. Fedchuk, L.I. Zubareva and T.L. Gridina: Antiviral Res. *46*, A60 (2000).
17 L.E. Puzis and V.P. Lozitsky: Acta Virol. *32*, 515–521 (1988).
18 G. Luo, A. Torri, W.E. Harte, S. Danetz, C. Cianci, L. Tiley, S. Day, D. Mullaney, K.L. Yu, C. Ouellet et al.: J. Virol. *71*, 4062–4070 (1997).

19   S.J. Plotch, B. O'Hara, J. Morin, O. Palant, J. LaRocque, J.D. Bloom, S.A. Lang Jr, M.J. DiGrandi, M. Bradley, R. Nilakantan et al.: J. Virol. 73, 140–151 (1999).

20   S. Shigeta: Drugs R & D 2, 153–164 (1999).

21   W.J. Hornback, J.E. Munroe, J. Tang and R.K. Sachs: Abstracts of the Interscience Conference on Antimicrobial Agents and Chemotherapy [abstract #950] 39, San Francisco, Sep 1999.

22   F.Y. Aoki, in: K.G. Nicholson, R.G. Webster and A.J. Hay (eds.): Textbook of influenza, Blackwell Science, Oxford 1998, 457–476.

23   F.G. Hayden and A.J. Hay: Curr. Top. Microbiol. Immunol. 176, 119–130 (1992).

24   F.G. Hayden, R.B. Belshe, R.D. Clover, A.J. Hay, M.G. Oakes and W. Soo: N. Engl. J. Med. 321, 1696–1702 (1989).

25   F.G. Hayden, J.M. Gwaltney Jr, R.L. van de Castle, K.F. Adams and B. Giordani: Antimicrob. Agents Chemother. 19, 226–233 (1981).

26   A.S. Monto and N.H. Arden: Clin. Infect. Dis. 15, 362–367 (1992).

27   Q. Tu, L.H. Pinto, G.X. Luo, M.A. Shaughnessy, D. Mullaney, S. Kurtz, M. Krystal and R.A. Lamb: J. Virol. 70, 4246–4252 (1996).

28   H. Ochiai, S. Sakai, T. Hirabayashi, Y. Shimizu and K. Terasawa: Antiviral Res. 27, 425–430 (1995).

29   R.A. Lamb and R.M. Krug, in: B.N. Fields, D.M. Knipe and P.M. Howley (eds.): Fields virology, Lippincott-Williams & Wilkins, Philadelphia 1996, 1353–1445.

30   L. Doan, B. Handa, N.A. Roberts and K. Klumpp: Biochemistry 38, 5612–5619 (1999).

31   J.E. Tomassini, M.E. Davies, J.C. Hastings, R. Lingham, M. Mojena, S.L. Raghoobar, S.B. Singh, J.S. Tkacz and M.A. Goetz: Antimicrob. Agents Chemother. 40, 1189–1193 (1996).

32   C. Cianci, T.D.Y. Chung, N. Meanwell, H. Putz, M. Hagen, R.J. Colonno, M. Krystal: Antiviral Chem. Chemother. 7, 353–360 (1996).

33   J. Tomassini, H. Selnick, M.E. Davies, M.E. Armstrong, J. Baldwin, M. Bourgeois, J. Hastings, D. Hazuda, J. Lewis, W. McClements et al: Antimicrob. Agents Chemother. 38, 2827–2837 (1994).

34   J.C. Hastings, H. Selnick, B. Wolanski and J.E. Tomassini: Antimicrob. Agents Chemother. 40, 1304–1307 (1996).

35   M. Tisdale, M. Ellis, K. Klumpp, S. Court and M. Ford: Antmicrob Agents Chemother 39, 2454–2458 (1995).

36   M. Tisdale, M. Ellis, S. Court and M. Ford: Antiviral Res. 20 (Suppl. 1), 100 (1993).

37   M. Tisdale, G. Appleyard, J.V. Tuttle, D.J. Nelson, S. Nusinoff-Lehrman, W. Al Nakib, J.N. Stables, D.J.M. Purifoy, K.L. Powell and G. Darby: Antiviral Chem. Chemother. 4, 281–287 (1993).

38   E.H. Nasser, A.K. Judd, A. Sanchez, D. Anastasiou and D.J. Bucher: J. Virol. 70, 8639–8644 (1996).

39   A.K. Judd, A. Sanchez, D.J. Bucher, J.H. Huffman, K. Bailey and R.W. Sidwell: Antimicrob. Agents Chemother. 41, 687–692 (1997).

40   C. Elster, E. Fourest, F. Baudin, K. Larsen, S. Cusack and R.W. Ruigrok: J. Gen. Virol. 75, 37–42 (1994).

41   B. Sha and M. Luo: Nat. Struct. Biol. 4, 239–244 (1997).

42   D.B. Olsen, F. Benseler, J.L. Cole, M.W. Stahlhut, R.E. Dempski, P.L. Darke and, L.C. Kuo: J. Biol. Chem. 271, 7435–7439 (1996).

43   T.D.Y. Chung, C. Cianci, M. Hagen, B. Terry, J.T. Matthews, M. Krystal and R.J. Colonno: Proc. Natl. Acad. Sci. USA 91, 2372–2376 (1994).

44   G. Luo, S. Danetz and M. Krystal: J. Gen. Virol. *78*, 2329–2333 (1997).

45   T. Abe, S. Suzuki, T. Hatta, K. Takai, T. Yokota and H. Takaku: Antivir. Chem. Chemother. *9*, 253–262 (1998).

46   T. Mizuta, M. Fujiwara, T. Hatta, T. Abe, N. Miyano-Kurosaki, S. Shigeta, T. Yokota and H. Takaku: Nat. Biotechnol. *17*, 583–587 (1999).

47   J.M. Colacino, D.C. Delong, J.R. Nelson, W.A. Spitzer, J. Tang, F. Victor and C.Y. Wu: Antimicrob. Agents Chemother. *34*, 2156–2163 (1990).

48   F.G. Hayden, A.R. Tunkel, J.J. Treanor, R.F. Betts, S. Allerheiligen and J. Harris: Antimicrob. Agents Chemother. *38*, 1178–1181 (1994).

49   B.E. Gilbert and V. Knight: Antimicrob. Agents Chemother. *30*, 201–205 (1986).

50   V. Knight and B. Gilbert: Eur. J. Clin. Microb. Infect. Dis. *7*, 721–731 (1988).

51   D.S. Stein, C.M. Creticos, G.G. Jackson, J.M. Bernstein, F.G. Hayden, G.M. Schiff and D.I. Bernstein: Antimicrob. Agents Chemother. *31*, 1285–1287 (1987).

52   F.G. Hayden, C.A. Sable, J.D. Connor and J. Lane: Antiviral Ther. *1*, 51–56 (1996).

53   P. Palese, K. Tobita, M. Ueda and R.W. Compans: Virology *61*, 397–410 (1974).

54   P.M. Colman, J.N. Varghese and W.G. Laver: Nature *303*, 41–44 (1983).

55   D.B. Mendel and R.W. Sidwell: Drug Resist Updates *1*, 184–189 (1998).

56   J.L. McKimm-Breschkin, T.J. Blick and A. Sahasrabudhe, in: L.E. Brown, A.W. Hampson and R.G. Webster (eds.): Options for the control of influenza III. Elsevier Science, Amsterdam 1996, 726–734.

57   H. Goto and Y. Kawaoka: Proc. Natl. Acad. Sci. USA *95*, 10224–10228 (1998).

58   C. Luo, E. Nobusawa and K. Nakajima: J. Gen. Virol. *80*, 2969–2976 (1999).

59   J.N. Varghese, W.G. Laver and P.M. Colman: Nature *303*, 35–40 (1983).

60   J.N. Varghese and P.M. Colman: J. Mol. Biol. *221*, 473–486 (1991).

61   J.N. Varghese, J.L. McKimm-Breschkin, J.B. Caldwell, A.A. Kortt and P.M. Colman: Proteins *14*, 327–332 (1992).

62   P. Meindl and H. Tuppy: Hoppe Seylers Z. Physiol. Chem. *350*, 1088–1092 (1969).

63   P. Palese and J.L. Schulman, in: J.S. Oxford (ed.): Chemoprophylaxis and virus infections of the upper respiratory tract, vol. 1, CRC Press, Boca Raton, FL 1977, 189–205.

64   P. Meindl, G. Bodo, P. Palese, J. Schulman and H. Tuppy: Virology *58*, 457–463 (1974).

65   P. Palese and R.W. Compans: J. Gen. Virol. *33*, 159–163 (1976).

66   M. von Itzstein, W.Y. Wu, G.B. Kok, M.S. Pegg, J.C. Dyason, B. Jin, T. Van Phan, M.L. Smythe, H.F. White, S.W. Oliver et al.: Nature *363*, 418–423 (1993).

67   S. Newman, J. Brown, M. Pickford, S. Fayinka and L. Cass: Abstracts of the Interscience Conference on Antimicrobial Agents and Chemotherapy [abstract H134] *37*, 237 (1997).

68   C.U. Kim, W. Lew, M.A. Williams, H. Liu, L. Zhang, S. Swaminathan, N. Bischofberger, M.S. Chen, D.B. Mendel, C.Y. Tai et al.: J. Am. Chem. Soc. *119*, 681–690 (1997).

69   W. Li, P.A. Escarpe, E.J. Eisenberg, K.C. Cundy, C. Sweet, K.J. Jakeman, J. Mersonn, W. Lew, M. Williams, L. Zhang et al.: Antimicrob. Agents Chemother. *42*, 647–653 (1998).

70   D.B. Mendel, C.Y. Tai, P.A. Escarpe, W. Li, R.W. Sidwell, J.H. Huffman, C. Sweet, K.J. Jakeman, J. Merson, S.A. Lacy et al: Antimicrob. Agents Chemother. *42*, 640–646 (1998).

71   F.G. Hayden and B.S. Rollins: Antiviral Res. *34*, A86 (1997).

72   I.A. Leneva, N. Roberts, E.A. Govorkova, O.G. Golubeva and R.G. Webster: Antiviral Res. *48*, 101–115 (2000).

73   S. Bantia, P. Chand, C. Parker, S. Ananth, L. Horn, P. Kotian, A. Dehghani, Y. Kattan, T. Lin, T. Hutchinson et al.: Abstracts of the Interscience Conference on Antimicrobial Agents and Chemotherapy [abstract 947] *39*, 323 (1999).

74   J.H. Huffman, A. Morrison, V. Stowell, D.L. Barnard, K. Bush and R.W. Sidwell: Abstracts of the Interscience Conference on Antimicrobial Agents and Chemotherapy 39, 322–323 (1999).

75   S. Bantia, P. Chand, C. Parker, S. Ananth, L. Horn, P. Kotian, A. Dehghani, Y. Kattan, T. Lin, T. Hutchinson et al.: Abstracts of the Interscience Conference on Antimicrobial Agents and Chemotherapy [abstract 948] 39, 323 (1999).

76   R.W. Sidwell, J.H. Huffman, K.W. Bailey, P.A. Bemis, T. Coogan, K. Bush and Y.S. Babu: Abstracts of the Interscience Conference on Antimicrobial Agents and Chemotherapy 39, 323 (1999).

77   P.W. Smith, J.E. Robinson, D.N. Evans, S.L. Sollis, P.D. Howes, N. Trivedi and R.C. Bethell: Bioorg. Med. Chem. Lett. 9, 601–604 (1999).

78   P.S. Jones, P.W. Smith, G.W. Hardy, P.D. Howes, R.J. Upton and R.C. Bethell: Bioorg. Med. Chem. Lett. 9, 605–610 (1999).

79   C. Holzer, M. von Iztstein, B. Jin, M. Pegg, W. Stewart and W.-Y. Wu: Glycocon. J. 10, 40–44 (1993).

80   P.W. Smith, N. Trivedi, P.D. Howes, S.L. Sollis, G. Rahim, R.C. Bethell and S. Lynn: Bioorg. Med. Chem. Lett. 9, 611–614 (1999).

81   J.S. Oxford and R. Lambkin: Drug Discovery Today 3, 448–456 (1998).

82   L.V. Gubareva, C.R. Penn and R.G. Webster: Virology 212, 323–330 (1995).

83   J.M. Woods, R.C. Bethell, J.A.V. Coates, N. Healy, S.A. Hiscox, B.A. Pearson, D.M. Ryan, J. Ticehurst, J. Tilling, S.M. Walcott et al.: Antimicrob. Agents Chemother. 37, 1473–1479 (1993).

84   E.A. Govorkova, G. Murti, B. Meignier, C. de Taisne and R.G. Webster: J. Virol. 70, 5519–5524 (1996).

85   T. Ito, Y. Suzuki, A. Takada, A. Kawamoto, K. Otsuki, H. Masada, M. Yamada, T. Suzuki, H. Kida and Y. Kawaoka: J. Virol. 71, 3357–3362 (1997).

86   L.V. Gubareva, M.N. Matrosovch, M.K. Brenner, R.C. Bethell and R.G. Webster: J. Infect. Dis. 178, 1257–1262 (1998).

87   J.L. McKimm-Breschkin, T.J. Blick, A. Sahasrabudhe, T. Tiong, D. Marshall, G.J. Hart, R.C. Bethell and C.R. Penn: Antimicrob. Agents Chemother. 40, 40–46 (1996).

88   J.S. Oxford, I.S. Logan and C.W. Potter: Ann. NY Acad. Sci. 173, 300–313 (1970).

89   L.V. Gubareva, R. Bethell, G.J. Hart, K.G. Murti, C.R. Penn and R.G. Webster: J. Virol. 70, 1818–1827 (1996).

90   C.R. Penn, J.M. Barnett, R.C. Bethell, R. Fenton, K.L. Gearing, N. Healy and A.J. Jowett, in: L.E. Brown, A.W. Hampson and R. Webster (eds.): Options for the control of influenza III, Elsevier Science, Amsterdam 1996, 735–740.

91   A. Sahasrabudhe, T. Blick and J. McKimm-Breschkin, in: L.E. Brown, A.W. Hampson and R.G. Webster (eds.): Options for the control of influenza III, Elsevier Science, Amsterdam 1996, 748–752.

92   C.Y. Tai, P.A. Escarpe, R.W. Sidwell, M.A. Williams, W. Lew, H. Wu, C.U. Kim and D.B. Mendel: Antimicrob. Agents Chemother. 42, 3234–3241 (1998).

93   S. Bantia, S. Ananth, L. Horn, C. Parker, U. Gulati, P. Chand, Y. Babu and G. Air: Antiviral Res. 46, A60 (2000).

94   K.A. Staschke, J.M. Colacino, A.J. Baxter, G.M. Air, A. Bansal, W.J. Hornback, J.E. Munroe and W.G. Laver: Virology 214, 642–646 (1995).

95   L.V. Gubareva, M.J. Robinson, R.C. Bethell and R.G. Webster: J. Virol. 71, 3385–3390 (1997).

96   J. Carr, J. Ives, N. Roberts, L. Kelly, R. Lambkin, J. Oxford, C.Y.Tai, D. Mendel and F. Hayden: Antiviral Res. *46*, A59 (2000).

97   L.V. Gubareva, C.Y. Tai, D.B. Mendel, J. Ives, J. Carr, N.A. Roberts and F.G. Hayden: Antiviral Res. *46*, A59 (2000).

98   Z.M. Wang, C.Y. Tai and D.B. Mendel: Antiviral Res. [abstract 80] *46*, A60 (2000).

99   Z.M. Wang, C.Y. Tai and D.B. Mendel: Antiviral Res. [abstract 81] *46*, A60 (2000).

100   S. Raut, J. Hurd, R.J. Cureton, G. Blandford and R.B. Heath: J. Med. Microbiol. *8*, 127–136 (1975).

101   P.R. Wyde, R.B. Couch, B.F. Mackler, T.R. Cate and B.M. Levy: Infect. Immun. *15*, 221–229 (1977).

102   M.D. Ryan, J. Ticehurst, M.H. Dempsey and C.R. Penn: Antimicrob. Agents Chemother. *38*, 2270–2275 (1994).

103   R.W. Sidwell, J.H. Huffman, D.L. Barnard, K.W. Bailey, M-H. Wong, A. Morrison, T. Syndergaard and C.U. Kim: Antiviral Res. 37, 107–120 (1998).

104   M.D. Ryan, J. Ticehurst and M.H. Dempsey: Antimicrob. Agents Chemother. *39*, 2583–2584 (1995).

105   R.J. Fenton, I. Owens, P. Morley and C.R. Penn: Options for the Control of Influenza III [abstract], Cairns, Australia, 4–9 May 1996.

106   R.W. Sidwell, R.A. Burger, J.H. Huffman, K.W. Bailey and R.P. Warren: Abstracts of the Interscience Conference on Antimicrobial Agents and Chemotherapy 38, 335 (1998).

107   G. He, J. Massarella and P. Ward: Clin. Pharmacokinet. *37*, 471–484 (1999).

108   E.J. Eisenberg, A. Bidgood and K.C. Cundy: Antimicrob. Agents Chemother. *41*, 1949–1952 (1997).

109   M.J. Daniel, J.M. Barnett and B.A. Pearson: Clin. Pharmacokinet. *36* (Suppl. 1), 41–50 (1999).

110   L. Cass, J. Brown, M. Pickford, S. Fayinka , S.P. Newman, C.J. Johansson and A. Bye: Clin. Pharmacokinet. *36* (Suppl. 1), 21–31 (1999).

111   A. Webster, M. Boyce, S. Edmundson and I. Miller: Clin. Pharmacokinet. *36* (Suppl. 1), 51–58 (1999).

112   J.J. Treanor, F.G. Hayden, P.S. Vrooman, R. Barbarash, R. Bettis, D. Riff, S. Singh, N. Kinnersley, P. Ward and R.G. Mills: JAMA *283*, 1016–1024 (2000).

113   C. Efthymiopoulos, P. Barrington, J. Patel, A. Harker, A. Harris, E.K. Hussey and A. Bye: Abstracts of the Interscience Conference on Antimicrobial Agents and Chemotherapy *34*, 265 (1994).

114   R.J. Malcolmson and J.K. Embleton: Pharm. Sci. Tech. Today *1*, 394–398 (1998).

115   K.G. Neilsen, M. Skov, B. Klug, M. Ifversen and H. Bisgaard: Eur. Respir. J. *10*, 2105–2109 (1997).

116   D.P. Calfee, A.W. Peng, E.K. Hussey, M. Lobo and F.G. Hayden: Antiviral Ther. *4*, 143–149 (1999).

117   M. Kurowski, J. Barrett, E. Waalberg, N.V. Nagaraja, H. Derendorf and H. Wiltshire: Interscience Conference on Antimicrobial Agents and Chemotherapy, Toronto, Canada, 17–20 Sep 2000.

118   F.G. Hayden, J.J. Treanor, R.F. Betts, M. Lobo, J.D. Esinhart and E.K. Hussey: JAMA *275*, 295–299 (1996).

119   F.G. Hayden, J.T. Treanor, R.S. Fritz, M. Lobo, R.F. Betts, M. Miller, N. Kinnersley, R.G. Mills, P. Ward and S.E. Straus: JAMA *282*, 1240–1246 (1999).

120   F.G. Hayden, M. Lobo, E.K. Hussy and C.U. Eason, in: L.E. Brown, A.W. Hampson and

R.G. Webster (eds.): Options for the control of influenza III, Elsevier Science, Amsterdam 1996, 718–725.

121   F.G. Hayden, L. Jennings, R. Robson, G. Schiff, H. Jackson, B. Rana, G. McClelland, D. Ipe, N. Roberts and P. Ward: Antiviral Ther. *5*, 205–213 (2000).

122   F.G. Hayden, J.J. Treanor, R. Qu and C.L. Fowler: 9th ICID [abstract #80.018], Buenos Aires, 10–13 Apr 2000.

123   F.G. Hayden, R.S. Fritz, M. Lobo, G. Alvord, W. Strober and S.E. Straus: J. Clin. Invest. *101*, 643–649 (1998).

124   F.G. Hayden, R.L. Atmar, M. Schilling, C. Johnson, D. Poretz, D. Parr, L. Huson, P. Ward, R.G. Mills and the Oseltamivir Study Group: N. Engl. J. Med. *341*, 1336–1343 (1999).

125   MIST (Management of Influenza in the Southern Hemisphere Trialists) Study Group: Lancet *352*, 1877–1881 (1998).

126   D. Fleming, M. Mäkelä, K. Pauksens, C. Man, A. Webster and O. Keene: 36th IDSA, Denver, USA, 12–15 Nov 1998.

127   J. Lalezari, T. Klein, J. Stapleton, M. Elliott, N. Flack and O. Keene: 21st ICC, Birmingham, UK, 4–7 Jul 1999.

128   K.G. Nicholson, F.Y. Aoki, A.D.M.E. Osterhaus, S. Trottier, O. Carewicz, C.H. Mercier, A. Rode, N. Kinnersley, P. Ward and the Neuraminidase Inhibitor Flu Treatment Investigator Group: Lancet *355*, 1845–1850 (2000).

129   J.A. Hedrick, A. Barzilai, U. Behre, F.W. Henderson, J. Hammond, L. Reilly, O. Keene: Pediatr. Infect Dis. J. *19*, 410–417 (2000).

130   K. Reisinger, F. Hayden, R. Whitley, R. Dutkowski, D. Ipe, R. Mills and P. Ward: 10th ECCMID, Stockholm, 28–31 May 2000.

131   A.S. Monto, D.P. Robinson, M.L. Herlocher, J.M. Hinson Jr, M.J. Elliott and A. Crisp: JAMA *282*, 31–35 (1999).

132   V. De Bock, P. Peters, T. von Planta, M. Gibbens and P. Ward: Clin. Microbiol. Infect *6* (Suppl. 1), 140 (2000).

133   J. Oxford, H. Jackson, L. Huson and P. Ward: 2nd ISIRV, Cayman Islands, 10–12 Dec 1999.

134   F.G. Hayden, A.D.M.E. Osterhaus, J.J. Treanor, D.M. Fleming, F.Y. Aoki, K.G. Nicholson, A.M. Bohnen, H.M. Hirst, O. Keene and K. Wightman: N. Engl. J. Med. *337*, 874–880 (1997).

135   G. Yamey: BMJ *320*, 334 (2000).

136   A.M. McBean, J.D. Babish and J.L. Warren: Arch. Intern. Med. *153*, 2105–2111 (1993).

137   Pounsford JC: Eur. Respir. Rev. *4*, 82–84 (1994).

138   J. Ives, J. Carr, N.A. Roberts, C.Y. Tai, D.B. Mendel, L. Kelly, R. Lambkin and J. Oxford: J. Clin. Virol. [P-321] *18*, 251 (2000).

139   J. Ives, J. Carr, N.A. Roberts, C.Y. Tai, D.B. Mendel, L. Kelly, R. Lambkin and J. Oxford: J. Clin. Virol. [P-330] *18*, 255 (2000).

Antiviral Agents – Advances and Problems (E. Jucker, Ed.)
©2001 Birkhäuser Verlag, Basel (Switzerland)

Recent advances in prevention and treatment of hepatitis C virus infections

By Q. May Wang and Beverly A. Heinz

Infectious Diseases Research, Lilly Research Laboratories, Eli Lilly and Company, Indianapolis, IN 46285, USA

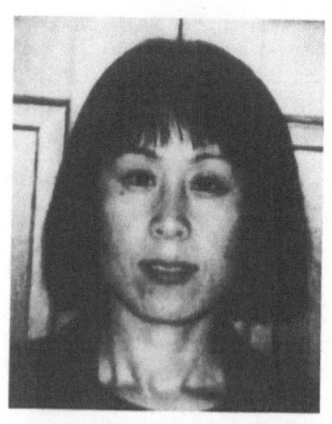

Q. May Wang

received her B.S. and M.S. degrees with a major in Biology from Shandong University, China. She earned her Ph.D. in Biochemistry from Purdue University, Indiana and then had post-doctoral training at Indiana University School of Medicine. Dr. Wang joined Lilly Research Laboratories as a Senior Biochemist in 1995.

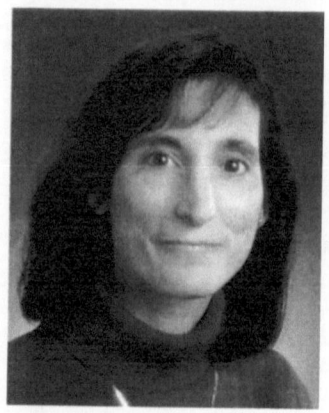

Beverly A. Heinz

earned a B.S. in Biology from Rensselaer Polytechnic Institute in Troy, New York, and her M.S. and Ph.D. degrees from the Department of Bacteriology at the University of Wisconsin-Madison. She then completed four years of post-doctoral training at the Institute for Molecular Virology at UW-Madison. In 1990, Dr. Heinz joined Lilly Research Laboratories as a Senior Virologist working in the field of antiviral drug discovery.

Summary

Hepatitis C virus (HCV) is the leading cause of chronic hepatitis in humans. As members of the flavivirus family, HCVs are a group of small single-stranded, positive-sense RNA viruses. Upon translation of the genome, a polyprotein precursor is synthesized and further processed by both cellular and viral proteases to generate functional viral proteins. Treatment options are currently limited to the administration of α-interferon alone or in combination with ribavirin. Unfortunately, these approaches are characterized by relatively poor efficacy and an unfavorable side-effect profile. Therefore, intensive effort is directed at the discovery of novel molecules to treat this disease. These new approaches include the development of prophylactic and therapeutic vaccines, the identification of interferons with improved pharmacokinetic characteristics, and the discovery of novel drugs designed to inhibit the function of three major viral proteins: protease, helicase and polymerase. Finally, the HCV RNA genome itself, particularly the IRES element, is being actively exploited as an antiviral target using antisense molecules and catalytic ribozymes. This review summarizes the most recent findings in each of these areas. Although not intended to be comprehensive, it should serve as a first resource for those individuals who desire updated information in this rapidly changing field.

Contents

Keywords
Hepatitis, hepatitis C virus, interferon, ribavirin, antiviral inhibitors, IRES, protease inhibitors.

Glossary of abbreviations
ALT, aminotransferase levels; CTL, cytotoxic T lymphocyte; HCC, hepatocellular carcinoma; HCV, hepatitis C virus; IFN, interferon; IMPDH, inosine monophosphate dehydrogenase; IRES, internal ribosome entry site; NS, nonstructural; NTR, non-translated region; ORF, open reading frame; PTB, polypyrimidine tract binding; SAR: structure-activity relationship.

1   Introduction

Hepatitis C virus (HCV) was first identified in 1989 as the etiologic agent of non-A, non-B hepatitis [1] and is currently recognized as the leading cause of chronic liver disease worldwide. In contrast to hepatitis B virus infection, in which only about 5% of adult infections become chronic, more than 80% of HCV-infected patients develop chronic hepatitis. Moreover, 20–50% of those persistently infected with HCV will develop liver cirrhosis and hepatocellular carcinoma (HCC) [2]. It is estimated that there are 10,000 deaths in the USA per year due to chronic liver failure or HCC [3]. In addition, HCV disease is responsible for 25–50% of all liver transplants in US centers, and the recurrence of HCV infection following liver transplantation is universal [4]. Typically, HCV disease emerges after a 10–20 year period during which symptoms, if they exist at all, are mild and non-specific. Although the prevalence varies greatly among different countries, it has been estimated that up to 170 million people (3% of the world's population), are infected with HCV [5]. A recent study in the USA found that 65% of all HCV-infected persons are 30 to 49 years old [6].

The modes of HCV transmission include blood transfusion, occupational exposure and injection drug abuse. In addition, there are a large number of cases that continue to be attributed to unknown risk factors; these most likely result from incidental parenteral exposure to contaminated objects, such as sharing razors or toothbrushes. The frequency of sexual transmission of HCV appears to be low, except in cases of co-infection with HIV [7]. Current views on the epidemiology of HCV were recently summarized [8].

1.1   Pathogenesis

HCV disease typically begins with an acute infection which resembles other forms of acute viral hepatitis, beginning with malaise, nausea and right upper quadrant pain. Although the mean incubation period to onset of symptoms is ~7 weeks, HCV RNA is detectable in serum within 1–2 weeks. After several weeks, serum alanine aminotransferase (ALT) levels increase. Only about a third of patients will develop jaundice or other symptoms; the majority of infections are subclinical.

In at least 85% of cases, the HCV infection becomes chronic (for review see [9]). Symptoms seen in these patients, such as nausea, anorexia and dark urine, are generally mild and nonspecific, and serum ALT levels tend to fluctuate between elevated and normal. The major serious complication of chronic HCV infection, which can take from 1 to 30 years to develop, is cirrhosis. The development of cirrhosis is characterized by the symptoms of end-stage liver disease, including severe fatigue, muscle weakness and jaundice. Cirrhosis caused by HCV infection is currently the most frequent cause of liver transplantation in the USA and western Europe. In addition, chronic HCV infection is a major cause of hepatocellular carcinoma, a disease for which treatments are inadequate. The molecular relationship between HCV infection and hepatocarcinogenesis was recently reviewed [10]. Finally, several nonhepatic manifestations of HCV infection are known as well, including arthritis, glomerulonephritis, essential mixed cryoglobulinemia, and porphyria cutanea tarda [11].

The pathogenesis of HCV infection is believed to have a basis in immunological injury, involving both humoral and cellular factors (reviewed in [12]). In these models, liver cell damage is caused by soluble cytotoxic mediators and the activation of inflammatory cells. A role for apoptosis has been proposed as well (summarized in [13]). Unfortunately, research in these areas is hampered by the lack of a cell culture virus replication system and a small animal model for infection.

1.2   Infectious agent

The HCV virion is composed of a lipid bilayer with two species of membrane glycoprotein (E1 and E2) surrounding a nucleocapsid. The genome, as shown in Figure 1, consists of one piece of single-stranded, positive-sense RNA containing approximately 9500 nucleotides encoding a single open reading frame (ORF). The plus-strand RNA is replicated *via* a negative-stranded intermediate. Although HCV cannot yet be replicated reliably in cell culture, transcripts encoding the plus-sense RNA have been shown to be infectious in the chimpanzee animal model [14, 15]. The overall genome sequence and organization of HCV, as well as its apparent method of replication, most closely resemble the family *Flaviviridae*. This family of viruses contains the classic flaviviruses, such as the yellow fever and dengue fever

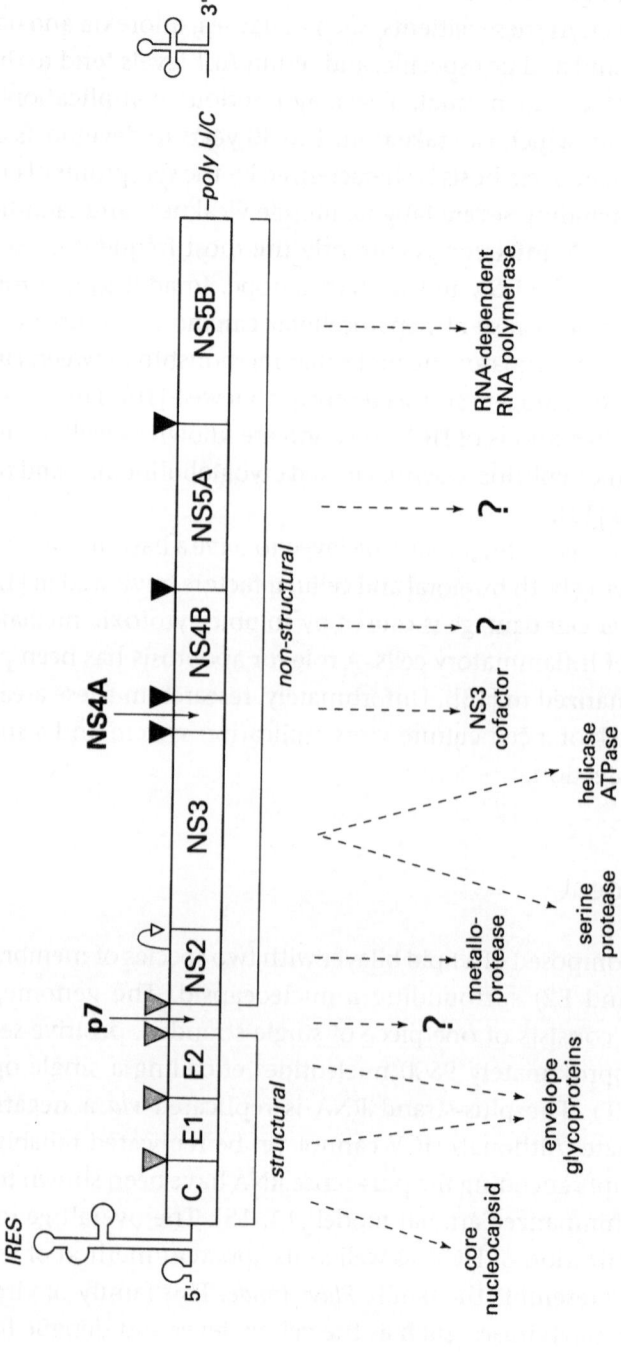

Fig. 1
Schematic of HCV genome organization and processing of viral proteins. Boxes represent the coding regions; stem-loop structures represent the 5'- and 3'-NTRs. Cleavages mediated by host signal peptidase are indicated by grey triangles. NS3 serine protease cleavage sites are designated by black triangles. Self-cleavage at the NS2/NS3 junction is shown by a curved arrow. Proteins whose function is unknown are indicated by a question mark.

viruses, and the pestiviruses, including bovine viral diarrhea and hog cholera viruses. Recently, HCV was classified as a separate genus within this family with the name "Hepacivirus" [16]. Phylogenetic analyses have classified HCV into six major genotypes, numbered 1–6. There is a strong association with geographic distribution and HCV genotype; for example, genotype 1a is most common in North America and Europe, whereas genotypes 1b and 2 predominate in Asia [17]. Additionally, genotype 1b has been associated with more severe disease recurrence following liver transplantation than non-1b genotypes [18].

The ORF of HCV is preceded by a highly conserved 5'-nontranslated region (5'-NTR), approximately 342 nucleotides in length, whose folded structure plays at least two critical roles in virus replication. First, in its anti-sense form it controls the initiation of transcription of positive-strand RNA synthesis. Second, it governs translation of the viral polyprotein *via* an embedded IRES (internal ribosome entry site) element at approximately nucleotides #42–345 of the 5'-NTR. The translation of HCV occurs *via* a cap-independent mechanism. The IRES element functions by directing internal entry of the 40S ribosome subunits to the viral RNA at the site of the initiating AUG without scanning [19]. Thus, the HCV translation is similar to that of all picornaviral (e.g., poliovirus) and certain cellular mRNAs, such as those encoding the immunoglobulin heavy chain binding protein (BiP) and the vascular epithelial growth factor [20].

The HCV ORF translates into a single polyprotein precursor that is cleaved co- and post-translationally by both host cellular and virus-encoded proteases [21], releasing three structural and at least six nonstructural (NS) viral proteins (Fig. 1). Cleavages directed by the host cell signal peptidase produce the structural proteins, including the nucleocapsid known as core protein, two envelope proteins, E1 and E2, and a small membrane-associated protein of unknown function called p7. Signal sequences within this region direct its secretion into the endoplasmic reticulum (ER) [22]. It is known that E1 and E2 are glycosylated. The remaining six nonstructural proteins are processed by viral proteases. These include: a cis-active metalloprotease comprising the NS2 and the adjacent NS3 sequences (which cleaves the NS2/3 junction) [23], a multifunctional NS3 (containing serine protease, NTPase and unwinding helicase activities (reviewed in [24] and [25])), auxiliary factor NS4A, a cofactor for NS3 protease [26], two proteins of unknown function, NS4B and NS5A, and an RNA-dependent RNA polymerase called NS5B [27].

Downstream of the ORF is a stretch of approximately 240 bases known as the 3'-NTR. The 3'-NTR consists of three elements: a 30- to 40-nucleotide region that is poorly conserved among different genotypes, a 20- to 200-nucleotide polypyrimidine (poly U/C) tract, and a highly conserved 98-nucleotide sequence termed the 3'X region. Both the poly U/C tract and the 3'X region have been found to be essential for HCV infection in the chimpanzee model [28]. The function of the poly U/C tract is not known but is likely to be important because similar tracts are found in the untranslated regions (generally 5') of other positive-strand RNA viruses, such as cardioviruses. Additionally, the HCV poly U/C tract has been found to bind two cellular proteins: the polypyrimidine tract-binding protein, PTB, and a smaller protein known as p35 [29]. The role of the 3'X region has been explored in more detail. As determined by computer modeling and enzymatic and chemical probing, the 3'X region has been shown to form stable secondary structures [30–32]. The 3'X RNA forms a three-stem-loop structure and, like the poly U/C tract and the IRES element [33], also binds to PTB [29, 34]. The 3'X region plays a role in initiation of the synthesis of minus-strand RNA as well as the regulation of IRES-dependent translation from the 5' end of HCV RNA [35].

In infected patients, HCV tends to exist as quasi-species of closely related but distinct viral populations. This genetic heterogeneity is caused by the low fidelity of the RNA-dependent RNA polymerase which permits spontaneous nucleotide substitutions at a rate of about 10^{-2} to 10^{-3} substitutions per nucleotide per year [36]. The production of HCV quasi-species has been documented in hepatocytes, peripheral blood mononuclear cells and ascitic fluid of patients with late-stage chronic HCV [37]. As a result, therapies for HCV infection will likely be hindered by the development of viral escape mutants resistant to antiviral drugs and vaccines.

1.3   Cell culture systems

Although numerous cell-based replication assays for HCV have been reported (see [38] for review), none has yet proven to be practical and readily reproducible. This shortcoming has severely limited the possible molecular studies of HCV replication and evaluation of antiviral molecules. The majority of these approaches rely on reverse transcriptase -PCR to monitor the production of minute amounts of plus- and minus-strand RNA. Nevertheless, evidence of mutational changes in the genome of HCV during culture in hepatocytes and cell lines [39, 40] strongly suggests that HCV can replicate at a low level *in vitro*. Perhaps the most encouraging cell-based assay was recently reported by Lohmann et al. [41]. This system uses neomycin selection of hepatoma cells transfected with a bicistronic transcript encoding a subgenomic replicon of HCV lacking the structural proteins. Sufficient levels of viral RNA and protein were synthesized to permit detection by Northern blots and radioisotopic labeling, respectively. Confirmation of the significance of these results awaits reproduction of the work by other groups.

In addition, there have been recent efforts to determine the cellular receptor used by HCV during infection. The E2 glycoprotein is thought to be responsible for initiating virus attachment to its receptor [42]. Both CD81 [43] and the low density lipoprotein (LDL) receptor [44] have been implicated as the HCV receptor on target cells. In a recent study of the specificity of interaction between E2 and CD81, various forms of E2 were compared for ability to bind CD81 [45]. The authors demonstrated that monomeric rather than aggregated E2 preferentially bound to CD81, and that intracellular forms of E2 had a higher affinity for CD81 than did secreted forms. A deeper understanding of how HCV interacts with the cellular receptor must await the development of a robust cell-based viral replication assay.

1.4 Animal models

To date, chimpanzees remain the only species other than humans with known susceptibility to HCV infection. Infection in chimpanzees closely resembles that seen in humans where there is an acute phase of the disease, a host immune response, and long-term sequelae such as cirrhosis and HCC. Because the chimpanzee can be infected by injecting cDNA-derived full-length transcripts directly into the liver [14, 15], the critical role played by viral proteins or RNA structures in determining infectivity can be evaluated [46]. In addition, the chimpanzee model illustrates the basic features of pathogenesis and immunology of HCV infection (reviewed in [47]). Because the use of chimpanzees is quite limited due to high cost and low availability, alternative animal models have been intensively explored. Experimental HCV infection has been reported in tupaias (tree shrews), a species closely related to primates [48], and in immunodeficient mice [reviewed in 49]. So far, the suitability of these animal models as a replacement for the chimpanzee has not been demonstrated unequivocally.

2 Prophylactic and therapeutic vaccines for HCV

Chronic HCV infections occur at high rates despite the induction of specific humoral and cellular immune responses elicited by the host. Thus, there is a pressing need to develop new vaccination strategies. Designing a prophylactic vaccine for HCV is problematic in several respects: low levels of viremia, the existence of quasi-species due to high genetic variability in the E1 and E2 glycoproteins, and the lack of a convenient animal model. Nevertheless, there has been some encouraging progress in this area.

Vaccine candidates include recombinant subunit proteins and nucleic acids. For example, chimpanzees vaccinated with recombinant envelope proteins developed high serum titers of anti-E2 antibodies and were protected against subsequent challenge with a homologous virus [50]. Even in the cases when complete protection was not provided, the resulting infection with a challenge virus produced beneficial results (lower viremia and minimal liver disease). It has been proposed that a vaccine composed of a recombinant form of several HCV proteins including the envelope glycoprotein, should provide protection against infection by different genotypes by priming cross-neutralizing anti-envelope antibodies and wide helper and inflammatory CD4[+] T-cell responses [51]. However, experience with HIV suggests that a multifaceted approach of vaccination together with antivirals may be necessary to maximize the inhibitory effect. A review of the clinical and economic issues concerning prophylactic use of immunoglobulin was recently published [52]. DNA vaccines that express viral antigens intracellularly can also serve as an immune system stimulant, especially for cytotoxic T-lymphocyte (CTL) responses. The nucleic acid may be introduced by direct injection or *via* a gene therapy approach. For a more complete discussion of the issues involved in the different vaccination strategies for HCV, see [53].

Currently, there are many commercial approaches underway to develop an effective HCV vaccine, some using novel methods to stimulate the immune system. Only a few examples will be described here. First, work is underway to develop technologies that deliver therapeutic proteins to stimulate a CTL response to HCV [54]. In this approach, two proteins (PA and LFn) can be inserted into the cell membrane and form a pore, facilitating the entry of peptides or protein antigens into the cytoplasm. Antigens are processed and displayed on the cell surface, eliciting a CTL response and inducing the production of cellular cytokines. Second, many novel approaches are underway to improve engineered vaccines for HCV, including epitope enhancement and the presence of cytokines in the adjuvant [55]. Clinical trials with proprietary adjuvants are underway to test vaccines that may be suitable for both prophylactic and therapeutic use [56]. In a third example, a series of vaccines is being based on proprietary immunostimulatory DNA sequences [57]. These sequences, when administered with viral antigens, are thought to redirect the immune system to elicit a CTL response instead of a humoral immune response. Pre-clinical work is underway. Similarly, an immunotherapeutic vaccine that purportedly stimulates CD4+ and CD8+ T-cells to react to HCV-infected cells is under development; clinical trials are planned for the year 2000 [58]. Fourth, an effort is underway to develop recombinant vaccine candidates based on the E1 protein of HCV 1b [59]. Pre-clinical studies in chimpanzees chronically infected with HCV indicate that the vaccine does produce antibodies to E1, resulting in the elimination of HCV antigens from the liver, restoration of normal liver enzymes and improved liver histology. Alternate approaches include DNA immunization with chimeric viruses such as Hepatitis B virus [60] and adenovirus [61], and passive immunization with immunoglobulin from HCV-infected individuals, intended for post-exposure prophylaxis and the prevention of re-infection following liver transplant [62]. In summary, much effort is underway to design and test novel prophylactic and therapeutic approaches.

3   Antiviral treatment for HCV infection

As discussed above, prevention of HCV by prophylactic vaccines has been problematic due to the presence of large numbers of HCV genotypes and subtypes. Therefore, selective inhibition of HCV replication by immune modulators or by synthetic molecules could be a very effective approach to the treatment of HCV infection. Because the clinical importance of HCV has only been recognized in recent years, the development of small-molecule therapies targeting the HCV RNA genome or proteins is still at a relatively early stage. To date, the approved treatments for chronic HCV infection consist of either interferon alone or a combination of interferon and ribavirin. The following sections summarize the interferon treatments currently available and other ongoing pre-clinical antiviral approaches.

3.1   Current treatments

In the USA, interferon-α (IFNα) was the first approved treatment for chronic HCV infections. Belonging to a group of immunomodulatory proteins also termed cytokines, IFNs are involved in the human immune defense process and can be produced/secreted by host cells following viral infections. The antiviral mechanism associated with IFNs has not been clearly defined. However, it has been proposed that IFNs act *via* a cascade of events: by binding to their specific cellular receptors, they activate certain enzymes regulating protein synthesis, and eventually initiate antiviral responses [63]. In this regard, at least two cellular enzymes are known to be activated by IFN [63]: 2',5'-oligo-adenylate synthetase (OAS) and RNA-dependent protein kinase (PKR). OAS is an enzyme responsible for the synthesis of adenylate oligomer; its activation by IFN causes viral RNA degradation. PKR is a serine/threonine protein kinase that phosphorylates initiation factor eIF2A. When PKR is activated by IFN, it will phosphorylate eIF2A, resulting in the inhibition of both mRNA translation initiation and viral replication.

The first pilot study using recombinant IFNα for treatment of chronic HCV infection was carried out in 1986 by Hoofnagle and colleagues [64]. Since then, various clinical trials have been conducted to optimize IFNα treatment of HCV-infected patients [63]. It has been concluded that approximately 40% of treated patients had an initial response to IFN therapy, and about 70% of these responders relapsed after the treatment had ended (for review see [63, 65]). Overall, the long-term response to IFNα occurred in only 10–30% of patients [66]. Interestingly, patients infected with HCV genotype 1 consistently showed a poorer response to IFNα than did the other major genotypes [63, 65]. Such a low sensitivity to IFNα might be correlated to a sequence termed the IFN-sensitivity determining region (ISDR) within the HCV NS5A gene; however, these data are highly controversial [67]. In addition, response to IFN treatment might be affected by other factors such as patient's age, ethnic differences and duration of infection [63]. Since HCV exists *in vivo* as a population of heterogeneous quasi-species, the degree of quasi-species diversity might affect a patient's response to IFN treatment. Various side-effects have been observed in patients treated with IFNα. Most patients develop a severe flu-like syndrome, with symptoms such as fever, fatigue, muscle aches and headache; some also develop more severe side effects such as depression, nausea, weight loss and diarrhea [63].

Due to the low response rate and frequent relapse associated with the IFNα monotherapy, a combination therapy of IFNα and ribavirin was explored. Ribavirin is a known antiviral agent with a broad spectrum of activity against several pathogenic DNA and RNA viruses [63, 68]. This molecule, 1-β-D-ribo-furanosyl-1,2,4-triazole-3-carboxamide, is a nucleoside guanosine analogue containing a modified base. Although the inhibitory mechanism for ribavirin is not clearly understood, it has been proposed that this molecule inhibits inosine monophosphate dehydrogenase (see below), leading to a decreased intracellular pool of guanosine triphosphate [63]. This indirectly suppresses viral RNA synthesis. Other hypothesized mechanisms of action include the direct inhibition of viral RNA-dependent RNA polymerase and the prevention of efficient translation of viral transcripts [63].

Ribavirin has been successfully used for treatment of pneumonia caused by respiratory syncytial virus infection [63, 68]. When this broad spectrum antiviral agent was used in combination with IFNα, the overall response rate increased to ~40% [69, 70]. It has been shown that the combination therapy is most effective for treatment of patients who relapsed from previous IFN treatment. Unfortunately, additional side-effects have been described in the combination treatment [69, 70]. The most significant effect was reported to be hemolytic anemia due to the accumulation of ribavirin in erythrocytes.

3.2   Emerging therapies

Efforts to improve current IFN treatments are still ongoing. In this regard, a major advance is the recent development of a pegylated version of IFNα by several groups. The pegylated IFNα is generated through modification of the lysine residues of the IFNα protein by polyethylene glycol. As compared to the native IFNα form, pegylated IFNα demonstrated improved pharmacokinetic features including an increased half-life in circulation, delayed clear-

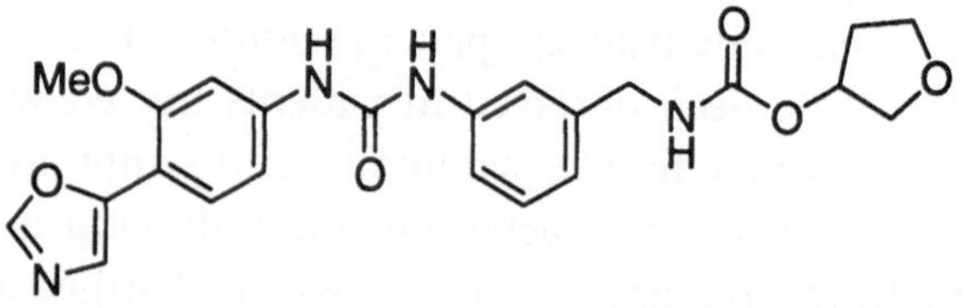

Fig. 2
VX-497

ance and reduced immunogenicity [71–73]. Therefore, the major advantage of the pegylated IFNα over the unmodified form is its properties *in vivo*, which may allow lower and less frequent doses and thus fewer side-effects. For example, the current dosage of IFNα for HCV treatment is 3 MIU administered subcutaneously or intramuscularly three times a week for 12 months, while the pegylated IFN-a could be injected once per week for the same period [73, 74]. Currently, therapeutic use of pegylated IFNα in combination with ribavirin is in phase III trials in the US and Europe.

Another emerging therapy is use of an inhibitor of cellular inosine monophosphate dehydrogenase (IMPDH) to treat HCV infections. This inhibitor, designated VX-497 (Fig. 2), was developed using structure-based drug design. VX-497 is an active site inhibitor of IMPDH and is currently in phase II clinical trials [75]. *In vitro* studies suggested that this inhibitor exerts its effects on lymphocyte migration and proliferation, and thus might prevent both virus proliferation and liver inflammation.

In a recent announcement, clinical trials have been initiated for a novel small compound that specifically inhibits a key replication activity of HCV [76]. However, no information was given regarding the compound's structure, mechanism of inhibition, or the specific target that this compound might inhibit.

3.3 Antiviral approaches in clinical and pre-clinical development

Parallel to the activities and efforts mentioned above, considerable energy has been devoted to development of specific antiviral compounds targeting the HCV genome and proteins encoded by the virus. The most recent significant advances in this regard include the identification of antisense RNAs and catalytic RNA molecules (ribozymes) that cleave the HCV genome. In addition, antiviral compounds targeting important viral enzymes such as protease, helicase, and polymerase have been discovered in recent years. Detailed information regarding progress in each of these approaches is given below.

3.3.1 Antiviral agents targeting the HCV genome

Because the sequence and structure of the HCV 5'-NTR are critical for viability and well conserved among genotypes, this region is an attractive target for the development of antivirals. The highly structured IRES in the HCV 5'-NTR controls cap-independent initiation of translation by directing ribosomes to the authentic initiation AUG upstream of the ORF. This function requires the interaction of viral RNA with proteins of cellular and, possibly, viral origin [77]. An interesting feature of the HCV IRES is that it apparently extends past the AUG into the nucleotide sequence of the core protein [78, 79]. In fact, it has been reported that the HCV core protein interacts with the 5'-NTR of the genome and modulates translation [80]. Moreover, the RNA replication signals present at the 5' terminus may also extend into the IRES element [77]. A comprehensive summary of the structure and function of the HCV IRES was recently published [81].

In the current model, the 5'-NTR folds into four structural domains, named I through IV (Fig. 3a). Domain I consists of a small stem-loop near the 5' terminus that is not critical for translation [78]. Domains II and III contain complex secondary structures. The base of Domain III forms an essential RNA pseudoknot [82]. Domain IV consists of a small stem-loop including the initiation AUG and the first 11 nucleotides of the ORF. In a recent study, chemical and enzymatic probing of the IRES in solution under various ionic conditions demonstrated that the RNA has a unique and stable three-dimensional structure at physiological salt concentrations; this folding is dependent on divalent metal ions [83]. The HCV IRES is unique in that 40S ribosomal subunits bind directly to the RNA in the absence of all initiation factors [84], including eIF4A, which is required for ribosomal attachment to capped mRNAs and the picornaviral IRES [85]. Thus, the HCV IRES first recruits the translational components, then orients the components to permit a productive interaction leading to initiation. In this way, translation initiation in HCV is similar to that of prokaryotes. The site of interaction between the IRES and p25, a component of the 40S ribosomal subunit, has been mapped using

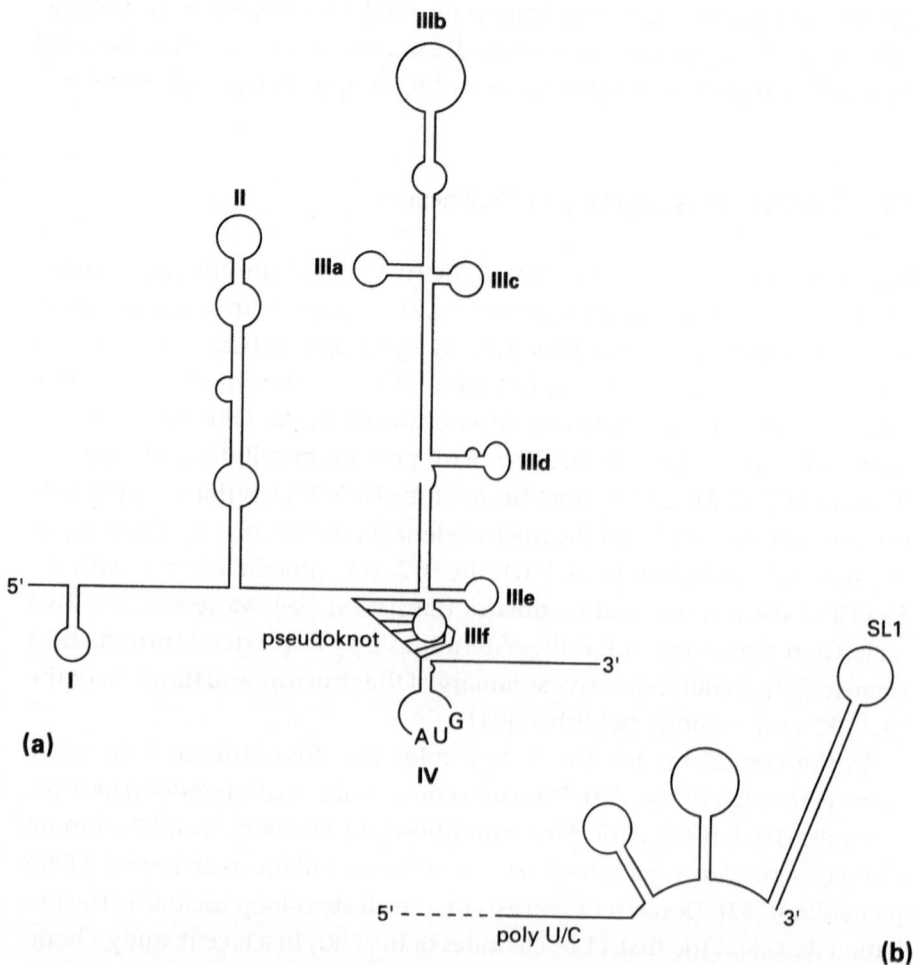

(a)

(b)

Fig. 3
Secondary and tertiary structure of the 5'- and 3'-NTRs of HCV. (a): Structure of the 3'-UTR as described in references 77, 86, and 87. Major stem-loop domains are indicated I-IV. Base-pairs involving stem-loop IIIf to form a pseudoknot structure are shown. The initiation AUG codon is indicated on stem-loop IV. (b): Secondary structure of the 98 nucleotides comprising the 3'X region of the HCV genome as identified in reference 32. The major stem-loop (SL I) is indicated.

UV cross-linking studies [86]. A detailed description of translation initiation by HCV was recently published [87].

The 98 nucleotides of the 3'X region of the 3'-NTR also fold into a conserved, stable secondary structure containing three stem-loops (Fig. 3b) [32].

This model was confirmed by chemical and enzymatic probing and temperature-dependent UV spectroscopy [32]. There is increasing evidence that the 5' and 3' termini of HCV RNA interact in ways that modulate transcription and translation [34, 88, 89].

There are many efforts underway to develop antivirals that target the 5'-NTR of HCV. Nucleic acids, in the form of antisense oligonucleotides or ribozymes, have been extensively explored in model systems. In cell culture-based assays, these molecules can be delivered in two ways: *via* liposome-mediated uptake from an extracellular source, or *via* intracellular generation using a gene therapy approach. Gene therapy using adenoviral vectors is particularly applicable to HCV infection because they can express the transgene in slowly dividing cells such as hepatocytes [90].

The use of antisense oligonucleotides against HCV has recently been investigated. The inhibitory effects of antisense molecules can be based on inhibiting translation, the induction of RNAse-H, or the inhibition of RNA splicing [91]. In recent studies, antisense oligonucleotides have been shown to inhibit HCV gene expression in *in vitro* translation assays and in transformed hepatocytes expressing the core protein [92, 93]. In addition, some of these oligonucleotides demonstrated dose-dependent inhibition of a luciferase reporter protein fused to the HCV IRES expressed in the livers of BALB/C mice [94]. The primary shortcoming of antisense molecules as therapeutic agents derives from their sensitivity to degradation by nucleases in serum. As a result, considerable effort has been devoted to identifying chemical modifications that enhance stability. Early work with phosphorothioate oligonucleotides resulted in enhanced stability but an unfavorable toxicity profile, including immune cell stimulation, complement activation and the abnormal induction of blood clotting [92]. In subsequent studies, various chemical modifications have succeeded in maximizing potency and specificity while improving half-life and toxicity profiles [91]. More recent developments suggest that a 2'-O-methoxyethyl-modified oligonucleotide may represent the next generation of antisense therapeutic agents [92]. A clinical trial to test safety and efficacy of this class of antisense oligonucleotide was recently announced [95].

A second antiviral approach based on a nucleic acid therapeutic agent is the use of hammerhead ribozymes directed against the HCV 5'-NTR [see 96 for review of antiviral ribozymes]. In surrogate cell culture systems, cleavage of this critical region results in the inhibition of IRES-driven protein translation [97]. This inhibition caused decreased infectivity in cell culture of an infectious HCV-poliovirus chimera [98]. Phase I clinical trials of a ribozyme for HCV are currently underway [99]. In other experimental approaches, the inhibition of translation results from ribozymes delivered *via* adenoviral gene therapy in cultured cells [100] and in a transgenic mouse model [101]. Similarly, the hairpin ribozymes are being developed as a potential gene therapy for HCV [102]. In this approach, a single therapeutic vector expresses several ribozymes targeting conserved regions of the viral genome.

In addition to nucleic acid-based approaches, several companies are screening the HCV IRES using libraries of small molecules. Ligand binding can be detected using a biochemical approach (that is, inhibition of translation of a reporter gene) or *via* biophysical methods. To date, no small-sized molecules have been reported as effective inhibitors targeting HCV IRES.

An additional strategy to target the HCV RNA genome is suggested by the interaction of RNA-binding proteins of cellular origin [103]. These include PTB and the La autoantigen, which have been found to bind specifically *in vitro* to either the 5'-NTR and/or 3'-NTR regions of the genome [33, 34, 104]. The relevance of these interactions was strengthened by a recent report showing that the La protein present in cytoplasmic extracts from human liver biopsies could interact specifically with the poly U/C tract of the 3'-NTR [105]. The significance of this presence is not certain, however. Unlike translation of the picornaviral IRES, PTB and La are apparently not required for the initiation of translation on the HCV IRES [84]. It is likely that a clear understanding of the role for these RNA-binding proteins will not be possible until a robust HCV replication system becomes available.

3.3.2 Antiviral agents targeting HCV proteins

As shown in Figure 1, the entire HCV genome encodes at least ten viral proteins in the following order: C-E1-E2-p7-NS2-NS3-NS4A-NS4B-NS5A-NS5B [106–109]. The six NS proteins are believed to be non-structural and involved in the viral genome replication process. In principle, each of these viral encoded proteins could serve as potential targets for antiviral therapy, assuming they are essential for viral replication and/or infection. However, the roles of some of the HCV nonstructural proteins, such as NS4B and NS5A, are not fully understood and thus no functional assays are available for these potential targets [67, 107, 110]. Consequently, development of antiviral agents that specifically interact with these viral proteins has been greatly hampered.

On the other hand, nonstructural proteins, such as NS3 and NS5B, have been studied extensively and their functions have been elucidated [106–113]. Various functional assays have been developed, which allow the measurement of their enzymatic activity in the presence of candidate antiviral compounds. As discussed below, several novel compounds demonstrating inhibitory activity against these enzymes have been identified and viewed as potential anti-HCV agents.

Development of NS3 protease inhibitors
NS3 is a multi-functional enzyme with the protease activity constrained in the N-terminal 180 amino acids and the RNA unwinding helicase and ATPase activity in the C-terminal 451 amino acids [106–109]. Sequence and structural analyses of the N-terminal domain of the NS3 protein have revealed that it represents a chymotrypsin-type serine protease with its catalytic triad identified as His-Asp-Ser [16, 26, 114]. The NS3 serine protease is responsible for generation of four mature viral proteins including NS4A, NS4B, NS5A and NS5B, which are the key components of the HCV replication complex [106–109]. It has been found that the catalytic activity of NS3 protease is stimulated by NS4A through formation of a stable complex between the two proteins [26, 115]. Recently, it has been shown that NS3 serine protease is essential for HCV replication and infection in the chimpanzee model [46]. Taken together, these observations indicate that the HCV NS3 protease, especially complexed with the NS4A cofactor, is one of the most attractive targets for chemotherapeutic intervention [24, 110, 111, 113].

Generation of active HCV NS3 protease in different recombinant systems has been reported widely (for review see [107]). Additionally, various accurate and convenient assays that employ small peptides derived from the NS3 processing sites as substrates have become available. Furthermore, the crystal structures for the full-length NS3 protein and the protease domain, alone or complexed with the NS4A fragment, have been solved [26, 114, 116, 117]. These efforts have greatly facilitated identification of viral protease inhibitors through both large-scale screening and/or rational design approaches. To date, structurally divergent molecules that inhibit the HCV NS3 protease have been described. These molecules can be classified into two major groups: nonpeptidic and peptidic.

97

Table 1.
Nonpeptidic inhibitors for HCV NS3 serine protease

Inhibitor	Structure	Potency	Inhibition mechanism
Phenathrenequinone (Sch68631)		$IC_{50} = 7.7\ \mu M$	ND
Thiazolidine (RD46205)		$IC_{50} = 14\ \mu M$	Noncompetitive
THNB (RD24039)		$IC_{50} = 77\ \mu M$	Mixed
Halogenated benzanilide		$IC_{50} = 6.5\ \mu M$	Noncompetitive
Hemiketal lactone (Sch351633)		$IC_{50} = 25\ \mu M$	ND

Note: for a convenient comparison, inhibition potency of the indicated compound has been converted to molar concentrations. ND, not determined; THNB, 2,4,6-trihydroxy,3-nitrobenzamide.

As seen in Table 1, several nonpeptidic molecules have been reported to inhibit HCV NS3 protease activity. These include a quinone-type compound isolated from the microorganism *Streptomyces* sp (Sch68631) [118], a thiazolidine derivative (RD46205) [119], 2,4,6-trihydroxy-3-nitrobenzamides

Table 2.
Competitive peptidic inhibitors for HCV NS3 protease

Source	Structure	Inhibition potency	Refs.
5A/5B	D-D-I-V-P-C-OH	$IC_{50} = 71$ μM	[123]
5A/5B	Ac-D-D-I-V-P-C-OH	$IC_{50} = 28$ μM	[123]
5A/5B	Ac-D-d-I-V-P-C-OH	$IC_{50} = 4.0$ μM	[123]
5A/5B	Ac-D-d-I-V-P-Nva-OH	$IC_{50} = 17$ μM	[124]
5A/5B	Ac-D-d-I-V-P-Nva-H	$IC_{50} = 1.1$ μM	[124]
5A/5B	Ac-D-d-I-V-P-Nva-CONHBn	$IC_{50} = 0.64$ μM	[124]
4A/4B	Ac-D-E-M-E-E-C-OH	$IC_{50} = 1.01$ μM	[125]
4A/4B	Ac-D-E-Dif-D-Cha-C-OH	$IC_{50} = 0.05$ μM	[126]
4A/4B	Ac-D-Gla-L-I-Cha-C-OH	$IC_{50} = 0.0015$ μM	[126]

Note: d is for D-Aspartic acid. The followings represent modified amino acids: Nva, norvaline; Dif, 3,3-diphenylalanine; Gla, D-γ-carboxy glutamic acid, Cha, β-cyclohexylalanine

(RD24039) [120], halogenated benzanilides [121], and a hemiketal lactone isolated from the fungus *Penicillium griseofulvum* (Sch351633) [122]. All of these molecules displayed potencies in the low micromolar range against the NS3 protease *in vitro*. These data together with their inhibitory mechanisms are summarized in Table 1.

The peptidic inhibitors thus far described for HCV NS3 are summarized in Table 2. These inhibitors were designed to mimic the peptides that represent the NS3 cleavage sites on the viral polyprotein. Some of them were identical to the NS3 cleavage products of the peptide substrates; thus they served as reversible competitive inhibitors for the viral protease. For example, a hexapeptide DDIVPC-OH, corresponding to the N-terminal cleavage product of the peptide derived from the NS5A/5B site for NS3 protease, was able to inhibit NS3 protease with an IC_{50} of 71 μM and K_i of 14 μM [123]. Potency was enhanced slightly by capping this peptide with an acetyl group at the N-terminus (Tab. 2). Further structure-activity relationship (SAR) studies revealed that replacement of P5 glutamic acid with the isomeric D-counterpart could enhance the potency several fold, while various modifications of the P1 cysteine side chain resulted in less potent compounds [124]. When norvaline was introduced into the P1 position, the resulting peptide Ac-DdIVP-Nva-OH exhibited improved inhibitory activity (Tab. 2). In a parallel investigation, NS3 inhibition by the products of peptide substrates derived from the NS4A/4B and NS4B/5A site was also observed [125]. A detailed SAR study was conducted on the hexapeptide Ac-DEMEEC-OH using a combinatorial chemistry approach [126]. After a sequential optimization at positions P2 through P5, several potent inhibitors with low-nanomolar IC_{50} were identified as summarized in Table 2 [126]. Of these, peptide Ac-D-Gla-L-I-Cha-C-OH demonstrated an IC_{50} of 1.5 nM against the purified HCV NS3 protease [126].

Similar to the approaches employed for other serine proteases, peptide analogues containing various electrophilic carbonyl groups that could serve as warheads to attack the active site serine hydroxyl group were also developed [124]. To date, aldehyde, α-ketoamide and fluorine-containing carbonyl derivatives have been explored [124]. However, these modifications to the core peptides provide only a marginal improvement in potency (Tab. 2). The most potent compound in this series is the modified peptide Ac-DdIVP-Nva-CONHBn with an IC_{50} of 0.64 µM; unfortunately, this compound lacks specificity in that it also inhibits human and porcine elastase efficiently [124]. In addition, synthesis of cyclic biphenyl ethers based on a tetrapeptide inhibitor Ac-Dif-Glu-Cha-Cys-OH has been recently reported [127]; however, no biological data are currently available for these peptidic ether analogues.

In addition to the small peptides mentioned above, a panel of macromolecular inhibitors for HCV NS3 has been disclosed. In general, these molecules are protein ligands which inhibit HCV NS3 protease through its direct binding to the viral enzyme. For example, a group of minimized antibody-like proteins, also termed minibodies, were identified through a phage-displayed synthetic repertoire. They could bind and inactivate the NS3 protease selectively with low micromolar IC_{50} and kinetic values [128–130]. Additionally, selective NS3 protease inhibitors have been designed and synthesized on the basis of eglin c protein [131]. Eglin c, a 70 amino acid protein isolated from leeches, is a well-known potent inhibitor of several serine proteases including chemotrypsin and subtilisin [132]. Several engineered eglin c mutant proteins demonstrated nanomolar potency against HCV NS3 [131]. In addition to identifying potent ligand inhbitors, these studies have provided information that will be useful for designing more potent and smaller-sized antivirals [130].

Development of HCV ATPase/helicase inhibitors

As discussed above, the C-terminal portion of the HCV NS3 protein defines an ATP-dependent helicase activity which is independent of the protease domain located at the N-terminus. Because the HCV helicase domain contains a conserved motif -DECH- box, it has been classified into the RNA heli-

Table 3.
HCV NS3 helicase inhibitors.

Piperidine derivatives	Heterocyclic carboxamide
$IC_{50} = 7\ \mu M$	$IC_{50} = 0.7\ \mu M$

case superfamily II (for review see [133, 134]). It is believed that HCV helicase activity is responsible for RNA unwinding during the viral replication process and its essential role has been demonstrated in the chimpanzee model [46, 107]. Due to its importance in the viral life cycle, great attention has been given to this enzyme. Generation of active recombinant HCV helicase proteins, assay development and biochemical characterization studies have been extensively described in the literature (for review see [107, 109]). In addition, the crystal structure for the HCV helicase domain, first described in 1998 [134–136], is expected to have a positive impact on the design and development of selective HCV ATPase/helicase inhibitors.

The development of specific inhibitors against the HCV helicase and/or ATPase activity has lagged behind our basic understanding of this enzyme; to date, only a few small-molecule inhibitors have been reported. Two closely related compounds, piperidine derivatives and heterocyclic substituted carboxamides, have been claimed to inhibit HCV helicase *in vitro* [137–139]. As summarized in Table 3, both compounds showed low micromolar IC_{50}s against HCV helicase activity. Macromolecular inhibitors that block HCV helicase activity have also been reported. For example, RNA aptamers rich in secondary structures were found to interact with the NS3 protein and thus inhibited both the protease and helicase activities of NS3 [140].

The ATPase activity of the HCV NS3 protein, which is required for its unwinding helicase activity, has also been viewed as a target suitable for antiviral therapy. In this regard, two compounds were recently reported to inhibit the NS3 ATPase activity. These two molecules, paclitaxel and trifluoperazine, inhibited the NS3 ATPase activity by interacting with the enzyme's ATP binding site [141]. Paclitaxel, an antimitotic agent isolated from the western yew plant, inhibited the NS3 ATPase activity competitively with an IC_{50} determined to be 17 µM, and trifluoperazine, a calmodulin antagonist, inactivated the viral ATPase by a noncompetitive mechanism with an IC_{50} of 105 µM [141]. On the other hand, paclitaxel and trifluoperazine are known for their interaction with the ATP-binding sites of other proteins, which suggested that their inhibitory activity against HCV NS3 ATPase activity was not specific.

Development of HCV polymerase inhibitors
The NS5B protein encoded by the HCV genome is associated with the RNA-dependent RNA polymerase activity [21, 142]. Recombinant NS5B expressed in both bacterial and insect cells demonstrated RNA synthesis activity using either homopolymeric RNAs or the HCV RNA genome as templates [142–144]. In the viral life cycle, the NS5B protein might assume the responsibility for viral genome replication by interacting with other viral and cellular proteins (for review see [112]). The viral polymerase has been proposed as the key component of the viral replicase complex and its essential function in HCV infection has been confirmed in the chimpanzee model [46]. Recently, several groups solved the X-ray crystallographic structure of the HCV NS5B [145–147].

HCV NS5B polymerase has also been considered an attractive target for antiviral therapy due to its critical role in viral replication and the lack of any known cellular counterparts. Notwithstanding the quantity of biochemical and structural information available for this viral polymerase, there have been no specific inhibitors that target the HCV NS5B reported so far. Nevertheless, it is noteworthy that several groups have examined the effects of known polymerase inhibitors and antiviral agents on HCV NS5B polymerase activity *in vitro*. NS5B activity was not sensitive to phosphonoacetic acid and phosphonoformic acid, inhibitors for DNA-dependent DNA polymerase and reverse transcriptases [148–150]. It has also been found that certain triphosphates of deoxynucleotide analogues which are active against other viral polymerases, such as AZT and 3TC, do not significantly inhibit the NS5B activity [148–150].

On the other hand, the presence of cerulenin and gliotoxin resulted in moderate inhibition of HCV NS5B activity [148, 151]. Interestingly, both cerulenin, a specific inhibitor of lipid and sterol biosynthesis, and gliotoxin, a fungal metabolite, have been reported to inhibit other viral RNA-dependent

RNA polymerases [148, 152]. In addition, transition state metals such as Ni^{2+} and Zn^{2+} could inhibit the NS5B RNA synthesis activity with IC_{50} in low micromolar range [150, 151]. It was proposed that these inhibitory metals compete with the required divalent cation Mg^{2+} for binding to the enzyme [150]. Certain positively charged polymers such as heparin and polylysine could also inhibit HCV NS5B polymerase activity *in vitro* [150]. However, their inhibition mechanism has not been clearly defined.

More recently, several groups reported that purified HCV NS5B polymerase is capable of synthesizing RNA using a primer-independent *de novo* mechanism of initiation [153–155]. It is generally accepted that a *de novo* RNA initiation pathway is likely to be the mode of viral RNA genome replication that takes place in infected cells. Therefore, NS5B polymerase assays developed based on this function might promote the discovery of novel inhibitors that specifically block the initiation step.

Inhibitor development for other HCV proteins and enzymes
In the absence of an efficient cell culture system for HCV replication, antiviral research targeting HCV proteins with no known function or with no functional assay available, such as NS4B and NS5A, has been hindered. Consequently, there have been no specific inhibitors reported for these proteins to date.

It is worth mentioning that NS4A, a cofactor for the NS3 serine protease, could be an interesting target for antiviral development [24, 107, 109]. It has been proposed that a direct interaction between NS3 and the NS4A cofactor might be important for NS3 proteolytic activity [26, 115]. From this point of view, inhibitors that block the protein-protein interaction between NS3 and NS4A would have the potential to interfere with viral polyprotein processing catalyzed by NS3 protease [26, 109, 115]. Several peptides derived from NS4A demonstrated inhibitory activity against HCV NS3 protease activity *in vitro* with low micromolar IC_{50} values [110, 156]. They apparently inhibited the NS3 enzyme by competing with the cofactor NS4A for binding to the enzyme [110].

In addition to the viral proteins discussed above, HCV NS2 protein is also of particular interest. No known cellular homologues of NS2 have been identified. Its N-terminal portion is responsible for membrane association, and its C-terminus together with NS3 is believed to catalyze the cleavage of NS2/3 site on the viral polyprotein ([107] for review). Unlike the NS3 serine protease, the catalytic mechanism of the NS2/3 protease has not been clearly defined. It functions either as a metalloprotease requiring metals such as Zn^{2+} for activity or as a cysteine protease [157, 158]. Interestingly, cleavage product-derived peptides or peptides resembling the NS2/3 cleavage site did not inhibit the NS2/3 protease activity, while peptides derived from NS4A were found to inactivate NS2/3 activity with K_i values as low as 3 µM [159].

4   Conclusions

As the major cause of chronic hepatitis in humans, HCV is closely associated with cirrhosis and hepatocellular carcinoma. At present, no effective prophylactic vaccines or antivirals are available for either prevention or treatment of HCV-related infections. The major challenges for vaccine development include the existence of divergent HCV genotypes and quasi-species and the induction of persistence despite the presence of specific immune responses. Current treatment options, which are limited to interferon alone or in combination with ribavirin, provide only limited efficacy and/or unfavorable side effects for a large proportion of patients. Unfortunately, the lack of an efficient cell culture system and a convenient animal model to study HCV replication and *in vivo* infection has greatly impeded efforts to develop HCV-specific antivirals. In spite of these obstacles, two different approaches have been intensively explored in recent years. One approach is to target well-characterized HCV enzymes and the other is to target the HCV RNA genome itself.

To date, peptidic inhibitors active in the nanomolar range for HCV NS3 protease have been described. However, the non-peptidic inhibitors identified thus far demonstrated only moderate activity. It is hoped that extensive SAR studies based on these core structures may result in more potent compounds. As compared to the NS3 protease, developments of specific inhibitors against the HCV polymerase and helicase are proceeding at a much slower rate. The expectation is that the availability of their crystal structures will facilitate identification of novel inhibitors against these enzymes. On the other hand, significant progress has been made in developing inhibitors that target the HCV genome. In this regard, two molecules targeting the HCV IRES have recently entered phase I clinical trials: an antisense oligonucleotide, ISIS 14803 [95], and a catalytic hammerhead ribozyme,

LY466700 [99]. This progress provides optimism that an effective antiviral agent will emerge within the next few years for treatment of HCV infections.

Acknowledgment

The authors would like to thank Dr. Joseph Colacino for reviewing this paper and providing helpful suggestions.

References

1   Choo Q.-L., G. Kuo, A.J. Weiner, R.L. Overby, D.W. Bradley and M. Houghton: Science *244*, 359 (1989).

2   Saito I., T. Miyamura, A. Ohbayashi, H. Harada, T. Katayama, S. Kikuchi, Y. Watanabe, S. Koi, M. Onji, Y. Ohta et al.: Proc. Natl. Acad. Sci. USA *87*, 6547 (1990).

3   Consensus Development Panel. National Institutes of Health Consensus Development Conference Panel statement: Hepatology *26*, Suppl. 1, 2S (1997).

4   Berenguer, M. and T.L. Wright: Proc. Assoc. Amer. Phys. *110*, 98 (1998).

5   World Health Organization: Weekly Epidemiological Record *72*, 65 (1997).

6   Alter, M., D. Kruszon-Moran, O.V. Nainan, G.M. McQuillan, F. Gao, L.A. Moyer, R.A. Kaslow and H.S. Margolis: New Engl. J. Med. *341*, 556 (1999).

7   Wright, T., H. Hollander, X. Pu et al.: Hepatology *20*, 1152 (1994).

8   Thomas, D.L.: Curr Top Microbiol Immunol. *242*, 25 (2000).

9   Hoofnagle, J.H.: Hepatology *26*, 15S (1997).

10   Hayashi, J., H. Aoki, Y. Arakawa and O. Hino: Intervirology *42*, 205 (1999).

11   Hadziyannis, S.J.: J. Viral Hepatitis *4*, 9 (1997).

12   Cerny, A. and F.V. Chisari: Hepatology *30*, 595 (1999).

13   Lau, J.Y.N., X. Xie, M.M.C. Lai and P.C. Wu: Seminars in Liver Disease *18*, 169 (1998).

14   Kolykhalov, A.A, A.A. Agapov, K.J. Blight, K. Mihalik, S.M. Feinstone and C.M. Rice: Science *277*, 570 (1997).

15   Yanagi, M., R.H. Purcell, S.U. Emerson and J. Bukh: Proc. Natl. Acad. Sci. USA *97*, 8738 (1997).

16   Miller, R.H. and R.H. Purcell: Proc. Natl Acad. Sci. USA *87*, 2057 (1990).

17   Mizokami M. and E. Orito: Intervirology *42*, 159 (1999).

18   Gordon, F.D., J.J. Poterucha, J. Germer, N.N. Zein, K.P. Batts, J.B. Gross Jr., R. Wiesner and D. Persing: Transplantation *63*, 1419 (1997).

19   Honda, M., E.A. Brown and S.M. Lemon: RNA *2*, 955 (1996).

20   Houdebine L.M. and J. Attal: Transgenic Res. *8*, 157 (1999).

21   Major, M.E. and S.M. Feinstone: Hepatology *25*, 1527 (1997).

22   Hijikata, M., H. Mizushima, Y. Tanji, Y. Komoda, Y. Hirowatari, T. Akagi et al.: Proc. Natl. Acad. Sci. USA *90*, 10773 (1993).

23   Grakoui A., D.W. McCourt, C. Wychowski, S.M. Feinstone and C.M. Rice: Proc. Natl. Acad. Sci. USA *90*, 10583 (1993).

24   Kwong A.D., J.L. Kim, G. Rao, D. Lipovsek and S.A. Raybuck: Antiviral Res. *41*, 67 (1999).

25   Kwong, A.D., J.L. Kim and C. Lin: Curr. Top. Microbiol. Immunol. *242*, 171 (2000).

26   Kim, J.L., K.A. Morgenstern, C. Lin, T. Fox, M.D. Dwyer, J.A. Landro et al.: Cell *87*, 343 (1996).

27   DeFrancesco, R., S.E. Behrens, L. Tomei, S. Altamura and J. Jiricny: Meth. Enzymol. *275*, 58 (1996).

28   Yanagi, M., M.St. Claire, S.U. Emerson, R.H. Purcell and J. Bukh: Proc. Natl. Acad. Sci. USA *96*, 2291 (1999).

29   Luo G.: Virology *256*, 105 (1999).

30   Kolykhalov, A.A., S.M. Feinstone and C.M. Rice: J. Virol. *70*, 3363 (1996).

31   Tanaka, T., N. Kato, M.-J. Cho, K. Sugiyama and K. Shimotohno: J. Virol. *70*, 3307 (1996).

32   Blight K.J. and C.M. Rice: J. Virol. *71*, 7345 (1997).

33   Ali, N. and A. Siddiqui: J. Virol. *69*, 6367 (1995).

34   Tsuchihara, K., T. Tanaka, M. Hijikata, S. Kuge, H. Toyoda, A. Nomoto, N. Yamamoto and K. Shimotohno: J. Virol. *71*, 6720 (1997).

35   Ito, T., S.M. Tahara and M.M.C. Lai: J. Virol. *72*, 8789 (1998).

36   Fang, J.W.S., V. Chow and J.Y.N. Lau: Clin. Liver Dis. *1*, 493 (1997).

37   Hsu, C.-W., C.-T. Yeh, P. G.-C. Chen and Y.-F. Liaw: J. Infect. Dis. *180*, 992 (1999).

38   Kato, N. and K. Shimotohno: Curr. Top. Microbiol. Immunol. *242*, 261 (2000).

39   Rumin, S., P. Berthillon, E. Tanaka, K. Kiyosawa, M.-A. Trabaud, T. Bizollon, C. Gouillat, P. Gripon, C. Guguen-Guillouzo, G. Inchauspe et al.: J. Gen. Virology *80*, 3007 (1999).

40   Kato, N., M. Ikeda, T. Mizutani, K. Sugiyama, M. Noguchi, S. Hirohashi and K. Shimotohno: Jpn. J. Cancer Res. *87*, 787 (1996).

41   Lohmann, V., F. Korner, J.-O. Koch, U. Herian, L. Theilmenn and R. Bartenschlager: Science *285*, 110 (1999).

42   Rosa, D., S. Campagnoli, C. Moretto, E. Guenzi, L. Cousens, M. Chin, C. Dong, A.J. Weiner, J.Y.N. Lau, Q.-L. Choo et al.: Proc. Natl. Acad. Sci. USA *93*, 1759 (1996) .

43   Pileri, P., Y. Uematsu, S. Campagnoli, G. Galli, F. Falugi, R. Petracca, A.J. Weiner, M. Houghton, D. Rosa, G. Grandi et al.: Science *282*, 938 (1998).

44   Agnello, V., G. Abel, M. Elfahal, G. B. Knight and Q.-X. Zhang: Proc. Natl. Acad. Sci. USA *96*, 12766 (1999).

45   Flint, M., J. Dubuisson, C. Maidens, R. Harrop, G.R. Guile, P. Borrow and J.A. McKeating: J. Virol. *74*, 702 (2000).

46   Kolykhalov A., K. Mihalik, S.M. Feinstone and C.M. Rice: 6th Intl Symposium on HCV. A40 (1999).

47   Walker, C.M.: Springer Semin. Immunopathol. *19*, 85 (1997).

48   Xie, Z.-C., J.-I. Riezu-Boj, J.-J. Lasarte, J. Guillen, J.-H. Su, M.-P. Civeira and J. Prieto: Virology *244*, 513 (1998).

49   Schinazi, R.F., E. Ilan, P.L. Black, X. Yao and S. Dagan: Antiviral Chem. Chemother. *10*, 99 (1999).

50   Choo, Q.-L., G. Kuo, R. Ralston, A.J. Weiner, D.Y. Chien, G. Van Nest, J. Han, K. Berger, K. Thudium, C. Kuo et al.: Proc. Natl. Acad. Sci. USA *91*, 1294 (1994).

51   Abrignani, S. and D. Rosa: Clin. Diag. Virol. *10*, 181 (1998).

52   Piazza, M., L. Sagliocca, G. Tosone, V. Guadagnino, M.A. Stazi, R. Orlando, G. Borgia, D. Rosa, S. Abrignani, F. Palumbo et al.: BioDrugs *12*, 291 (1999).

53   Houghton, M.: Curr. Top. Microbiol. Immunol. *242*, 327 (2000).

54   AVANT Immunotherapeutics, 1999.

55   Berzofsky, J.A., J.D. Ahlers, M.A. Derby, C.D. Pendleton, T. Arichi and I.M. Belyakov: Immunological Reviews *170*, 151 (1999).

56   Chiron Press Release, February 16, 1998.

57   IMSWorld R&D Focus, 9/30/99.

58   Pharmaprojects, Record No. 028455, 1999.

59   IMSWorld R&D Focus, 9/6/99.

60   R & D Insight, p. 15–16, Accession No. 11242, September 15, 1999.

61   R & D Insight, p. 21–23, Accession No. 4742, September 15, 1999.

62   R & D Insight, p. 1–2, Accession No. 4347, November 10, 1999.

63   Damen, M. and D. Bresters, in: H.W. Reesink (ed.): Curr. Stud. Hematol. Blood Transf. Karger Publishers 1998, Basel.

64   Hoofnagle, J.H., K.D. Mullen, D.B. Jones, V. Rustgi, A. Di Bisceglie, M. Peters, J.G. Waggoner, Y. Park and E.A. Jones: N. Engl. J. Med. *315*, 1575 (1986).

65   Davis, G.L. and J.H. Hoofnagle: Hepatology *6*, 1038 (1986).

66   Houghton, M., in: B.N. Fields et al. (eds.): Fields Virology. Raven Publishers 1996, Philadelphia.

67   Pawlotsky, J.M. and G. Germanidis: J. Viral Hepatitis *6*, 343 (1999).

68   Rankin, J.T. Jr., S.B. Eppes, J.B. Antczak and W.K. Joklik: Virology *168*, 147 (1989).

69   Christie, J.M. and R.W. Chapman: Hosp Med. *60*, 357 (1999).

70   Slater, M.J. and B.E. Clarke: Exp. Opin. Ther. Patents *6*, 739 (1996).

71   Hoffmann-La Roche, EP809996, 1997.

72   Hoffmann-La Roche, WO9964016, 1997.

73   Schering-Plough Press Release, Nov. 9, 1999.

74   Pharmaceutical News Daily, Jan. 7, 2000.

75   Wright, T., M.L. Shiffman, S. Knox, E. Ette, R.S. Kauffman and J. Alam: AASLD Meeting, a990 (1999).

76   Pharmaceutical News Daily, Feb. 29, 2000.

77   Lemon, S.M. and M. Honda: Seminars in Virology *8*, 274 (1997).

78   Honda, M., L-H. Ping, R.C.A. Rijnbrand, E. Amphlett, B. Clarke, D. Rowlands and S.M. Lemon: Virology *222*, 31 (1996).

79   Honda, M., R. Rijnbrand, G. Abell, D. Kim and S.M. Lemon: J. Virol. *73*, 4941 (1999).

80   Shimoike, T., S. Mimori, H. Tani, Y. Matsuura and T. Miyamura: J. Virol. *73*, 9718 (1999).

81   Rijnbrand, R.C.A. and S.M. Lemon: Curr. Top. Microbiol. Immunol. *242*, 85 (2000).

82   Wang, C., S.Y. Le, N. Ali and A. Siddiqui: RNA *1*, 526 (1995).

83   Kieft, J.S., K. Zhou, R. Jubin, M.G. Murray, J.Y.N. Lau and J.A. Doudna: J. Mol. Biol. *292*, 513 (1999).

84   Pestova, T.V., I.N. Shatsky, S.P. Fletcher, R.J. Jackson and C.U.T. Hellen: Genes Dev. *12*, 67 (1998).

85   Pestova, T.V., C.U.T. Hellen and I.N. Shatsky: Mol. Cell Biol. *16*, 6859 (1996).

86   Fukushi, S., M. Okada, T. Kageyama, F.B. Hoshino and K. Katayama:Virus Genes *19*, 153 (1999).

87   Hellen, C.U.T. and T.V. Pestova: J. Viral Hep. *6*, 79 (1999).

88   Ito, T. and M.M.C. Lai: Virology *254*, 288 (1999).

89   Ito, T., S.M. Tahara and M.M.C. Lai: J. Virol. *72*, 8789 (1998).

90   Connelly, S.: Curr. Opinion in Molec. Therapeutics *1*, 565 (1999).

91   Caselmann, W.H., S. Eisenhardt and M. Alt: Intervirology *40*, 394 (1997).

92 Brown-Driver, V., T. Eto, E. Lesnik, K.P. Anderson and R.C. Hanecak: Antisense & Nucleic Acid Drug Dev. *9*, 145 (1999).

93 Wakita, T., D. Moradpour, K. Tokushihge and J.R. Wands: J. Med. Virology *57*, 217 (1999).

94 Zhang, H., R. Hanecak, V. Brown-Driver, R. Azad, B. Conklin, M.C. Fox and K.P. Anderson: Antimicrob. Agents Chemother. *43*, 347 (1999).

95 ISIS Press Release, March 1, 2000.

96 Menke, A. and G. Hobom: Molec. Biotechnol. *8*, 17 (1997).

97 Sakamoto, N., C.H. Wu and G.Y. Wu: J. Clin. Invest. *98*, 2720 (1996).

98 Macejak, D.G., K.L. Jensen, S.F. Jamison, K. Domenico, E.C. Roberts, N. Chaudhary, I. von Carlowitz, L. Bellon, M.J. Tong, A. Conrad et al.: Hepatology *31*, 769 (2000).

99 RPI Press Release, February 16, 2000.

100 Lieber, A., C.Y. He, S.J. Polyak, D.R. Gretch, D. Barr and M.A. Kay: J. Virol. *70*, 8782 (1996).

101 Lieber, A. and M.A. Kay: J. Virol. *70*, 3153 (1996).

102 R & D Insight, p. 3–4, Accession No. 11542, February 17, 1999.

103 Yen, J.H., S.C. Chang, C.R. Hu, S.C. Chu, S.S. Lin, Y.S. Hsieh and M.F. Chang: Virology *208*, 723 (1995).

104 Ali, N. and A. Siddiqui: Proc. Natl. Acad. Sci. USA *94*, 2249 (1997).

105 Spangberg, K. Goobar-Larsson, M. Wahren-Herlenius and S. Schwartz: J. Human Virol. *2*, 296 (1999).

106 Clarke, B.: J. Gen. Virol. *78*, 2397 (1997).

107 Reed, K.E. and C.M. Rice, in: H.W. Reesink (ed.): Curr. Stud. Hematol. Blood Transf. Karger Publishers 1998, Basel.

108 Suzuki, R., T. Suzuki, K. Ishii, Y. Matsuura and T. Miyamura: Intervirology *42*, 145 (1999).

109 Littlejohn, M., S. Locarnini and A. Bartholomeusz: Antiviral Therapy *3*, 83 (1999).

110 Walker, M.A.: Drug Discov. Today *4*, 518 (1999).

111 Shoemaker, K.R.: Curr. Opin. Anti-infect. Invest. *1*, 559 (1999).

112 Hagedorn, C.H., E.H. van Beers and C. De Staercke: Curr. Top. Microbiol. Immunol. *242*, 225 (2000).

113 Bartenschlager, R.: Viral Hepat. *6*, 165 (1999).

114 Love, R.A., H.E. Parge, J.A. Wickersham, Z. Hostomsky, N. Habuka, E.W. Moomaw, T. Adachi and Z. Hostomska: Cell *87*, 331 (1996).

115 Bartenschlager, R., V. Lohmann, T. Wilkinson, J.O. Koch: J. Virol. *69*, 7519 (1995).

116 Yan, Y., Y. Li, S. Munshi, V. Sardana, J.L. Cole, M. Sardana, C. Steinkuehler, L. Tomei, R. De Francesco, L.C. Kuo and Z. Chen: Protein Sci. *7*, 837 (1998).

117 Yao, N., P. Reichert, S.S. Taremi, W.W. Prosise and P.C. Weber: Structure Fold Des. *7*, 1353 (1999).

118 Chu, M., R. Mierzwa, I. Truumees, A. King, M. Patel, R. Berrie, A. Hart, N. Butkiewicz, B. Mahapatra, T.M. Chan and M.S. Puar: Tetrahedron Lett. *37*, 7229 (1996).

119 Sudo, K., Y. Matsumoto, M. Matsushima, M. Fujiwara, K. Konno, K. Shimotohno, S. Shigeta and T. Yokota: Biochem. Biophys. Res. Commun. *238*, 643 (1997).

120 Sudo, K., Y. Matsumoto, M. Matsushima, K. Konno, K. Shimotohno, S. Shigeta and T. Yokota: Antiviral Chem. Chemother. *8*, 541 (1997).

121 Kakiuchi, N., Y. Komoda, K. Komoda, N. Takeshita, S. Okada, T. Tani and K. Shimotohno: FEBS Lett. *421*, 217 (1998).

122 Chu, M., R. Mierzwa, L. He, A. King, M. Patel, J. Pichardo, A. Hart, N. Butkiewicz and M.S. Puar: Bioorg. Med. Chem. Lett. *9*, 1949 (1999).

123   Llinas-Brunet, M., M. Bailey, G. Fazal, S. Goulet, T. Halmos, S. Laplante, R. Maurice, M. Poirier, M. Poupart, D. Thibeault et al.: Bioorg. Med. Chem. Lett. *8*, 1713 (1998).

124   Llinas-Brunet, M., M. Bailey, R. Ddziel, G. Fazal, V. Gorys, S. Goulet, T. Halmos, R. Maurice, M. Poirier, M. Poupart et al.: Bioorg. Med. Chem. Lett. *8*, 2719 (1998).

125   Steinkuhler, C., G. Biasiol, M. Brunetti, A. Urbani, U. Koch, R. Cortese, A. Pessi and R. De Francesco: Biochemistry *37*, 8899 (1998).

126   Ingallinella, P., S. Altamura, E. Bianchi, M. Taliani, R. Ingenito, R. Cortese, R. De Francesco, C. Steinkuhler and A. Pessi: Biochemistry *37*, 8906 (1998).

127   Marchetti, A., J.M. Ontoria and V.G. Matassa: Synlett, SI, 1000 (1999).

128   Dimasi, N., F. Martin, C. Volpari, M. Brunetti, G. Biasiol, S. Altamura, R. Cortese, R. De Francesco, C. Steinkuhler and M. Sollazzo: J Virol. *71*, 7461 (1997) .

129   Martin, F., C. Volpari, C. Steinkuhler, N. Dimasi, M. Brunetti, G. Biasiol, S. Altamura, R. Cortese, R. De Francesco and M. Sollazzo: Protein Eng. *10*, 607 (1997).

130   Martin, F., C. Steinkuhler, M. Brunetti, A. Pessi, R. Cortese, R. De Francesco and M. Sollazzo: Protein Eng. *12*, 1005 (1999).

131   Martin, F., N. Dimasi, C. Volpari, C. Perrera, S. Di Marco, M. Brunetti, C. Steinkuhler, R. De Francesco and M. Sollazzo: Biochemistry *37*, 11459 (1998).

132   Qasim, M.A., P.J. Ganz, C.W. Saunders, K.S. Bateman, M.N. James and M. Laskowski Jr.: Biochemistry *36*, 1598 (1997).

133   de la Cruz, J., D. Kressler and P. Linder: TIPS *24*, 192 (1999).

134   Kadare, G. and A. Heanni: J. Virol. *71*, 2583 (1997).

135   Cho, H.S., N.C. Ha, L.W. Kang, K.M. Chung, S.H. Back, S.K. Jang and B.H. Oh: J. Biol. Chem. *273*, 15045 (1998).

136   Kim, J.L., K.A. Morgenstern, J.P. Griffith, M.D. Dwyer, J.A. Thomson, M.A. Murcko, C. Lin and P.R. Caron: Structure *6*, 89 (1998).

137   Viropharma Inc. WO9736554 (1997).

138   Viropharma Inc. WO9736866 (1997).

139   Clarke, B.E. and M.J. Slater: Exp. Opin. Ther. Patents *7*, 979 (1997).

140   Kumar, P.K., K. Machida, P.T. Urvil, N. Kakiuchi, D. Vishnuvardhan, K. Shimotohno, K. Taira and S. Nishikawa: Virology *237*, 270 (1997).

141   Borowski, P., R. Kuehl, O. Mueller, L.H. Hwang, J. Schulze Zur Wiesch and H. Schmitz: Eur. J. Biochem. *266*, 715 (1999).

142   Behrens, S.E., L. Tomei and R. De Francesco: EMBO J. *15*, 12 (1996).

143   Lohmann, V., F. Korner, U. Herian and R. Bartenschlager: J. Virol. *71*, 8416 (1997).

144   Oh, J.W., T. Ito and M.M. Lai: J. Virol. *73*, 7694 (1999).

145   Ago, H., T. Adachi, A. Yoshida, M. Yamamoto, N. Habuka, K. Yatsunami and M. Miyano: Structure Fold Des. *7*, 1417 (1999).

146   Bressanelli, S., L. Tomei, A. Roussel, I. Incitti, R.L. Vitale, M. Mathieu, R. De Francesco and F.A. Rey: Proc. Natl. Acad. Sci. USA *96*, 13034 (1999).

147   Lesburg, C.A., M.B. Cable, E. Ferrari, Z. Hong, A.F. Mannarino and P.C. Weber: Nat. Struct. Biol. *6*, 937 (1999).

148   Lohmann, V., A. Roos, F. Korner, J.O. Koch and R. Bartenschlager: Virology *249*, 108 (1998).

149   Ishii, K., Y. Tanaka, C.C. Yap, H. Aizaki, Y. Matsuura and T. Miyamura: Hepatology *29*, 1227 (1999).

150   Johnson, R.B., X.L. Sun, M.A. Hockman, E.C. Villarreal, M. Wakulchik and Q.M. Wang: Arch. Biochem. Biophys.; in press (2000).

151   Ferrari, E., J. Wright-Minogue, J.W. Fang, B.M. Baroudy, J.Y. Lau and Z. Hong: J. Virol. *73*, 1649 (1999).

152   Rodriguez, P.L. and L. Carrasco: J Virol. *66*, 1971 (1992).

153   Luo, G., R.K. Hamatake, D.M. Mathis, J. Racela, K.L. Rigat, J. Lemm and R.J. Colonno: J. Virol. *74*, 851 (2000).

154   Sun, X.L., R.B. Johnson, M.A. Hockman and Q.M. Wang: Biochem. Biophys. Res. Commun. *268*, 798 (2000).

155   Zhong, W., A.S. Uss, E. Ferrari, J.Y. Lau and Z. Hong: J. Virol. *74*, 2017 (2000).

156   Schering Corp. WO9743310 (1997).

157   Wu, Z., N. Yao, H.V. Le and P.C. Weber: TIPS *23*, 92 (1998).

158   Gorbalenya, A.E. and E.J. Snijder: Perspect Drug Discov. Des. *6*, 64 (1996).

159   Darke, P.L., A.R. Jacobs, L. Waxman and L.C. Kuo: J. Biol. Chem. *274*, 34511 (1999).

Antiviral Agents – Advances and Problems (E. Jucker, Ed.)
©2001 Birkhäuser Verlag, Basel (Switzerland)

Drug discovery and development of antiviral agents for the treatment of chronic hepatitis B virus infection

By Kirk A. Staschke and Joseph M. Colacino

Infectious Diseases Research
Lilly Research Laboratories
Indianapolis, IN, USA

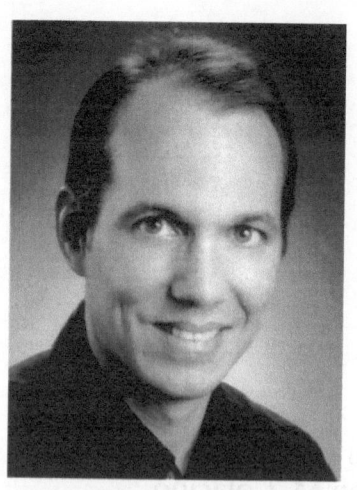

Kirk A. Staschke

was raised in New London, Ohio. He received a B.S. in Biochemistry from Ohio State University in 1989 after which he joined the Virology Research Division of Lilly Research Laboratories as an Associate Biochemist. In 1997, he was promoted to his current position of Assistant Senior Virologist in Infectious Diseases Research. In addition, since 1996, he has been a graduate student in the Department of Biochemistry and Molecular Biology at the Indiana University School of Medicine.

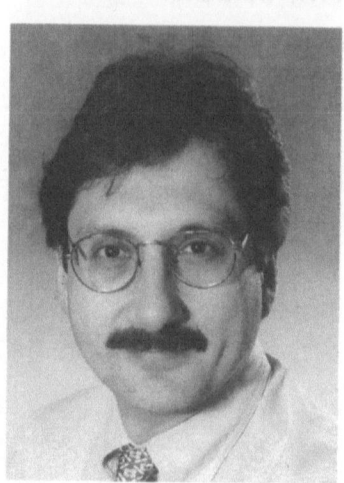

Joseph M. Colacino

is currently Director of Virology at the Lilly Research Laboratories, Eli Lilly and Company, in Indianapolis, Indiana. He received his BA from the University of Connecticut in Storrs and the MS degree from Southern Connecticut State University in New Haven. Colacino received his Ph.D. degree from Cornell Graduate School of Medical Sciences, Sloan-Kettering Division, New York City. After a post-doctoral fellowship at the Louisiana State University Medical Center, Shreveport, Colacino accepted a position as senior virologist with Lilly in 1989. His research has been in the areas of influenza virus, hepatitis B virus, HIV, and, most recently, hepatitis C virus.

Summary

A safe and effective vaccine for hepatitis B virus (HBV) has been available for nearly twenty years and currently campaigns to provide universal vaccination in developing countries are underway. Nevertheless, chronic HBV infection remains a leading cause of chronic hepatitis worldwide and there is a strong need for safe and effective antiviral therapies. Attempts to identify and develop antiviral agents to treat chronic HBV infection remains focused on nucleoside analogs such as 3TC (lamivudine), adefovir dipivoxil, (bis-POM

PMEA), and others. However, advances in our understanding of the molecular biology of HBV and the development of new assays for HBV polymerase activity, such as the reconstitution of active HBV polymerase in vitro, should facilitate large screening efforts for non-nucleoside reverse transcriptase inhibitors. Recent advances have furthered our understanding of clinical resistance to lamivudine, have provided new approaches to treatment, and have offered new perspectives on the major challenges to the identification and development of antiviral agents for chronic HBV infection. Here, in an update to our previous review article that appeared in this series [59a], we focus on recent advances that have occurred in the areas of virus structure and replication, in vitro viral polymerase assays, cell culture systems, and animal models.

Contents

Keywords

acyclovir, animal models, antiviral agents, antisense, ara-AMP, cell culture assay systems, combination therapy, conjugated nucleosides, DNA polymerase, famciclovir, fialuridine, FIAU, ganciclovir, gene therapy, hepatitis B virus, lamivudine, 3TC, *L*-nucleoside analogs, lobucavir, nucleoside analogs, penciclovir, prodrugs, pyrophosphate analogs, resistance, reverse transcriptase, ribozymes, virus replication, virus structure

Glossary of abbreviations

ACV, 9-(2-hydroxyethoxymethyl)guanine (acyclovir); ACV-MP, 5′-monophosphate of acyclovir; ACV-TP, 5′-triphosphate of acyclovir; ara-A, 9-β-*D*-arabinofuranosyladenine; ara-AMP, 5′-monophosphate of 9-β-*D*-arabinofuranosyladenine; AZT, 3′-azido-3′-deoxythymidine; bis-POM PMEA, bis[(pivaloyloxy)methyl] derivative of PMEA (GS-840); CCC DNA, covalently closed circular DNA; CC_{50}, cytotoxic concentration, 50%; CDG, carbocyclic analog of 2′-deoxyguanosine; CMV, cytomegalovirus infection; CTL, cytotoxic T lymphocyte; DAPD, (−)-β-*D*-2,6-diaminopurine dioxolane; ddA, 2′,3′-dideoxyadenine; ddC, 2′,3′-dideoxycytidine; ddCMP, 5′-monophosphate of ddC; ddI, 2',3'-dideoxyinosine; d4C, 3'-deoxy-2',3'-didehydrocytidine; d4T, 3'-deoxy-2',3'-dide-hydrothymidine; dGTP, the 5'-triphosphate of deoxyguanosine; DHBV, duck hepatitis B virus; dTTP, 5'-triphosphate of thymidine; DXG, dioxolane guanosine; EC_{50}, effective concentration, 50%; EC_{90}, effective concentration, 90%; FEAU, 2'-deoxy-2'-fluoro-1-β-D-arabinofuranosyl-5-ethyluracil; FIAC, 2'-deoxy-2'-fluoro-1-β-D-arabinofuranosyl-5-iodocytosine; FIAU, 2'-deoxy-2'-fluoro-1-β-D-arabinofuranosyl-5-iodouracil (fialuridine); FIAU-TP, 5'-triphosphate of FIAU; FLG, 2',3'-dideoxy-3'-fluoroguanosine; FLT, 3'-deoxy-3'-fluorothymidine; FMAU, 2'-deoxy-2'-fluoro-1-β-D-arabinofuranosyl-5-methyluracil; FTC, (–)-cis-5-fluoro-1-[2-(hydroxymethyl)-1,3-oxathio-lan-5-yl]cytosine; GCV, ganciclovir; (9-(1,3-dihydroxy-2-propoxymethyl)guanine); GSHV, gro-und squirrel hepatitis virus; HBcAg, hepatitis B virus c (or core) antigen; HBeAg, hepatitis B virus e (or envelope) antigen; HBsAg, hepatitis B virus s (or surface) antigen; HBV, hepatitis B virus; HIV, human immunodeficiency virus; HPMPC, (S)-1-(3-hydroxy-2-phosphonylmethoxypro-pyl)cytosine (cidofovir); IC_{50}, inhibitory concentration, 50%; IFN, interferon; L-FMAU, the L enantiomer of FMAU; L-HSA, lactosaminated human serum albumin; NAC, N-acetyl-L-cysteine; NBDNJ, N-butyldeoxynojirimycin; OLT, orthotopic liver transplantation; PAA, phosphonoace-tic acid; PFA, phosphonoformic acid (foscarnet); PMEA, 9-2-phosphonylmethoxyethyladenine; RNP, ribonucleoprotein; SI, selective index; 3TC, (2R, 5S) 1-[2-(hydroxymethyl)-1,3-oxathiolane-5-yl]cytosine (lamivudine; (–)BCH-189); WHV, woodchuck hepatitis virus

1 Introduction

Human hepatitis B virus (HBV) is the leading cause of chronic hepatitis throughout the world. According to the World Health Organization Execu-tive Summary (World Health Report, 1996), current estimates are that 5% of the world's population, or over 350 million people, are chronically infected with HBV, and in the United States, there are up to 1 million chronic carri-ers. The risk of acquiring HBV as a result of blood transfusions is estimated to be 1 in 63 000 [257].

Despite the existence of a safe and effective vaccine and efforts to provide universal vaccination in developing countries [220a], the worldwide preva-lence of HBV has not declined significantly [194]. A three-vaccine series is 88% effective in preventing HBV infection [239, 319] but, for the millions of chronically infected individuals, there is no effective treatment to clear the virus and limit the high risk of liver diseases associated with long term infec-tion – chronic hepatitis, cirrhosis, and hepatocellular carcinoma. Moreover, in the United States, HBV incidence increased by 37% from 1993 to 1995 to 6.3 cases/100 000 as a result of missed opportunities to vaccinate high-risk people [72]. In a study conducted at Johns Hopkins, it was determined that

23% of health care workers there were unvaccinated [290]. Additionally, a decreased response rate to the vaccine is observed among the elderly, smokers or obese individuals [239, 319] and protective antibody titers decline with time since vaccination [140, 213]. Since it will take at least a generation for the pool of chronic carriers to decrease, there are enough patients already infected who will benefit from effective treatment.

The current level of satisfaction in the treatment of this disease remains low. The only approved treatment are interferon alpha (IFN-α) (reviewed in [318]), lamivudine (epivir; 3TC) [140a], and, in some countries, thymosin α1 (zadaxin; Doctor's Guide, March 17, 1999 (http://pslgroup.com/dg/edfe2. htm)). Several forms of human IFN have been developed for use in humans including lymphoblastoid IFN, natural IFN-α, recombinant human IFN-α, recombinant human IFN-α2b, IFN-β and interferon γ. Although IFN initially had much promise, with increased use and evaluation, the limitations of this approach have become apparent. IFN must be given subcutaneously or by intramuscular injection and only 30–40% of the patients respond in the most optimal population. In those patients who fail therapy, higher doses and longer treatments of IFN do not improve the clinical outcome. There are numerous side-effects associated with IFN therapy including fatigue, fever and chills, muscle aches and pains, anorexia, abdominal pains and cramps, hair loss, bone marrow suppression, dizziness and vertigo, diarrhea, anxiety, psychosis, and autoimmune conditions [126]. Zadaxin or thymosin α1, an immunodulatory peptide, has been evaluated in combination with interferon or lamivudine. However, the clinical response rate for zadaxin was found to be variable [204a, b]. In a recent Phase III multicenter, radomized, double-blind, and placebo-controlled study, a total of 12 (25%) patients treated with thymosin α1 and six (13%) given placebo showed a sustained loss of HBV DNA with a corresponding loss of HBeAg during or following the 12 month study period. These results were not statistically significant ($p < 0.11$) and did not confirm treatment efficacy observed in previous clinical trials [204c].

Lamivudine (3TC) is now in widespread use clinically for the treatment of chronic HBV infection. While initially, resistance to 3TC was only observed in immunocompromised patients, as will be discussed below, it is now clear that resistance occurs in many patients including immunocompetent individuals undergoing sustained long-term therapy.

Since the sequelae of uncontrolled HBV infection, which can include chronicity, cirrhosis of the liver, and hepatocellular carcinoma, can be dire with a severe and debilitating impact on the quality of life, there is a compelling need for the development of drugs which can effectively control ongoing viral replication and treat the disease. Of the greatest immediate promise for the treatment of chronic HBV are nucleoside analogs, including among others, lamivudine, famciclovir, and GS-840 (bis-POM PMEA), which possess anti-HBV activity *in vitro* and *in vivo*. Of these agents, lamivudine, as will be discussed in greater detail, has undergone the most extensive evaluation.

An ideal profile for an anti-HBV agent would include a small molecule which can be delivered by oral administration as a single, low, daily dose. The compound must be selective and specific for the inhibition of HBV DNA replication without affecting host functions and must be non-toxic after long-term administration (>3 months). There are several problems associated with current approaches to anti-HBV therapy: 1) Extra-hepatic (lymphoid) and extra-hepatocyte (bile-duct cells) reservoirs of HBV which may necessitate the delivery of antiviral drugs to these sites; 2) The emergence of resistance. Variants of HBV resistant to famciclovir and lamivudine have been documented; 3) The persistence of covalently closed circular (CCC) viral DNA which leads to viral rebound following the cessation of most, if not all, current investigational therapies; and 4) Immunological tolerance in the existing pool of chronic HBV carriers must be broken in order to clear the virus through immune mechanisms following suppressive antiviral therapy. Because of these challenges, it is likely that combination chemotherapy (e.g., nucleoside analog + IFN; nucleoside analog + other immunomodulatory agent; nucleoside analog A + nucleoside analog B) will be necessary for the successful treatment and clearance of chronic HBV infection.

HBV can be transmitted vertically or horizontally through sexual contact or blood products. In most cases of horizontal transmission, infection of adults with HBV results in a self-limiting disease that is often sub-clinical with spontaneous clearance of infected hepatocytes within a few weeks of infection (reviewed in [139]). However, a small number (5–10%) of individuals will become chronically infected with HBV and it is this group that is at risk for developing cirrhosis of the liver and hepatocellular carcinoma. The positive correlation between active replication of HBV and liver cell damage has been established [128, 171, 233]. Successful antiviral therapy for HBV would be targeted to these individuals and have the immediate goals of inhibiting viral replication, clearing infected liver cells, and diminishing or eliminating the development of sequelae associated with long-term infection. It has been documented that antiviral therapy can bring about the disappearance of HBeAg from the serum with subsequent seroconversion to anti-HBe [28].

In order to consider approaches to the chemotherapeutic intervention of chronic HBV infection, an understanding of the virus structure and replication strategy is necessary. A brief consideration of these topics is provided below. For a more thorough treatment of basic hepatitis B virology, excellent review articles by Ganem and Varmus [104], Chisari et al. [48], Levine [168], Scaglioni et al. [244], Ganem [103], and more recently [258a], among others, are available.

2   Hepatitis B virus structure

HBV belongs to the hepadnaviridae family of viruses which includes woodchuck hepatitis virus (WHV), duck hepatitis B virus (DHBV), and ground squirrel hepatitis virus (GSHV). As the name of this family implies, these viruses are hepatotropic and have a DNA genome. In the serum, infectious HBV is spherical but non-infectious rod-like structures made up of the surface antigen (HBsAg) can be identified. The infectious spherical form, or Dane particle, is approximately 42 nm in diameter. The Dane particle contains a partially double-stranded DNA genome, the minus-strand of which is approximately 3200 nucleotides in length while the positive strand can vary from 1700 to 2800 nucleotides, depending on the subtype of the virus. Consequently, between 50 and 85% of the genome is double-stranded. The DNA genome is contained in a nucleocapsid of 22 to 25 nm in diameter which consists of the viral core antigen (HBcAg). Surrounding the viral core is a lipid envelope which is approximately 7 nm thick and is derived from the host cell membrane. Within the viral envelope can be found the viral surface antigen (HBsAg).

Although the cellular receptor for avian and mamalian hepadnavirus attachment has not been unequivocally identified, there is evidence that a domain of HBsAg is involved in attachment to the host cell. Although there has been much recent effort in this area [102a, 156a,b, 170a,b, 240a, 296a], expression of a putative receptor in cultured cells allowing for efficient virus uptake and replication has not been demonstrated.

The viral genome contains four overlapping genes which encode the various viral proteins. These are the 1) surface proteins consisting of the envelope glycoproteins pre-S1, pre-S2, and S, all of which are encoded by a single gene using alternative translation start sites; 2) the polymerase (P) gene, which contains the entire S gene sequence; 3) the core protein (HBcAg); and 4) the X protein which is not a constituent of the virus particle. The e antigen (HBeAg), which is found circulating in the serum and is diagnostic for chronic infection, is processed from the core antigen and, like the X protein, is not found in the virus particle.

3   Hepatitis B virus replication

The replication cycle of hepadnaviruses is illustrated schematically in Figure 1. Upon binding of HBV to the hepatocyte, the virus enters the cell by a pH-independent mechanism [113, 147]. Once in the nucleus of the infected cell, the partially double-stranded DNA genome is converted to a fully double-stranded covalently closed circular (CCC) form. CCC DNA serves as the template for transcription of the RNA pre-genome by host cell RNA polymerase II. The RNA pre-genome, which is terminally redundant and longer-than-genome in length serves two functions: 1) it is the messenger RNA for translation of the viral polymerase and core proteins; and 2) it serves as the template for reverse transcription of minus-strand DNA [280].

HBV encodes a multi-functional polymerase which contains both RNA- and DNA-dependent DNA polymerase activities and an RNaseH activity which was recently cloned and expressed in *E. coli* [166]. Additionally, HBV polymerase has the unique ability to serve as the primer for reverse transcription of the RNA pre-genome [161, 308, 312, 331]. In contrast to the reverse transcriptases of HIV and other retroviruses which are proteolytically processed from a polyprotein precursor, the polymerase of HBV is translated from a polycistronic viral RNA template, the RNA pre-genome, from an internal AUG codon [39, 256]. The reverse transcriptase (RT) domain of HBV and other hepadnaviral polymerases share amino acid sequence homology with that of retroviruses, including HIV [144, 231, 296]. As does the reverse transcriptase of HIV, HBV RT contains a conserved YMDD motif [224], the two aspartate residues of which are two of the three amino acids which make up the carboxylate triad that is involved in nucleotide binding within the cat-

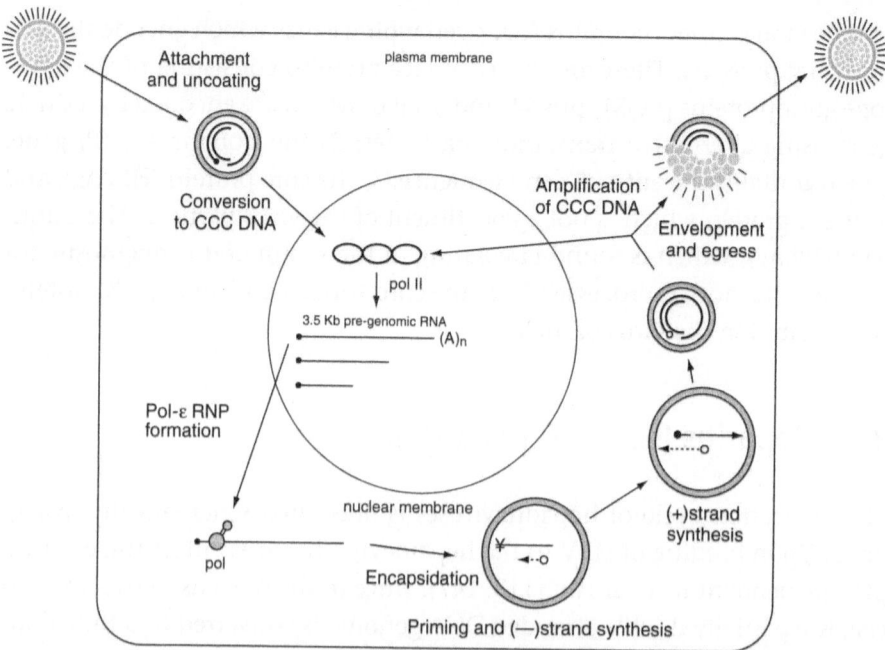

Fig. 1
The replication cycle of HBV in a permissive cell. Key targets for antiviral chemotherapy are indicated. Two virus replication pathways are shown: 1) the egress of the infectious and enveloped virion from the cell to infect other hepatocytes and, 2) the intracellular recycling of the covalently closed circular (CCC) DNA back to the nucleus.

alytic site of the enzyme. As will be discussed in greater detail below, mutations in this motif are associated with HIV- and HBV-resistance to the nucleoside analog, lamivudine.

The viral polymerase together with several proteins of host cell origin including hsp90 [134], p23 [135], and a 65 kDa protein [221], forms a ribonucleoprotein (RNP) complex with a stem-loop structure (ε) at the 5' end of the RNA pre-genome. The interacting domains of the HBV polymerase and hsp90 have been mapped [48a,b]. This stem-loop structure serves as the signal for packaging of pre-genomic RNA into nucleocapsids and as the template for the initiation of reverse transcription. Additionally, the polymerase-ε complex may be involved in activating the viral polymerase [286].

For duck hepatitis B virus (DHBV), a four nucleotide primer, with the sequence 5'-G-T-A-A-3', is synthesized using the bulge-loop of ε as the template. Following the synthesis of this primer DNA, the first of three intra-molecular template switches occurs and the short primer DNA is translocated to a direct repeat (DR1) which is located at the 3'-end of pre-genomic RNA and from which minus-strand synthesis resumes. Whether the same form of the viral polymerase is involved in the synthesis of both primer DNA and minus-strands is not known. The RNaseH activity of the viral polymerase is responsible for degrading the pre-genomic RNA, which is now hybridized to minus-strand DNA. Degradation of the RNA is complete except for a short stretch at the 5' end (16–18 nucleotides) which functions as the primer for the synthesis of the complementary plus-strand viral DNA. This primer RNA is then translocated to another direct repeat region (DR2) where the synthesis of plus-strand DNA is initiated. Failure to translocate (*in situ* priming) leads to the synthesis of a double-stranded linear form of the viral genome which is often seen in tissue culture. A third template switch enables the synthesis of the partially double-stranded DNA genome which is found in mature, infectious virus particles.

The nucleocapsid of the hepadnavirus, now containing the partially double-stranded DNA genome, acquires an envelope which is derived from the host cell membrane and which contains the surface antigen associated with the mature and infectious virus particle. As an alternative to this pathway, the encapsidated virus, rather than exiting the infected cell, can recycle back to the nucleus. This results in the amplification of intranuclear CCC DNA and it is estimated that each infected hepatocyte harbors 30–50 copies of this form of the viral DNA. These alternative pathways appear to be regulated by the level of HBsAg present in the infected cell.

4   Cell culture assay systems

The study of HBV replication and efforts to discover and evaluate anti-HBV agents have been hampered by the lack of useful *in vitro* infection systems. Although it has been demonstrated that primary duck hepatocytes can be infected with DHBV, cultured cells are only susceptible to infection for a few days and multiple rounds of virus replication do not occur [300]. Apparently, primary hepatocytes must be kept in the differentiated state in order to maintain infectability [102]. In studies using dimethyl sulfoxide in the cell culture medium, primary hepatocytes could be maintained in the differentiated state and were permissive for the spread of DHBV [102, 230]. The infection of primary duck hepatocytes with DHBV has been used to evaluate the efficacy and elucidate the mechanism of antiviral activity of a number of compounds including the carbocyclic analog of 2'-deoxyguanosine [95], suramin [223] and various 2',3'-dideoxynucleoside analogs [164]. Mammalian primary hepatocytes have also been cultured for use in hepadnavirus infection studies. For example, woodchuck hepatitis virus (WHV) and ground squirrel hepatitis virus (GSHV) were shown to replicate in primary hepatocytes obtained from woodchucks [3] and HBV has been shown to replicate in primary hepatocytes obtained from human liver tissue and cultured with or without dimethyl sulfoxide [111, 237]. Recently, treatment of virions with V8 protease to expose a fusion domain of the HBsAg was shown to promote virus entry into human hepatoblastoma cells [185]. This approach provides an HBV infection system which may prove to be useful for the study of the complete virus infection cycle and for the identification of antiviral agents in cell culture.

Since HBV is only infectious to primary hepatocytes and because of the difficulties, both logistical and technical, of culturing primary hepatocytes, alternative *in vitro* systems for the study of HBV replication, utilizing continuous cell lines, have been sought and developed. Through the efforts of several groups, human hepatocellular carcinoma cell lines which have been transfected with cloned, tandemly repeated multimers of the viral genome have yielded cell lines which transiently or constitutively replicate HBV [37, 260, 281, 299, 323]. Such cell lines can produce complete HBV particles which are infectious in chimpanzees [2]. Additionally, a human hepatoblastoma cell line (HepG2) was transfected with cloned DHBV DNA and cell lines which produce infectious viral particles indistinguishable from authentic DHBV were derived [101]. Importantly, these cell lines have been used for the evaluation of agents potentially useful as inhibitors of HBV replication [150, 160, 303, 325]. Recently, further efforts have resulted in the development of a cell culture system for the inducible expression of HBV in stably transfected hepatoblastoma cells which may prove to be useful for the study of HBV replication in a synchronized fashion and for the large-scale screening of compounds for the identification of inhibitors of viral replication [157].

The efficacy and selectivity of antiviral agents *in vitro* is usually determined using one of the above cell culture systems. Anti-HBV activity is customarily expressed as the EC_{50} or IC_{50}, i.e., the effective or inhibitory concentration of compound (μM) required to inhibit viral replication by 50% or HBV polymerase activity by 50%, respectively. Since HBV is not cytopathic in cell culture, virus replication can not be monitored visually. Rather, Southern blot analysis of intracellular viral DNA replicative intermediates (relaxed circular, single-stranded, double-stranded) and dot-blot or PCR analysis of viral DNA in virions released into the cell culture medium are used to compare the extent of viral replication in the presence of test compound to that found in the "no-drug" control. Cytotoxicity of a test compound can be assessed using one of various methods such as trypan blue dye exclusion, ^3H-thymidine uptake, MTT, or visual cell counting and is expressed as the concentration (μM) of compound required to inhibit cell growth by 50% (CC_{50}). The selectivity index (SI) is then determined by dividing the CC_{50} by the EC_{50} or EC_{90}.

5 Hepadnavirus polymerase assay systems

Most attempts at the chemotherapeutic intervention of HBV infection have been directed at the viral polymerase. Historically, assays to identify specific inhibitors of the HBV polymerase have been limited to the endogenous viral DNA polymerase. In these assays, extracellular virions are collected from infected patient serum or cell culture fluid, permeabilized with a non-ionic detergent, and provided with exogenously added nucleotide triphosphates, one or more of which is radiolabeled, in order to fill in the single stranded region of the genome using the minus-strand DNA as template. This approach, although not useful in a high-throughput format, has been used to evaluate pyrophosphate analogs and triphosphate forms of known nucleoside analog inhibitors of hepadnavirus replication.

Attempts to understand the other activities of HBV polymerase, including RNA-dependent DNA polymerase and RNaseH, until now have not been successful because the viral polymerase is tightly associated with the viral core and is not functional when separated from the whole virion. However, DHBV reverse transcriptase has recently been expressed in an active form in a cell-free translation system [133, 308, 309] and in yeast [285]. For a long time, efforts to express enzymatically active human HBV DNA polymerase in heterologous systems were unsuccessful. However, active HBV polymerase has been expressed in xenopus oocytes [259] and in a recombinant baculovirus system either alone [161] or in combination with the core protein [258c]. Now, human HBV polymerase has been expressed in active form in a Ty1-his3AI retroelement of yeast [230a]. These new systems will allow further evaluation and a more complete understanding of the mechanism of anti-HBV activity of known inhibitors [272, 333]. It is hoped that these new molecular systems will facilitate large screening efforts and aid in the identification of novel inhibitors of the viral polymerase.

6   Animal models

A number of animal models are available for the study of HBV replication and pathogenesis *in vivo*. One such model, infection of chimpanzees with HBV is not often used because of the endangered status of these animals and the high cost of each study. Infection of woodchucks with WHV is a well characterized model [153, 287a]. Woodchucks chronically infected with WHV can undergo all of the sequelae, including cirrhosis and hepatocellular carcinoma, that can occur in humans as a result of a chronic infection. Hence the woodchuck model is considered to be a powerfully predictive model of HBV infection. Lesser known models of hepatitis B virus infection have also been described including the infection of the Indian palm tree squirrel with tree squirrel hepatitis virus [199], a virus similar to HBV first identified in the tree squirrel [83, 84], and infection of Wistar rats by intravenous injection of HBV [326]. Offering the potential for new mammalian models of hepadnavirus replication, nonhuman primate hepadnaviruses were isolated from wooley monkeys [160a] and a captive gibbon [160b].

Another well-characterized model is infection of ducks with DHBV (reviewed by [334]) which is a widely used model for the evaluation of antiviral compounds. A number of agents, including phosphonoformate (foscarnet; [265]), adenine arabinoside [121], acyclovir and suramin [297], dideoxycytidine [143] and various other dideoxynucleoside analogs [164] have reduced transiently the levels of serum DHBV DNA and endogenous DHBV DNA polymerase in this model of infection. Treatment with acyclovir followed by suramin injection [297] and orally administered carbocyclic deoxyguanosine [95] have resulted in a prolonged inhibition of DHBV DNA synthesis in infected ducks. However, the duck model of infection is not as predictive as the woodchuck model for a number of reasons. These include differences between avian and mammalian metabolism, leading to differences in pharmacokinetics of test compounds, and differences between avian and mammalian immune systems.

Important for the consideration of these animal models are differences between the various members of the hepadnavirus family. At the nucleotide level, WHV displays approximately 70% homology to HBV whereas DHBV is only 40% homologous [294]. Additionally, unlike that of WHV or HBV, the genome of DHBV does not encode an X protein. The X protein, while not essential for replication in tissue culture [25], is necessary for WHV infectivity *in vivo* [332]. Therefore, it may also be assumed that the X protein plays a role in the *in vivo* infectivity of HBV. More recently, the X protein has been shown to activate Src tyrosine kinases and promote a high level of virus replication [145a]. Therefore, results with the duck model of infection must be interpreted cautiously.

The above *in vivo* models are useful in providing a means of evaluating test compounds for efficacy in treating an *in vivo* infection in which the virus undergoes its complete life cycle. Additionally, these models enable the systematic study of drug pharmacokinetics (including absorption, distribution, metabolism, and excretion) as well as drug toxicity. Other animal models have become available in which the virus does not undergo the complete life cycle. These include transgenic mice which express the complete genomes of WHV [120] or HBV and from which infectious virus particles can be isolated [6, 82]. More recently a model in which nude mice bearing HBV-producing tumors was developed and used for the evaluation of (–) cis-5-fluoro-1-[2-(hydroxymethyl)-1,3-oxathiolan-5-yl]cytosine [(–)FTC] [62]. Although these models are not appropriate for the examination of every stage of the virus replication cycle, they do provide relatively easy and economical *in vivo* test systems useful for resolving initial questions of efficacy and toxicity.

7   Antivirals for hepatitis B virus infection

The various points in the HBV replication cycle (Fig. 1), such as virus attachment and entry, uncoating, DNA replication, virus assembly, envelopment, and egress from the infected cell, represent potential targets for chemotherapeutic intervention. However, despite intensive efforts on the part of many academic and pharmaceutical laboratories to investigate other targets for anti-HBV chemotherapy, the most promising compounds are directed at the replication of viral DNA and of these, virtually all are nucleoside analogs. The following is a discussion of the most extensively studied nucleoside analogs and other inhibitors of HBV replication that have been or may be considered for clinical evaluation.

7.1   D-nucleoside analogs

7.1.1 Ara-AMP

Vidarabine (**1**; 9-β-D-arabinofuranosyladenine; Ara-A) is the parent compound of ara-AMP, its monophosphorylated and more water soluble metabolite. Ara-A and Ara-AMP are inhibitors of HBV replication *in vitro* [150, 303, 325] and in the duck model of HBV infection [121], presumably by acting as inhibitors of viral DNA polymerase in their triphosphate forms [32]. Ara-AMP was initially found to be effective in lowering serum levels of HBV and inducing prolonged remissions of disease [17, 129, 225, 258, 315]. However, in a subsequent randomized controlled study, Ara-AMP, given for 1 month, did not result in clinical or serological remissions in HBV disease, but did result in a high frequency of adverse advents [130]. In a further study, ten patients were treated with three 10-day courses of therapy during three successive months in an effort to maximize drug efficacy while minimizing any adverse advents [131]. The drug was administered intravenously at a dosage of 10 mg/kg/day. In chronically infected males, treatment resulted in a dramatic decrease in the serum levels of HBV DNA and DNA polymerase activity, although viral DNA was detectable in all of the patients and rebounded to pre-treatment levels soon after therapy was discontinued [131]. In this study, treatment with Ara-AMP was associated with appreciable neuromuscular toxicity. Thus it was concluded that, although Ara-AMP is a potent inhibitor of HBV replication, treatment with this drug does not result in a long-term clinical benefit and is associated with toxicity that limits its clinical utility. In other studies, severe and, in some cases, fatal neurological toxicities associated with Ara-AMP therapy have been reported [79, 227, 241]. While no longer considered as a monotherapy, efforts to target ara-AMP to the liver by

(1) Ara-A

(2) AZT

(3) ddl

(4) ddA

(5) ddC

(6) d4T

(7) d4C

(8) ddAPR

conjugation to lactosaminated serum albumin or poly-L-lysine have been well documented and will be discussed below.

7.1.2 Dideoxynucleoside analogs

Dideoxynucleoside analogs lack hydroxyl groups at both the 2' and 3' positions of the sugar moiety. The lack of a 3'-OH results in the inability to form

3'-5' phosphodiester linkages in the nascent DNA chain when these analogs are used as alternate substrates by DNA polymerase. Thus the DNA chain is terminated at the point of dideoxynucleotide incorporation. Considering the similarity between the reverse transcriptase domains of retroviruses and hepadnaviruses, along with the anti-retroviral activity of dideoxynucleoside analogs such as 3'-azido-2',3'-dideoxythymidine (2; AZT) and 2',3'-dideoxy-inosine (3; ddI), members of this class of compounds have been studied for use in the treatment of chronic HBV infection. A number of dideoxynucleo-side analogs have shown moderate activity against HBV replication in cell culture. In one study, 2',3'-dideoxyadenosine (4; ddA), 2',3'-dideoxycytidine (5; ddC), 2',3'-dideoxy-2',3'-didehydrothymidine (6; d4T), and 2',3'-dideoxy-2',3'-didehydrocytidine (7; d4C) inhibited HBV DNA synthesis in virus-pro-ducing human hepatoblastoma cells (HB611) with EC_{50} values ranging from 0.76 µg/ml (ddC) to 44.7 µg/ml (d4T) [325]. Other modified pyrimidine nucleosides including 2',3'-dideoxy-3'-fluorothymidine (FddT), 3'-fluoro-5-methyl-deoxycytidine (FddMeC), 3'-chloro-5-methyl-deoxycytidine (Cld-dMeC), 3'-amino-5-methyl-deoxycytidine (AddMeC), and d4T showed impressive anti-HBV activity in another virus producing hepatoblastoma cell line (HepG2.2.15) with EC_{50} values ranging from 0.54 µM (FddMeC) to 1.49 µM (ClddMeC) [197].

Various purine and pyrimidine dideoxynucleoside analogs have been evaluated in the duck model of HBV infection. Chronically infected duck-lings were treated with ddA or ddAPR (8; 2,6-diaminopurine-2',3'-dideoxy-riboside) at a dosage of 10 mg/kg twice daily by intramuscular injection. In animals treated with ddAPR, a rapid (within 1 week) clearance of virus was observed. In contrast, DHBV was not cleared in animals treated with ddA [164]. In another study, six chronically infected ducks were treated with AZT at dosages of 0.5 mg/kg or 5 mg/kg three times daily for 10 days given by intraperitoneal injection. No suppression of DHBV replication was observed in any of the treated animals, as determined by quantification of viral DNA levels in hepatocytes. In contrast to these results, ddC, at a dosage of 11 mg/m^2 given every 6 h by intravenous injection, appeared to be effective in suppressing levels of DHBV DNA and DNA polymerase in chronically infected ducks [143]. In a recent study, 2',3'-dideoxy-3'-fluoroguanosine (9; FLG) strongly suppressed serum DHBV DNA at doses as low as 1 mg/kg/day given twice daily by intraperitoneal injection for 7 to 10 days. Virus repli-cation, however, resumed upon discontinuation of treatment. In these same studies, 2',3'-dideoxy-3'-fluorothymidine (**10**; FLT) had no activity [180].

In a recent clinical study, six patients positive for both HIV and HBV were treated with ddI. Although ddI appeared to be well-tolerated in all patients, results from this study demonstrated that ddI had no significant antiviral effect in patients with chronic HBV infection [33]. The effect of AZT on viral replication in chronic HBsAg positive patients was also investigated. When 200 mgs of AZT were given orally, four times a day for 1 week, serum HBV DNA polymerase activity was reduced significantly in seven patients. A dose-response effect was also observed in patients receiving progressively lower doses of AZT [21]. Based on these results, it was concluded that, in contradistinction to results obtained in the duck model as discussed above, AZT may be of value in infected patients who do not respond to interferon alpha or in those who have high initial levels of HBV prior to the start of interferon therapy [21].

7.1.3 Dioxolanes

Various nucleoside analogs in the 3'-oxa series, which contain an oxygen in place of the 3' carbon of the ribose ring, have shown anti-HBV activity. Of particular interest is DAPD (**11**; (–)-β-D-2,6-diaminopurine dioxolane). In human hepatoblastoma cells (HepG2.2.15), DAPD inhibited HBV replication with an EC_{50} of approximately 0.1 μM with no observable toxicity at concentrations up to 300 μM. Recently it has been shown that DAPD was almost equally effective against a lamivudine resistant HBV variant containing the M550V substitution in the YMDD motif of the viral polymerase (see discussion below) as against the wild type virus [324a]. The deaminated metabolite of DAPD, dioxolane guanosine (**12**; DXG) also showed anti-HBV activity with an EC_{50} of approximately 1 μM and no observable toxicity up to 100 μM [254]. DAPD appeared to be relatively non-toxic but, at a concentration of 10 μM, did cause a slight elevation of lactic acid (an indication of possible mitochondrial dysfunction) in cultured cells [65]. In woodchucks, DAPD had an oral bioavailability of 3.7–8.2% but the apparent bioavailability of DXG, subsequent to the administration of its aminated precursor DAPD, was considerably greater [232]. Pharmacokinetic studies indicated that the half-life of DAPD in rats after intravenous administration was 0.37 hours due to its rapid conversion to DXG. The half-life of DXG is 1.6 hours in monkeys. The oral bioavailability was determined to be approximately 30% [43a].

Another dioxolane compound, (+)-β-D-1,3-dioxolane-5-fluorocytidine (**13**; β-D-FDOC) was shown to have more potent anti-HBV activity in culture than did (–)FTC, L-FddC, L-ddC, or ddC [255]. Efficacy studies in animal models of HBV infection would facilitate the determination of the clinical potential of these compounds as anti-HBV agents.

7.1.4 BMS-200,475

Recently, BMS-200,475 (entecavir; **14**), a new carbocyclic, cyclopentyl guanine analog in which the oxygen in the furanose ring is replaced with an exocyclic double bond, has shown potent activity against HBV *in vitro* [23, 138] and against WHV in the woodchuck model of infection [61]. This compound is more efficiently phosphorylated in HepG2 cells than is lamivudine, penciclovir, ganciclovir, acyclovir, or lobucavir [323a]. The compound is a selective inhibitor of HBV DNA polymerase with a K_i of 0.0012 µM [137a] and was found to inhibit the priming, reverse transcription and DNA-dependent DNA synthesis activities of HBV replication [258c]. Furthermore, mechanistic studies have shown that the triphosphate of entecavir is a nonobligate DNA chain terminator causing the polymerase to stall 2 to 3 nucleotides downstream following incorporation sites [258b]. In recent studies, entecavir was active against HBV with an EC_{50} of 0.004 µM and a CC_{50} of 30 µM (SI approximately 8000) in HepG2.2.15 cells but was not active against HIV-1, influenza, human cytomegalovirus, herpes simplex virus type 1, or varicella zoster virus [23, 138]. Importantly, BMS-200,475 did not inhibit the replication of mitochondrial DNA [138]. In the woodchuck model, oral doses of BMS-200,475 as low as 0.02 mg/kg once a day for 4 weeks resulted in a dramatic suppression of WHV replication [61]. Very recently, long term therapy of chronically infected woodchucks with entecavir proved to be highly effective. After treatment for at least 14 months, nine of ten animals were WHV DNA negative by PCR and the tenth animal showed a 6 log10 reduction in viral DNA. Importantly, treatment with entecavir led to a decrease of WHV CCC DNA to undectable levels and appeared to prevent the development of fatal hepatocellular carcinoma [61a]. Entecavir is currently being evaluated in clinical studies [223a].

(9) FLG

(10) FLT

(11) DAPD

(12) DXG

(13) FDOC

(14) BMS-200,475

(15) CDG

(16) Ribavirin

7.1.5 Carbodeoxyguanosine

The carbocyclic analog of 2'-deoxyguanosine (**15**; CDG), is a potent inhibitor of HBV replication in cell culture as determined by decreases in DNA polymerase activity associated with extracellular virus, secreted HBV DNA, and intracellular DNA replicative intermediates [228, 229]. CDG was found to incorporate into internucleotide positions within cellular DNA and was a competitive inhibitor of HBV DNA polymerase and DNA polymerase δ with respect to dGTP. However, the Ki for HBV DNA polymerase was 6-fold lower than that for DNA polymerase δ [229]. More recent mechanistic studies have demonstrated that the triphosphate of CDG inhibits the priming of DHBV DNA reverse transcription by 50% at a concentration of 0.5 μM in a cell-free system. This inhibition was more potent than that of acyclovir-triphosphate or penciclovir-triphosphate [68].

In primary duck hepatocytes, a 1-day treatment with CDG (1 to 10 ng/ml) resulted in a prolonged (at least 8 days) suppression of DHBV DNA replication. In congenitally infected ducklings, two oral doses of 100 ng/gram of body weight resulted in a delay of viral replication for up to 4 days [95]. In chronically infected ducks treated with CDG at a dosage of 10 μg/kg every other day, DHBV production was significantly suppressed during therapy, but virus was not completely eliminated in any of the animals during a 3-month treatment. Within a period of weeks to months after the cessation of therapy, virus replication returned in all hepatocytes [196]. The results of this study led to the conclusion that suppression of virus replication may not be sufficient to eliminate the virus and additional antiviral immune responses may be required. In addition, higher doses of CDG resulted in mild to moderate levels of liver injury. As the authors of this study indicated, this drug-induced injury along with virus-induced liver damage may have resulted in an increased rate of clearance of infected hepatocytes, the end-result being a more marked decrease in virus levels [196].

7.1.6 Ribavirin

Ribavirin, also known as virazole, (16; 1-β-D-ribofuranosyl-1,2,4-triazole-3-carboxamide), is a purine nucleoside analog with reported activity against a large number of DNA and RNA viruses [269]. Phosphorylation of ribavirin to the monophosphate by adenosine kinase [316] appears to be required for antiviral activity. Ribavirin-monophosphate is an inhibitor of inosine monophosphate dehydrogenase resulting in the selective decrease of intracellular pools of GTP [204, 278] and in most cases the *in vitro* antiviral activity of ribavirin can be reversed by the addition of guanosine [277]. The effect

(17) FIAC   (18) FIAU   (19) FMAU   (20) FEAU

of ribavirin against HBV has been studied *in vivo*. An early study demonstrated that in two HBsAg positive chimpanzees, ribavirin had no discernible effect on serum HBsAg levels [71]. More recently oral ribavirin at a dosage of 0.8 to 1.0 g/day was given alone or in conjunction with interferon beta to 24 patients with chronic active hepatitis. In most patients ribavirin alone or in combination with interferon beta reduced serum HBV DNA levels. In one patient receiving ribavirin alone, in two receiving interferon alone, and in two receiving the combination, HBeAg disappeared [141]. In another study, 18 chronically infected patients received between 800 and 1200 mgs of ribavirin per day for 24 weeks. Two patients became negative for HBV DNA and HBeAg. Additionally, HBV DNA levels remained below baseline for the duration of the 24 weeks of treatment and for the additional 24 weeks of follow up [98]. Taken together, these results indicate that ribavirin may have clinical utility, especially as an adjunct therapy with interferon or other treatment modalities. Indeed, the current standard of therapy for chronic hepatitis C virus infection is rebetron, which is a combination of interferon alpha-2b plus ribavirin in which ribavirin has an immunomodulatory effect to stimulate the Th1 arm of the immune response [283a].

7.1.7 Fialuridine

The 2'-fluorinated pyrimidine nucleoside analogs were first developed for their activity against herpes viruses [46, 49, 56, 96, 174, 183, 249, 251]. FIAC

(**17**; 1-2'-deoxy-2'-fluoro-1-β-D-arabinofuranosyl-5-iodocytosine) and FIAU (**18**; fialuridine; 1-2'-deoxy-2'-fluoro-1-β-D-arabinofuranosyl-5-iodouracil), the deaminated metabolite of FIAC, as well as other members of this group of nucleoside analogs, are preferentially monophosphorylated by herpes virus thymidine kinases [56, 154]. As a result, these compounds are more inhibitory to herpes viruses which contain a functional thymidine kinase than against herpes viruses which are thymidine kinase deficient [183]. Also, herpes viruses which are resistant to FIAC were less able to phosphorylate this nucleoside analog than were wild-type viruses and were less pathogenic in mice [57]. Various 2'-fluorinated pyrimidine nucleoside analogs have demonstrated activity against HBV *in vitro* [151, 273]. FIAU inhibited the replication of HBV and DHBV DNA in cell culture as determined by Southern blot analysis of replicative intermediates and PCR analysis of released virion DNA [273]. FIAU showed potent activity against DHBV in human hepatoblastoma cells but was relatively inactive against the same virus in chicken liver cells. It was determined that phosphorylated metabolites of FIAU accumulated in the human cells but not in the chicken cells, thus correlating anti-HBV activity with the levels of nucleoside analog phosphorylation [273], as has also been described for the anti-HBV activity of FLT [181]. The triphosphate of FIAC inhibits virion associated HBV DNA polymerase with an IC_{50} of 0.038 µM [114] and, in similar experiments, the triphosphate of FIAU was shown to inhibit endogenous DHBV DNA polymerase with an IC_{50} of 0.05 µM [250]. Using cell-free transcription and translation of DHBV reverse transcriptase, the triphosphate of FIAU was shown to inhibit the formation of primer DNA, which is required for the synthesis of full length minus-strand viral DNA, by 50% at a concentration of 0.66 µM [272].

In the woodchuck model of infection, FIAC, FMAU (**19**; 1-2'-deoxy-2'-fluoro-β-D-arabinofuranosyl-5-methyluracil) and FEAU (**20**; 1-2'-deoxy-2'-fluoro-β-D-arabinofuranosyl-5-ethyluracil) were effective in decreasing levels of serum WHV DNA but all three were shown to be toxic [93]. FMAU, at doses of 0.2 or 2.0 mg/kg/day for 5 days proved to be highly toxic and was associated with symptoms of CNS dysfunction. In Phase I trials, treatment of patients with FMAU resulted in serious CNS toxicity [1, 80]. These fluorinated pyrimidine nucleoside analogs were also active in chronically infected ducks but with less apparent toxicity than was seen in the woodchuck [94].

In clinical studies, FIAU was evaluated as a treatment for chronic HBV infection. Pilot studies with a 4-week course of oral FIAU treatment, demonstrated a significant inhibition of viral DNA replication, but the effect was not sustained [97]. Further trials with a longer treatment period were stopped after 12 weeks when signs of multi-organ toxicity involving muscle, nerve, liver, and pancreas appeared. Toxicity was delayed and included myopathy, lactic acidosis, peripheral neuropathy, pancreatitis, microvesicular fat infiltration of the liver, and liver failure resulting in five fatalities [198, 276].

Because of these clinical toxicities and considering the proposed mechanism of AZT-induced myopathy, the mechanism of FIAU-induced delayed toxicity is now thought to be mediated through mitochondrial dysfunction (reviewed in [55] and [125]). Consistent with this hypothesis, several groups have shown that treatment of cultured human liver cells with FIAU results in a concentration-dependent elevation of lactate levels [58, 64, 219] and ultrastructural changes in mitochondrial morphology [59, 64, 170]. These effects have been observed without a concomitant decrease in mitochondrial DNA abundance. The effect of FIAU on myotubules in culture prepared from human muscle biopsies was studied [260a]. Myotubules were treated with FIAU at concentrations of 0.01 μM to 100 μM for up to three weeks. Mitochondrial abnormalities were noted using electron microscopy. Importantly, three weeks after the removal of FIAU, the mitochondrial abnormalities were unchanged, in contrast to the effects induced by zidovudine which were reversible.

The nucleoside analog ddC, which is selectively toxic to mitochondria and which lacks a 3'-OH, also elevates lactate levels in cell culture but immediately reduces the abundance of mitochondrial DNA, most likely as a result of its ability to induce termination of nuclear and mitochondrial DNA elongation [41, 42]. In contrast to ddC, FIAU, which has an intact 3'-OH, is incorporated into DNA at internucleotide positions ([44, 59, 64, 109, 236], reviewed in [55]). In biochemical studies, it has been shown that the Ki of FIAU-TP for DNA polymerase γ, the polymerase which replicates mitochondrial DNA, is the lowest among the mammalian DNA polymerases. Moreover, FIAU-TP can be used as an alternative substrate in place of dTTP [169]. The degree of FIAU-induced toxicity has been correlated to the extent of its incorporation into DNA [145] as has been seen with ara-C [155]. Incorporation of FIAU into DNA may interfere with gene expression as indicated by studies demonstrating the potential for the presence of FIAU within duplex oligonucleotides to affect interactions between proteins and DNA [274]. Because of its severe toxicity, FIAU has been withdrawn from clinical development.

7.2 Acyclic nucleoside analogs

7.2.1 Acyclovir

Acyclovir (**21**; 9-(2-hydroxyethoxymethyl)guanine) is an analog of deoxy-guanosine which contains an acyclic sugar moiety and has been extensively studied as a selective inhibitor of various herpes viruses [76]. The triphosphate of this acyclic nucleoside analog (ACV-TP) has been shown to inhibit both endogenous HBV and WHV DNA polymerases with IC_{50} values of 0.9 µM and 0.7 µM, respectively [114]. Treatment of HBV-producing HB611 cells with ACV for 12 days resulted in a concentration-dependent reduction in HBV replicative DNA intermediates with an EC_{50} of 30 µg/ml [303]. Treatment of HBV-producing HepG2.2.15 cells with 50 µM ACV for 10 days led to a 90% reduction of HBV replicative DNA intermediates [150].

In vivo, viremia was immediately and stably reduced in ducks treated orally with ACV [297]. In a randomized, controlled trial, acyclovir was administered to chronically infected individuals as a continuous infusion at a dosage of 45 mg/kg/day for 28 days. At 12 months, four out of 15 treated patients sero-converted to anti-HBeAg, compared with one of 15 in the untreated group. Although ACV was well-tolerated and seroconversion in both groups was accompanied by an improvement in liver histology and a return to normal liver function tests, it was concluded that ACV is of no clinical benefit in chronic HBeAg carriers with stable disease [4]. Furthermore, in another study ACV did not enhance the antiviral effect of interferon or seroconversion to anti-HBeAg in chronic carriers [22]. Of interest is a recent study using wood-chucks which showed that treatment with ACV led to the termination of viral minus-strand DNA synthesis and the envelopment of arrested DNA intermediates into virion-like particles which were secreted from infected cells. This indicates that plus-strand viral DNA synthesis is not an obligate step in the replication cycle prior to secretion of the virus from the infected cell [287].

7.2.2 Ganciclovir

Ganciclovir (**22**; GCV; 9-(1,3-dihydroxy-2-propoxymethyl)guanine) is another acyclic guanosine nucleoside analog with potent activity against a number of human herpesviruses, especially, human cytomegalovirus [86].

(21) Acyclovir   (22) Ganciclovir

Ganciclovir is structurally similar to acyclovir but differs in having the functional equivalent of a 3'-OH group. This feature allows the incorporation of GCV into viral DNA without obligatory chain termination as occurs with acyclovir [234]. GCV has been widely used to treat severe, reactivated CMV infection after organ transplantation (reviewed in [18]). Considering this and since GCV has demonstrated activity against HBV in cell culture [151], against WHV in the woodchuck [153] and against DHBV in the duck [187, 310], this compound has been considered for use in the treatment of HBV following organ transplantation. In one clinical study designed to evaluate the safety and efficacy of GCV, nine patients with recurrent HBV infection after liver transplantation were treated with daily infusions of GCV for 24 weeks starting at an initial dosage of 5 mg/kg/day which was increased to 10 mg/kg/day [105]. In all of the patients, levels of serum HBV DNA decreased from those prior to treatment by a mean of 90% (range, 42% to 100%). In most of the patients, liver histology and function improved but HBsAg and HBeAg were present in serum and HBcAg was detectable in the liver. No major adverse events were described. Upon cessation of treatment, HBV DNA rose to pretreatment levels and recrudescence of disease occurred in all but one patient. In a heart transplant patient treated for HBV infection, GCV was well-tolerated and resulted in a remarkable improvement and normalization of liver function tests [5]. More recently, ganciclovir administered orally at 500 mg TID was able to suppress lamivudine-resistant virus [216a]. However, most results indicate that the clinical utility of GCV is limited by its poor bioavailability necessitating continuous infusion (reviewed in [127]), transient suppression of HBV DNA replication due to the inability to reduce levels of CCC DNA [187], and dose-limiting toxicities [35, 264]. Because of these considerations, greater focus has been directed to newer nucleoside analogs with improved pharmacokinetic profiles and increased antiviral potency.

(23) Penciclovir   (24) Famciclovir

7.2.3 Penciclovir and famciclovir

Penciclovir (**23**; (9-4-hydroxy-3-hydroxymethylbut-1-yl)guanine) is an acyclic nucleoside analog which is closely related to ganciclovir with the exception that the ether oxygen in the acyclic side chain is replaced with a methylene bridge [27]. This compound has an antiviral spectrum similar to that of ganciclovir but it is more active against herpes simplex and zoster viruses than against cytomegalovirus. Penciclovir has also shown activity against DHBV *in vitro* [262] and in congenitally infected ducks which were treated for 4 weeks at a dosage of 10 mg/kg/day administered by intraperitoneal injection [173]. At the end of 1 week, in seven of eight ducks levels of viremia were dramatically reduced and after 4 weeks, intrahepatic viral DNA, RNA, and protein levels were significantly reduced compared to those in control ducks. Significantly, levels of CCC DNA were reduced in the treated ducks [173]. The basis for the selective inhibition of HBV replication by penciclovir is at the level of viral DNA polymerase. The triphosphate of penciclovir, in particular the (R)-enantiomer, is a potent inhibitor of HBV reverse transcriptase *in vitro*, with an IC_{50} of 2.5 μM and a Ki of 0.03 μM [263]. Additionally, penciclovir was shown to be an inhibitor of the synthesis of minus-strand DHBV DNA in a cell-free system [68].

However, the poor bioavailability of penciclovir prompted the development of famciclovir (**24**; 9-[4-acetoxy-3-(acetoxymethyl)but-1-yl]-2-aminopurine), the prodrug of penciclovir. The major metabolic pathway of famciclovir is deacetylation at the 3 and 4 positions of the acyclic side chain followed by oxidation at the 6 position of the purine ring to yield the active metabolite, penciclovir [115]. In ducks infected with DHBV in ovo, famciclovir is effective in suppressing the replication of DHBV [298]. Case reports suggest that the drug is effective in patients with recurrent HBV after ortho-topic liver transplantation [26, 146]. With the exception of one case of pan-creatitis, in 50 patients using famciclovir for 30 days, only minimal side-effects were seen (reviewed in [248]). In the first report of a double-blind, con-trolled study of oral famciclovir for the treatment of chronic HBV infection, a drop of greater than 90% in HBV DNA levels was seen in six out of 11 patients receiving a 10-day course of therapy [190]. Recently a randomized, placebo-controlled study to evaluate a 12-month famciclovir treatment of patients with chronic HbeAg+ hepatitis B virus infection was conducted. Famciclovir at a dose of 500 mg three times daily gave only modest suppres-sion of viral replication but there was a significant improvement in liver his-tology at 1 year [70a]. However, resistance to famciclovir is associated with the L526M substitution in the B domain of the viral polymerase [156] and HBV variants that are resistant to lamivudine are cross-resistant to famciclovir [317a].

7.3   Phosphonate analogs and prodrugs

In efforts to identify nucleotide analogs which do not require the first phos-phorylation step for activation, phosphonates, which are analogs of mono-phosphates, have been developed for the treatment of viral infections. For a more thorough treatment of acyclic nucleoside phosphonates, including adefovir (PMEA) and cidofovir (HPMPC), we refer you to Naessens et al. [205]. Here we focus on PMEA (25; 9-2 phosphonylmethoxyethyl)adenine).

7.3.1 PMEA and bis-POM PMEA

PMEA has been shown to have activity against HBV in various cell culture systems and in primary duck hepatocytes infected with DHBV [117, 150, 325]. In human hepatoblastoma cells (HepG2.2.15), PMEA inhibited the replication of HBV DNA and release of virions from the cell with an EC_{50} of 0.7 μM while the 50% cytotoxic concentration (CC_{50}) of this compound was 150 μM (SI = 214). Using a recently developed, colorimetric PCR-based assay for the detection of extracellular HBV DNA, PMEA was shown to inhibit viral replication with an EC_{50} of 0.045 μg/ml and a selective index of 868.3 [279].

PMEA at 30 mg/kg/day was effective in decreasing serum levels of DHBV DNA in congenitally infected ducks [117].

The net negative charge of monophosphate analogs results in the poor penetration of these compounds into cells, thus limiting their utility as chemotherapeutic agents [172, 238]. Phosphonates, as monophosphate analogs, have the same limitation. Consequently, efforts to overcome this difficulty have included the development of membrane permeable prodrugs of the parent phosphonate analogs which can be cleaved intracellularly to release the active metabolite – the "pro-drug approach". The esterification of the neutral bis[(pivaloyloxy)methyl] (bis-POM) to biologically active nucleotide analogs has been described [81]. In one study, bis-POM PMEA (26) was administered orally to fasted male cynomolgus monkeys and levels of the active metabolite PMEA in the liver were significantly higher than those achieved with intravenous administration of PMEA itself [67]. Furthermore, bis-POM PMEA showed efficacy when given to 36 HIV-infected individuals for 14 days at a daily dosage of 125 mg [14]. In phase II clinical trials, in patients infected with wild type HBV, a 4 $\log_{10}$ reduction in serum HBV DNA was observed following a 12-week course of therapy with adefovir dipivoxil [104c]. Of interest, five patients with lamivudine-resistant HBV were treated with adefovir dipivoxil at dose of 5 to 30 mg daily. A reduction of two to four log10 in serum HBV DNA levels were seen in four of the patients and the fifth patient became negative for HBV DNA as determined by PCR [221a]. These clinical results are consistent with earlier laboratory findings in which PMEA remains active against lamivudine-resistant HBV in cell culture [98a].

7.3.2 Other prodrugs

The utility of various nucleoside analogs has been limited by a number of factors including, poor activation to the monophosphate, poor solubility, poor oral bioavailability, poor stability, or poor antiviral activity. In efforts to overcome these limitations, various prodrug moieties, which can be attached to nucleoside analogs in order to improve their overall biological activity, have been investigated. As an example, the aryloxyphosphoramidate derivatives of ddA and d4A were 100- to 1000-fold more active against HBV in cell culture than were the corresponding parent compounds [13]. Also, 1-O-octade-

(25) PMEA   (26) bis-POM PMEA

cyl-*sn*-glycero-3-phospho (ODG-P) and 1-O-hexadecyl-propanediol-3-phos-pho (HDP-P) derivatives of acyclovir were investigated. When compared to the parent acyclovir, ODG-P-acyclovir showed enhanced oral absorption in mice and both ODG-P-acyclovir and HDP-P-acyclovir displayed increased anti-HBV activity, greater than 15-fold and greater than 200-fold, respectively. Similarly, the ODG-P derivative of AZT was greater than 48-fold more active against HBV than was the parent AZT [132]. More recently, treatment of chronically infected woodchucks with ODG-P-acyclovir (10 mgs/kg BID for four weeks) resulted in a 95% reduction in WHV serum DNA while free acyclovir, had no effect [131a]. Although the suppression of WHV DNA by ODG-P-acyclovir was not sustained, these results indicate that various pro-drug approaches can be used to bypass the first activation step for nucleoside analogs that are poorly phosphorylated in liver cells.

Recently, the 5′-O-myristoyl derivatives of FLT and AZT were evaluated for anti-HBV activity in 2.2.15 cells [146a]. The 5′-O-(12-methoxydode-canoyl)ester derivatives of AZT and FLT inhibited HBV replication with an EC50 value of 2.7 μM and 2.8 μM, respectively. The AZT derivative displayed a CC50 of 727 uM while the FLT derivative had a CC_{50} value of 186 uM yielding selective indices of 269 and 66, respectively.

7.4   *L*-nucleoside analogs

L-nucleoside analogs are enantiomers of the conventional or "natural" β-*D*-nucleoside analogs and by definition have the same physicochemical properties but can differ dramatically in their biological effects such as antiviral activity or cytotoxicity. Synthesis of cis-nucleoside analogs with anti-HIV and anti-HBV activities results in mixtures of 1-β-D and 1-β-L stereoisomers and it has been observed that when these mixtures are separated, often the L-configuration nucleoside analogs have more potent anti-HBV activity than do the corresponding D-configuration analogs ([54, 74, 99]; reviewed in [69, 100]). Interest in this new class of nucleoside analogs has been bolstered by the success and imminent approval of lamivudine for the treatment of chronic HBV. In this review, we will focus on this L-configuration nucleoside analog and others which have been well-characterized.

7.4.1 Lamivudine

Lamivudine, also referred to as 3TC or (–) BCH-189 (27; (2R, 5S) 1-[2-(hydroxymethyl)-1,3-oxathiolane-5-yl]cytosine), is the single (–) enantiomer of the racemic mixture of 2'-deoxy-3'-thiacytidine. This compound, initially developed as a treatment for HIV infection, is also a potent inhibitor of HBV replication in vitro [38, 74] and in the chimpanzee and duck models of HBV infection [301]. In addition to inhibiting HIV reverse transcriptase [54], the triphosphate of lamivudine acts as a chain terminator for the synthesis of DNA by endogenous DHBV DNA polymerase [261]. Lamivudine is well absorbed after oral administration [327] and well-tolerated even when given for prolonged periods [73, 302]. It causes a rapid decrease in serum HBV DNA levels, clearance of HBeAg and, in some patients, decreases in serum aminotransferase. Within 4 weeks almost all patients treated orally with lamivudine at dosages of 25 to 100 mgs daily presented with greater than 90% reduction in serum HBV DNA. However, this suppression was transient in that viral DNA returned to pretreatment levels within 4 weeks of cessation of therapy [158]. In chronically infected patients treated orally with lamivudine for 6 months at a dosage of 25, 100, or 300 mgs daily, an improvement in liver histology without HBeAg seroconversion was observed [122]. In a study designed to assess subclinical mitochondrial toxicity, mitochondrial function was evaluated in 15 chronically infected patients who were treated with lamivudine for 24 weeks at dosages ranging form 25 to 300 mg/day. Quantification of the activity of mitochondrial enzymes in liver biopsies and use of the KICA (2-ketoisocap roic acid decarboxylation) breath test, which pro-

(27) 3TC (Lamivudine)   (28) FTC

vides early detection of impaired mitochondrial function, both revealed that lamivudine had no deleterious effects on mitochondrial function. Additionally, electron microscopic analysis of liver tissue revealed no abnormalities of mitochondrial structure [123].

In another trial, oral lamivudine at a dosage of 600 mgs daily for 12 months, showed good efficacy and was generally well-tolerated in 40 patients coinfected with both HIV and HBV. However, HBeAg and HBV DNA were still detectable in these patients, a situation which is predictive of viral rebound [20]. Other clinical trials have indicated that lamivudine may prove useful for the prevention of reinfection with HBV as often occurs following orthotopic liver transplantation [11, 110]. Overall, these trials indicate that elimination of chronic infection with a single inhibitor, such as lamivudine, may be difficult. Therefore, combination trials with lamivudine and IFNα are underway.

Lamivudine (known as epivir for HBV) has been approved by the FDA for use in chronic HBV infection [140a]. For more information regarding lamivudine, a number of review articles have recently been published [113a, 139a, 182a, 190a, 296b, 323b].

7.4.2 FTC

Another *L*-configuration nucleoside analog closely related to lamivudine is FTC (emitricitabine; **28**; (–)-*cis*-5-fluoro-1-[2-(hydroxymethyl)-1,3-oxathiolan-5-yl]cytosine) which contains a fluorine at the 5 position of the pyrimidine ring. The racemic mixture of this compound showed potent inhibition of HBV *in vitro* [74] and the triphosphate of *L*-FTC was more potent than that of *D*-FTC for the inhibition of HBV reverse transcriptase and for virion-associated DNA polymerase [69]. Similarly, the *L*-configuration was found to be much more potent (EC_{50} = 0.001 μM) than was the *D*-configuration (EC_{50} = 0.14 μM) against HBV replication in human hepatoblastoma cells and displayed minimal toxicity [99]. In addition, *L*-FTC has shown activity against HBV in primary human hepatocytes [63].

In a novel animal model using nude mice which bear HBV-producing tumors, oral treatment with *L*-FTC resulted in the reduction of serum HBV DNA levels and intracellular replicative DNA intermediates without decreasing tumor size [62]. More recently, naturally infected woodchucks were treated with *L*-FTC at dosages of 20 mg/kg or 30 mg/kg given intraperitoneally twice daily for 4 weeks [66]. In woodchucks receiving the 30 mg/kg b.i.d. dosage, levels of serum WHV DNA were reduced 20- to 150-fold (mean, 56-fold) and in woodchucks receiving the lower dosage, WHV DNA levels were reduced 6- to 49-fold (mean, 27-fold). In both groups, there were corresponding reductions in the levels of WHV DNA polymerase activity. One week after the cessation of treatment however, WHV returned to pretreatment levels in both groups. In these studies, increases in cytoplasmic lipid vacuoles were seen in woodchucks that received the 30 mg/kg b.i.d. dosage of *L*-FTC but this was not associated with any biochemical evidence of liver injury and *L*-FTC appeared to be well-tolerated in woodchucks when given for up to 25 days [66]. More recently, oral administration of emtricitabine to woodchucks was evaluated in a placebo-controlled study. A course of treatment for four weeks at dosages of 0.3 mg/kg/day to 30 mg/kg/day was found to significantly reduce viremia and intrahepatic WHV replication in a dose-dependent manner comparable to the potency of lamivudine. In this study, there was no evidence of drug-related toxicity [148a].

Early clinical studies indicate that emtricitabine is well tolerated and suppresses viral DNA replication by greater than 3 log 10 and is associated with normalization of serum ALT levels [296b]. Of note, HBV mutants that are resistant to lamivudine, have a decreased susceptibility to the antiviral activity of emtricitabine [156c]. For HIV, substitutions at amino acid residue 184 of the reverse transcriptase (analogous to position M550 of the HBV polymerase) confer resistance to both lamivudine and emtricitabine. Under selection with either drug, the initial change is frequently M184I which is subsequently replaced by M184V [104a].

(29) *L*-FMAU

7.4.3 *L*-FMAU

L-FMAU (**29**; 2′-fluoro-5-methyl-β-*L*-arabinofuranosyluracil) is the enantiomer of the well characterized FMAU. *L*-FMAU was found to have potent anti-HBV activity in human hepatoblastoma cells (EC$_{50}$ = 0.1 μM) and anti-Epstein-Barr virus activity in H1 lymphoma cells (EC$_{50}$ = 5 μM). The activity of *L*-FMAU against HBV, as determined by analysis of intracellular replicative DNA intermediates and released virion DNA, was greater than that of *D*-FMAU but against EBV, *L*-FMAU was less potent than was *D*-FMAU. *L*-FMAU, with a SI of greater than 2000 was much less toxic than was *D*-FMAU which displayed a SI of 25 [50]. *L*-FMAU was more potent against HBV than was either *L*-FEAU or *L*-FIAU (EC$_{50}$ >10 μM) [50, 188]. In further studies, *L*-FMAU did not inhibit the transcription of HBV RNA or HBV protein synthesis but did inhibit HBV DNA polymerase in a dose-dependent fashion, indicating a direct effect on the viral polymerase.

   L-FMAU was metabolized to the mono-, di-, and tri-phosphate forms in hepatoma cells but, nevertheless, was not incorporated into cellular DNA under experimental conditions in which incorporation of *D*-FMAU into DNA was readily detected [219, 324]. L-FMAU is phosphorylated by cytosolic thymidine kinase and mitochondrial deoxypyrimidine kinase as well as deoxycytidine kinase [178a]. It was found that the triphosphate of this analog inhibited DHBV DNA priming and reverse transcriptase activities [2a]. Although L-FMAU triphosphate is not a substrate for Epstein-Barr Virus DNA polymerase or cellular DNA polymerases, it was found to inhibit the elongation reaction as an uncompetitive inhibitor with respect to dNTPs or template-primer [155a]. Additionally L-FMAU triphosphate could not be used as a substrate by EBV DNA polymerase thus indicating a fundamentally different mechanism of antiviral activity against EBV and possibly against HBV [324].

The anti-HBV activities of D-FMAU and D-FIAU in woodchucks have been described. Both compounds displayed potent antiviral activity but had severe toxicities [93, 153, 289]. In contrast, L-FMAU was similarly effective but did not display any apparent toxicity. This compound was given orally to chronically infected woodchucks at a daily dose of 10 mg/kg for 12 weeks. Within 2 weeks, levels of serum WHV DNA decreased more than a 1000-fold and were undetectable for the remainder of the experiment. At the end of treatment, levels of WHV DNA replicative DNA intermediates were decreased more than 10-fold as compared to levels at pre-treatment or to those in untreated animals. Importantly, no signs of toxicity were observed in L-FMAU treated animals [288]. In the duck model of HBV infection, treatment of experimentally infected ducklings with L-FMAU (40 mgs/kgs/day for 5 days) resulted in a significant reduction of viremia which was sustained when therapy was prolonged for eight days [2a].

HBV variants which are resistant to lamivudine and contain the double substitution in the viral polymerase (L526M and M550V/I or A546V and M550V/I) are cross resistant to L-FMAU, although the degree of resistance is less than that seen with penciclovir [98a]. However, in another study L-FMAU showed similar activity when tested against a lamivudine-resistant virus containing the M550V substitution alone or when tested against wild-type virus [324a].

L-FMAU displayed a bioavailability of 59 to 64% in rats [321] and its pharmacokinetic profile was similar to that of D-FMAU except for the existence of non-renal clearance [320]. In a recent study, the pharmacokinetics of L-FMAU in woodchucks was reported and overall, its pharmacokinetic profile was similar to that seen in the rat with the exception of a slower elimination rate [317]. After an intravenous administration of 25 mg/kg, L-FMAU displayed a terminal phase half-life of 6.2 ± 2.0 h and its total clearance was characterized as moderate with an average of 0.23 ± 0.07 liter/h/kg. Clearance by the renal and non-renal route averaged 0.13 ± 0.08 and 0.10 ± 0.06 liter/h/kg, respectively. The bioavailability of L-FMAU in woodchucks was approximately 20%. Importantly, the concentration of L-FMAU in plasma remained above the previously reported in vitro EC_{50} for HBV for 24 h [317].

The severe toxicity of fialuridine (*D*-FIAU), which appears to be mediated by mitochondrial toxicity (reviewed in [55] and [125]), has focused attention on the potential for mitochondrial toxicity of other nucleoside analogs. Treatment of cells in culture with *D*-FIAU has been shown to result in increased levels of lactate in the medium [58, 64]. This is consistent with a deleterious effect on mitochondrial function causing cells to revert to anaerobic metabolism, the end-product of which is lactate. In experiments which compared *D*-FMAU, *D*-FIAU, and *L*-FMAU directly for the induction of lactate in human hepatoblastoma cells, both *D*-enantiomeric compounds, each at a concentration of 100 µM, were shown to increase lactate levels. In contrast, 100 or 200 µM *L*-FMAU had no effect on lactate levels, consistent with the notion that this compound is not inhibitory to mitochondrial function [219]. Taken together, the potent anti-HBV activity, the lack of incorporation into DNA, the lack of mitochondrial toxicity, the lack of toxicity in woodchucks, and the favorable pharmacokinetics of *L*-FMAU warrant further study of this novel nucleoside analog as a potential treatment for chronic HBV infection.

7.4.4 *L*-ddC and *L*-FddC

Other *L*-configuration nucleoside analogs that have recently been described are the *L*-enantiomers of ddC including *L*-ddC (**30**; 2′,3′-dideoxy-β-*L*-cytidine) and *L*-FddC (**31**; 2′,3′-dideoxy-β-*L*-5-fluorocytidine). These *L*-configuration nucleoside analogs are considerably more active against HBV than are the corresponding *D*-enantiomers and have decreased toxicities to B and T cell lines and human bone marrow progenitor cells [304]. *L*-FddC triphosphate was a more potent inhibitor of WHV DNA polymerase than was the triphosphate of the *D*-enantiomer [255]. In human hepatoblastoma cells, *L*-FddC inhibited HBV replication with an EC_{50} of 0.01 µM, 1000-fold more potent than *D*-FddC. Similarly, *L*-ddC, with an EC_{50} of 0.01 µM was 280-fold more active than was *D*-ddC [175]. In studies by one group, neither *L*-ddC nor *L*-FddC, at concentrations up to 100 µM, inhibited the replication of mitochondrial DNA [175] and the triphosphate of *L*-FddC was not an inhibitor of DNA polymerase γ [156]. However, studies by another group demonstrated that *L*-FddC caused a concentration-dependent increase in lactic acid and inhibited mitochondrial DNA replication in human hepatoblastoma

(30) *L*-ddC   (31) *L*-FddC   (32) *L*-d4C   (33) *L*-Fd4C

cells although it did not cause morphological changes in mitochondrial structure [65]. Further studies will be required to resolve these apparent differences.

In a cell-free system as described by Wang and Seeger [308], the triphosphate of *L*-FddC was shown to inhibit the synthesis of minus-strand DHBV DNA in a concentration-dependent manner [333]. Although, *L*-FddC had a long-lasting antiviral effect in primary hepatocyte cultures, in infected ducklings treated orally at a dosage of 50 mg/kg twice daily for 5 days, *L*-FddC displayed a potent (97% reduction) but transient suppression of DHBV DNA [333]. Whether these compounds will demonstrate potential clinical utility for the treatment of HBV infection will be dependent upon further evaluation in animal models of HBV infection.

7.4.5 *L*-d4C and *L*-Fd4C

Two newly described *L*-nucleoside analogs, 2′,3′-dideoxy-2′,3′-didehydro-β-*L*-cytidine (**32**; *L*-d4C) and 2′,3′-dideoxy-2′,3′-didehydro-β-*L*-5-fluorocytidine (**33**; *L*-Fd4C) have been shown to be potent inhibitors of HBV replication in virus-producing hepatoma cells [177]. As determined by analysis of intracellular replicative DNA intermediates, *L*-d4C inhibited HBV replication by 50% (EC_{50}) at a concentration of 0.008 μM and *L*-Fd4C displayed an EC_{50} of 0.002 μM. Both compounds inhibited the replication of CEM cells with CC_{50} values of 20 μM and 7 μM, respectively. Neither compound had an

NH$_2$

(34) Cytallene

appreciable effect on mitochondrial DNA content. These encouraging *in vitro* results will prompt further study of these compounds.

7.4.6 Cytallene

Cytallene (**34**; 1-(4'-hydroxy-1',2'-butadienyl)cytosine) is a recently described acyclic cytosine nucleoside analog with potent anti-HBV activity [330]. Although the racemic mixture of this compound was evaluated, the (+) and (–) enantiomers were tested separately for anti-HBV activity. The (+) enantiomer inhibited HBV replication by 50% (EC$_{50}$) at a concentration of >10 µM while the (–) enantiomer had an EC$_{50}$ of 0.08 µM as determined by Southern blot analysis of intracellular viral replicative DNA intermediates. The (–) enantiomer was toxic to CEM cells at 12 µM (CC$_{50}$), yielding a SI of 150, while the (+) enantiomer was toxic at >30 µM. Neither compound affected mitochondrial DNA levels.

7.4.7 *L*-dideoxypurine nucleoside analogs

Numerous purine β-*L*-2',3'-dideoxy nucleoside analogs have been evaluated for activity against HBV in cell culture. β-*L*-ddG, β-*L*-ddA, and derivatives of these analogs with modifications in the sugar, base, or both failed to demonstrate potent anti-HBV activity. However, β-*L*-d4A (the didehydro derivative of β-*L*-ddA) and the *N*-triphenylphosphine derivative of β-*L*-d4A did show selective activity with EC_{50} values of 0.1 μM and 1 μM, respectively, as determined by analysis of intracellular HBV replicative DNA intermediates [75]. None of these compounds, including β-*L*-d4A, decreased mitochondrial DNA abundance at concentrations up to 10 μM [75]. Other groups have reported similar findings for β-*L*-ddG [176, 191] and β-*L*-ddA [176].

7.5   Oxetanocins and derivatives

7.5.1 Oxetanocins

The oxetanocin nucleoside analogs include oxetanocin A (**35**; 9-(2-deoxy-2-hydroxymethyl-β-*D*-erythro-oxetanosyl)adenine), isolated from the filtrate of *Bacillus megaterium* [267], and oxetanocin G (**36**; 9-(2-deoxy-2-hydroxymethyl-β-*D*-erythro-oxetanosyl)guanine), which has been produced from oxetanocin A [268]. Oxetanocin A has been shown to inhibit HBV replication in human hepatoblastoma (HB611) cells with an EC_{50} of 16 μg/ml and a SI of 4.3 [303]. Oxetanocin G inhibited HBV replication in cell culture with an EC_{50} of 1.5 μM and a SI of greater than 667 [207]. The triphosphate of oxetanocin G was shown to inhibit endogenous HBV DNA polymerase and DNA polymerase α with IC_{50} values of 1.5 μM and 10.3 μM, respectively, and was incorporated into viral DNA but with a lower efficiency than that of dGTP. Additionally, using HIV-reverse transcriptase or DNA polymerase α, it was shown that DNA could be extended from the point of oxetanocin G incorporation [207].

Transgenic mice which carry an integrated HBV genome, were treated parenterally with oxetanocin G at a dosage of 15 mg/kg given twice daily. In treated animals, viral DNA synthesis in the liver was inhibited almost completely [206]. Treatment of woodchucks with oxetanocin G, at a dosage of 1 or 2 mgs/kg/day given orally for 5 days, resulted in only incomplete suppression of serum WHV DNA, levels of which returned to baseline values subsequent to cessation of therapy [137]. In this study, oxetanocin G appeared to be more toxic in woodchucks than was previously observed in rats or mice [210], an observation which points to species differences and the need for further *in vivo* evaluation concerning the toxicity of this and related compounds.

(35) Oxetanocin A

(36) Oxetanocin G

(37) Cyclobut A

(38) Cyclobut G (Lobucavir)

7.5.2 Carbocyclic oxetanocins

Cyclobut A (**37**) and cyclobut G (**38**) have a methylene bridge in place of the oxygen in the oxetanose ring and therefore are the carbocyclic analogs of the oxetanocins. These compounds have been widely studied for their broad spectrum of activity against various herpesviruses and have recently shown activity against HBV *in vitro*. Currently, the (–) enantiomer of cyclobut G (known as lobucavir) is undergoing clinical evaluation for the treatment of various herpesvirus infections in HIV-positive individuals (reviewed in [192]). The clinical development of lobucavir was halted because long term administration of this drug to rats and mice appeared to be associated with neoplasia [190a].

(39) PFA (Foscarnet)

7.6 Pyrophosphate analogs

7.6.1 Foscarnet

Foscarnet or phosphonoformate (39; PFA), is a pyrophosphate analog that lacks impressive anti-herpetic activity in cell culture but was shown to have potent antiherpetic activity when used topically in various animal models (reviewed in [78]). PFA, and the closely related phosphonoacetate (PAA) were shown to inhibit herpesvirus DNA polymerase [118, 193]. PAA binds to the pyrophosphate exchange site of DNA polymerase and blocks formation of the 3'-5'-phosphodiester linkage thus preventing further elongation of viral DNA [167]. Herpesvirus DNA polymerases were 50- to 150-fold more sensitive to the inhibition of PAA or PFA than was cellular DNA polymerase α (reviewed in [78]). It was later shown that PFA inhibited endogenous HBV DNA polymerase by 95% at a concentration of 500 μM. This inhibition was non-competitive with a Ki of 7.2 μM with respect to dTTP as the variable substrate [214]. More recently, PFA was found to have activity against endogenous DHBV DNA polymerase with an IC_{50} of 4 μM, whereas PAA had no activity [182]. Similarly, PAA was found also to be inactive against endogenous HBV DNA polymerase [119]. It should be noted that PFA, although an inhibitor of endogenous hepadnavirus DNA polymerase, does not interfere with priming of reverse transcription of the RNA pre-genome [308].

PFA was shown to be effective in the duck model of HBV infection. Ducks chronically infected with DHBV were treated for 10 days with foscarnet at a dosage of 50 mg/kg given intraperitoneally twice per day (low dose) or 250 mg/kg given in the same way (high dose). Treatment resulted in a dose-related decrease in the levels of serum and intrahepatic DHBV DNA but viral DNA rebounded to pre-treatment levels soon after the cessation of treatment [265]. In a clinical evaluation, patients with chronic HBV infection were treated with PFA given by continuous infusion at 0.15 mg/kg/minute for 7 days or 180 mg/kg/day given as three 60 mg/kg bolus injections per day. In all patients HBV DNA levels declined markedly but remained detectable. Furthermore, in all but one patient, HBV DNA levels returned to baseline within 1 month after cessation of therapy [10]. Significantly, treatment with PFA was associated with nausea, vomiting, and impaired renal function prompting dose reduction in three of eight patients [10]. Considering the inconvenience of administration, the toxicity, and the lack of efficacy of PFA, it is unlikely that this agent alone will prove to have clinical utility for the treatment of chronic HBV infection. Therefore, the use of foscarnet in combination with other modalities has been considered. For instance, it has been reported that the antiviral effects of foscarnet and ganciclovir in combination are additive against DHBV in culture [52], indicating a potential clinical utility for foscarnet in combination with other antiviral agents. However, the combination of ganciclovir and foscarnet did not demonstrate sustained efficacy for HBV recurrence after liver transplantation [270].

The conjugation of PFA with antiviral nucleoside analogs has been attempted with mixed results. Prompted by observations demonstrating the inhibition of HIV by AZT-PFA [240], it became apparent that conjugates of 2',3'-dideoxy-3'-thiacytidine (3TC; BCH-189; lamivudine) and PFA might be useful as inhibitors of HBV replication. New analogs in which the oxygen atom of the pseudoribose ring of BCH-189 was linked to the phosphorous atom of PFA were designed [40]. It was found that the anti-HIV and anti-DHBV activities of PFA-BCH-189 conjugates were much lower than those of the parent BCH-189. It was determined that poor uptake of the polar conjugates by the infected cells was the most likely explanation for the reduced antiviral activity. Thus the presence of the PFA moiety in the conjugate appears to reduce the antiviral activity of BCH-189.

7.7 Conjugated nucleosides targeted to the liver

Although evidence is available for the presence and possibly the replication of HBV in extrahepatic sites during chronic infection [162], HBV replication occurs predominantly within the liver parenchymal cells resulting in liver damage. Therefore, targeting antiviral agents, including nucleoside analogs, antisense oligonucleotides, or ribozymes, to the liver might improve antiviral efficacy and minimize toxicity to other organs. Such agents can be targeted to the liver by conjugating them to carriers which can be recognized by hepatocyte-specific receptors, such as the asialoglycoprotein receptor, also known as the Ashwell receptor [7]. The selection of a drug-carrier complex is determined by the following considerations as outlined by Meijer and Molema [201] and reviewed in Rensen et al. [235]: 1) passage of the drug-carrier complex through 100–105 nm fenestrae formed by the liver endothelial layer; 2) adequate drug loading; 3) target specificity within the whole organism including the lack of uptake by liver macrophages and other cell types; 4) lack of immunogenicity and toxicity of the drug-carrier complex; 5) release and retention of the active component, i.e., free drug, into the cytoplasm of the cell; and 6) and presence of the Ashwell receptor under disease conditions, especially during chronic HBV infection which has been shown to decrease the number of these receptors [31, 195, 242].

In light of these considerations, a lysosomotropic approach was taken in which ara-AMP or ACV monophosphate (ACV-MP) was coupled to lactosaminated human serum albumin (L-HSA), a neoglycoprotein which contains terminal galactosyl groups [88–90]. L-HSA is selectively taken up by hepatocytes via receptor mediated endocytosis after which it is degraded in lysosomes. When coupled to L-HSA, agents such as ara-AMP or ACV-MP are also carried selectively into the liver. In the woodchuck model of HBV infection, chronically infected animals were treated with free or conjugated ara-AMP or ACV-MP intravenously every day for 5 days. At a dosage of 10 mg/kg/day, unconjugated ara-AMP reduced viremia by 25-fold but virus replication resumed immediately upon discontinuation of treatment. A dosage of conjugated ara-AMP (equivalent to 1.5 mg/kg/day of free ara-AMP) resulted in a 25- to 125-fold decrease in serum levels of viral DNA, which in several woodchucks never rebounded to pre-treatment levels during a 9 to 64 day follow-up. Importantly, no effect on lymphocyte counts was observed as has been the case for unconjugated ara-AMP. In this model, neither free nor conjugated ACV-MP was effective [226]. These results indicated that conjugated ara-AMP was more effective and less toxic than unconjugated ara-AMP.

In another study, ara-AMP was conjugated to the naturally occurring polysaccharide, arabinogalactan. When chronically infected woodchucks were treated with daily injections of this conjugate for 14 days at a dose equivalent to 3 mg of ara-AMP/kg, serum levels of WHV DNA dropped and remained low for 42 days after discontinuation of therapy [77]. Similarly, treatment of chronically infected woodchucks with L-HSA conjugated to ddCMP at a dosage of 10.4 mg/kg (equivalent to 0.25 mg/kg of free ddC) resulted in a decrease in serum levels of WHV DNA without apparent toxicity [328].

In patients chronically infected with HBV, intravenous administration for 28 days of ara-AMP conjugated to L-HSA at dosages ranging from 34 to 53 mg/kg/day (equivalent to 1.5 to 2.3 mg/kg/day of free ara-AMP) resulted in a marked decline in serum levels of HBV DNA with an increase in viral DNA levels soon after cessation of treatment [34]. However, treatment with conjugated ara-AMP was not associated with the neurotoxicity typically seen with free ara-AMP. Treatment did result in an increase in serum alkaline phosphatase and platelet number, both of which returned to normal within 2 months after treatment [34]. A drawback to this approach is that the conjugate must be administered intravenously. This has prompted the development of agents conjugated to lactosaminated poly-L-lysine carriers which can be administered intramuscularly [90].

Efforts to target other antiviral agents to liver cells are now underway. *In vitro* experiments have pointed to the potential feasibility of targeting conjugated antisense oligonucleotides to infected liver cells. The results demonstrate that antisense complexes can be directed to the asialoglycoprotein receptors on HBV producing hepatoblastoma cells and inhibit HBV replication [208, 322].

7.8 Novel approaches

In addition to the nucleoside analogs as anti-HBV therapies, several other approaches to inhibit HBV replication have been described.

7.8.1 *Phyllanthus amarus*

Extracts from the plants *Phyllanthus amarus* and *Eclipta alba* have been used in traditional medicine for the treatment of jaundice and general liver problems [291]. Extracts of *P. amarus*, consisting of phyllanthin, hypophyllanthin, and triacontanal [282], have been shown to inhibit WHV endogenous DNA polymerase [305]. Recent experiments have suggested that *P. amarus* extracts have a bimodal mechanism of action inhibiting both HBV polymerase activity and HBV mRNA transcription [165], a process which is carried out by host cell RNA polymerase II. Treatment of chronic HBV carriers with *P. amarus* for 30 days resulted in a loss of HBsAg in 59% of patients as compared to 4% in placebo-treated control subjects [292]. More recently, in the duck model of HBV infection, extracts of *P. amarus* were used orally or intraperitoneally to treat congenitally infected ducklings. In contrast to results obtained in humans, *P. amarus* did not result in a reduction of circulating viral DNA in the serum or in an inhibition of viral replication in the liver [212]. These apparently discordant observations illustrate the difficulty in extrapolating results from the duck model of infection to the clinical situation.

7.8.2 *N*-acetyl-L-cysteine (NAC)

N-acetyl-L-cysteine (NAC) is a reactive oxygen intermediate scavenger and is routinely used to treat acetominophen-induced hepatotoxicity [271]. Recent work by Weiss et al. [313] showed that treatment of HBV producing cells with 3, 10, or 30 mM NAC for 48 hours resulted in a reduction of extracellular HBV DNA by 2.5, 10, and 50-fold, respectively. Importantly, NAC was not toxic at concentrations up to 30 mM and had no effect on HBV transcription or HBV replication, as determined by Southern blot analysis of HBV intracellular replicative DNA intermediates. It did, however, have a profound effect on HBsAg expression and, to a lesser extent, on the expression of HBc/eAg. Since HBsAg is known to be stabilized by several disulfide bonds, it was speculated that NAC may effect HBsAg oligomerization and thus virus assembly. Further studies are required to fully assess the utility of NAC as a therapy for HBV infection.

7.8.3 Analogs of myristic acid

Given the fact that preS1 of HBV [222] and both preS and sAg of DHBV [189] are covalently myristylated, several inhibitors of *N*-myristoyltransferase were tested for their ability to inhibit hepatitis B virus replication [220]. Of several analogs tested, 12-methoxydodecanoic acid showed the best activity. Treatment of HBV-producing HepG2.2.15 cells with 12-methoxydodecanoic acid resulted in a decrease in both extracellular HBV DNA (EC_{90} = 60 µM) and intracellular replicative DNA intermediates (EC_{90} = 90 µM) and the compound was cytotoxic at 378 µM yielding selective indices of 6.3 and 4.2, respectively. None of the analogs tested showed significant activity against DHBV in infected primary duck hepatocytes.

7.8.4 Destruxin B

The cyclodepsipeptide destruxin B (**40**) was shown to suppress the secretion of HBsAg from Hep3B cells with an EC_{50} of 0.5 µM [43]. In addition, destruxin B affected HBsAg production in transiently transfected Huh-7 cells. Destruxin B appeared to affect the steady state levels of HBsAg mRNA and showed no apparent toxicity. Since cyclodepsipeptides are known to exhibit a wide variety of biological activities, further mechanistic studies as well as HBV antiviral testing are needed.

7.8.5 Hypericin

Hypericin (**41**), an aromatic polycyclic anthrone isolated from the plant *Hypericum triquetrifolium* Turra (St. Johnswort), was reported to have anti-retroviral activity in mice infected with Friend leukemia virus or radiation leukemia virus [202]. Hypericin was also reported to inhibit HIV-1 replication in lymphocytes and purified HIV-1 reverse transcriptase [252]. Subsequently, hypericin and its analog, pseudohypericin, were shown to inactivate enveloped but not non-enveloped viruses [136, 184, 283, 284]. Accordingly, the use of hypericin as an inactivator of enveloped viruses in blood components and products has been considered [163].

Hypericin was found to be active against DHBV in cell culture. After a single 1-h incubation with 10 or 1 µg of hypericin per ml, cells which are stably transfected with a clone of DHBV stopped producing infectious virus for 5 days although non-infectious virus particles continued to be released into the cell culture medium. Biochemical studies of these particles, including Western blot analysis, indicated that the viral preS protein was present in covalently cross-linked aggregates, suggesting that hypericin inhibits a late step

(40) Destruxin B

(41) Hypericin

(42) NBDNJ

in viral morphogenesis [203]. The observation that hypericin did not inactivate DHBV, an enveloped virus, to any great extent [203], points to the possibility that the compound may have a unique mechanism of activity for
hepadnaviruses. Although hypericin has been clinically evaluated for the
treatment of AIDS, no such studies have been reported for the treatment of
chronic HBV infection.

7.8.6 Aucubin

The search for agents among traditional Oriental medicines useful for liver
ailments including viral hepatitis, has led to the isolation of aucubin, an iri-
doid glycoside from *Plantago asiatica* and *Aucuba japonica*. Aucubin, when
pre-incubated with β-glucosidase to yield the aglycone derivative, showed significant suppression of HBV DNA replication in HBV producing hepatoblas-

toma cells at concentrations below those causing cytotoxicity [36]. Studies to evaluate the efficacy of aucubin in animal models of HBV infection are underway [36].

7.8.7 N-butyldeoxynojirimycin

N-butyldeoxynojirimcyin (**42**; NBDNJ), an imino sugar, is a known inhibitor of α-glucosidase I which catalyzes the removal of terminal glucose residues from newly formed oligosaccharides [91]. NBDNJ has been shown to inhibit the replication of human immunodeficiency virus in cell culture by interfering with the normal processing of the viral envelope glycoprotein, gp120 [142]. As mentioned previously, HBV contains three envelope proteins, pre-S1, pre-S2, and S, all of which are N-glycosylated. Since the S antigen is common to all three, the isoforms of this protein share a common N-linked glycosylation site at amino acid position 146. The pre-S2 protein contains an additional N-linked glycosylation site at amino acid position 4 (reviewed in [103]). Considering their role in virus assembly and secretion from the host cell [29], inhibition of the normal glycan processing of these proteins would be expected to result in the suppression of the formation and release of infectious HBV. Treatment of HBV-producing hepatoblastoma cells with 500 or 1000 μg of NBDNJ per ml for 6 days completely suppressed the release of HBV into the cell culture supernatant [24]. When examined, treated cells were found to contain elevated levels of HBV DNA indicating that virus DNA replication was not inhibited whereas virus assembly and release were. In further studies, treatment of virus producing cells with NBDNJ resulted in the increased glycosylation of pre-S2 [200] and retention of this protein within lysosomes [186]. Taken together, these results point to the importance of the pre-S2 antigen in virus assembly and secretion from the infected cell and suggest that interference of the normal glycan processing of pre-S2 may represent a novel approach to the chemotherapeutic intervention of HBV infection.

The potential utility of this approach has been recently demonstrated using the woodchuck model of HBV infection. In woodchucks treated with apparently non-toxic doses of DBDNJ, there was a significant decrease in WHV viremia which was associated with hyperglucosylated glycan in the serum [23a].

7.8.8 CCC DNA inhibitors

Most of the approaches to the treatment of HBV infection, especially nucleoside analogs, do not result in the complete clearance of CCC DNA. With an intracellular half-life of 3–5 days as described for DHBV [51], the persistence of CCC DNA in the infected cell nucleus is thought to be the major reason for virus rebound after the cessation of antiviral therapy. Exploiting the differences between host cell chromosomal DNA and HBV DNA in terms of chromatin structure [209], agents such as inhibitors of topoisomerase and gyrase have been evaluated for their ability to affect the level and/or function of CCC DNA. The topoisomerase inhibitors, ellipticine, amsacrine, adriamycin, and mitozantrone and the DNA gyrase B inhibitor, coumermycin A1, inhibited DHBV DNA replication *in vitro*. By contrast, the gyrase inhibitors nalidixic acid and novobiocin demonstrated only partial inhibition [53]. Further studies in which courmerycin A1 was used in combination with ampligen (an immunomodulator and interferon inducer) and ganciclovir to treat congenitally infected ducklings revealed that DHBV DNA replication was inhibited but CCC DNA forms persisted. As expected, levels of viral DNA returned to baseline within 1 week after the cessation of therapy [211]. In other studies, the combination of ganciclovir and nalidixic acid, when given to infected ducks for 28 days, resulted in a decrease of replicative DNA intermediates, particularly the supercoiled CCC DNA, without evidence of hepatotoxicity [311]. More recently, treatment of HBV producing cells with the topoisomerase I inhibitor, camptothecin, a plant alkaloid derived from *Camptotheca acuminata*, resulted in the arrest of these cells in G2 and a concomitant increase in the replication of HBV DNA [218]. These apparently conflicting results call for further research into the biological activity of these compounds. Although there is clinical experience for camptothecin as a treatment for psoriasis and certain cancers, to our knowledge no controlled clinical evaluation of this or other compounds, which affect the level or function of CCC DNA, has been reported for the treatment of chronic HBV infection.

7.8.9 Antisense and ribozymes

Traditional approaches to the chemotherapeutic intervention of viral infections have relied on the inhibition of viral proteins, most notably virus-specific enzymes. For example, the phosphorylated metabolites of nucleoside analogs, such as those discussed here, target the hepadnavirus DNA polymerase. Another approach is to block the translation of virus specific "sense" mRNA by sequence-specific hybridization of exogenously added "antisense" oligodeoxynucleotides. In addition to hybrid arrest of translation of viral proteins, the mRNA in the sense:antisense hybrid molecule would, in some cases, be susceptible to degradation by the action of RNaseH thus preventing translation. This is known as the "antisense approach," the principle of which was first demonstrated by using a phosphodiester oligonucleotide to inhibit the replication of Rous sarcoma virus [275, 329]. It has been shown that antisense oligonucleotides which are directed against the message of HBsAg, inhibit the expression of this protein in cell culture [108]. More recently, in HBV-producing HepG2.2.15 cells it was demonstrated that a series of antisense oligonucleotides targeted to either HBV structural proteins or to the packaging signal (ε) inhibited HBV replication [152]. Of interest was the observation that antisense oligonucleotides directed to ε were the most potent inhibitors of viral replication.

Results demonstrating the efficacy of antisense oligonucleotides in the duck model of HBV infection are encouraging for the potential use of antisense oligonucleotides as a treatment modality for HBV infection. Treatment of DHBV infected ducklings with phosphorothioate-modified oligonucleotides directed to the 5' end of the pre-S gene administered intravenously at a dosage of 20 µg/gram of body weight per day for 10 days led to the abrogation of DHBV replication [215]. Specificity of this inhibition was shown by demonstrating that random oligodeoxynucleotides or oligonucleotides in the sense orientation had no effect on virus replication.

The use of antisense oligonucleotides as antiviral drugs is limited by a number of factors: 1) the polyanionic character of the molecule which hinders penetration into the cell; 2) the susceptibility of unmodified oligonucleotides to enzymatic degradation; 3) the poor bioavailability of these molecules which necessitates high dosages and parenteral administration; 4) the lack of tissue specificity; and 5) the relatively high cost and difficulty of bulk oligonucleotide synthesis. Much effort has been directed to address these issues (reviewed in [85]). For instance, modification of the sugar-phosphate backbone, the bases, or both has resulted in greater resistance to degradation. Additionally, conjugation of oligodeoxynucleotides to moieties, such as asialo-oromucoid, targets the oligodeoxynucleotide to the liver and increases the uptake of the polyanionic macromolecule into cells via the Ashwell receptor resulting in greater suppression of HBsAg synthesis [30, 322]. Importantly, much progress has been made in reducing the cost and turn-around time of bulk oligonucleotide synthesis. The clinical feasibility of this approach for the treatment of HBV infection has not yet been determined.

In further efforts to overcome the limitations of antisense chemotherapy, ribozymes, which are RNA molecules able to carry out sequence specific catalytic cleavage of target RNA molecules, have been considered as antivirals. Ribozymes can be targeted to the HBV RNA pre-genome [306] or to other viral mRNAs and therefore disrupt viral replication. In one study, a hammerhead-ribozyme targeted to the encapsidation signal (ε) led to efficient cleavage of HBV RNA *in vitro*. However, in co-transfection experiments using mutant ribozymes, it was shown that an antisense effect contributed significantly to the observed decrease of HBV pre-genomic RNA levels [19]. In another study, hairpin ribozymes were designed to target the HBV RNA pre-genome as well as mRNAs encoding HBsAg, viral polymerase, and X protein. Initially, the ability of each ribozyme to cleave the corresponding target RNA *in vitro* was demonstrated. Subsequently, the cDNA of each ribozyme was introduced into HBV producing cells using a retroviral expression vector and it was demonstrated that when unmodified ribozymes were co-expressed in these cells, the production of HBV particles was reduced by 66%. When ribozymes which were structurally modified to increase catalytic efficiency were co-expressed in these cells, HBV particle production was suppressed by 83% [314]. In more recent cell culture experiments, ribozymes that inhibit HBV replication by targeting the viral RNA in the S antigen and polymerase overlapping sequences were identified from a hairpin ribozyme library [335]. These "proof-of-principle experiments" point to possible use of ribozymes as inhibitors of HBV replication but the clinical potential of this approach cannot be assessed without the results of additional *in vivo* experiments.

8 Resistance

Retroviruses and hepadnaviruses both replicate through a reverse transcription step but the rate of silent mutations in the HBV genome is 100-fold less than that observed for retroviral genomes [106, 217]. The reasons for the relatively greater evolutionary stability of the HBV genome may be due, in part, to its compact nature and the presence of multiple overlapping reading frames [107]. Because there is no adequate *in vitro* infection system, laboratory experiments to address the emergence of drug-resistant HBV variants are not as technically feasible as they are for other viruses such as herpesviruses, retroviruses, or influenza. Consequently, the potential for the development of HBV resistance to antiviral agents was not appreciated until isolates of resistant virus could be obtained from patients undergoing antiviral therapy. However, it had been known that a mutation leading to the amino acid change, M184V, in the conserved YMDD motif of the active site of HIV-1 reverse transcriptase conferred resistance to lamivudine [253]. Using this knowledge, an analogous mutation was introduced into the reverse transcriptase of DHBV (M512V) using site-directed mutagenesis [87]. In transiently transfected cells, lamivudine was markedly less active against mutant virus than it was against wild-type virus. These mutations, and others, are schematically summarized in Figure 2 which provides a schematic comparison of the reverse transcriptase domains of HIV-1 and HBV (wild-type and drug-resistant variants). All of the mutations in drug-resistant variants of HBV reported thus far map to the "palm" sub-domain [148] which contains the active site of reverse transcriptase.

Resistance of HBV to lamivudine first appeared in several orthotopic liver transplantation (OLT) patients who received the drug either before or after OLT to prevent recurrent HBV infection. Despite an initial suppression of viral levels during therapy, the recurrence of HBV infection was observed between 1 and 9 months after OLT. Genetic characterization of viruses isolated following recurrence revealed a mutation in the polymerase gene leading to the amino acid alteration of methionine (M) to valine (V) or isoleucine (I) at position 550 (M550V; M550I) within the YMDD motif [16, 178, 295]. Resistance has also been described in OLT patients receiving long term oral famciclovir [8, 9] but in this case, amino acid alterations were not in the YMDD motif but rather at amino acid positions 519 (V519L) and 526 (L526M). It was also shown that endogenous DNA polymerase from famciclovir resistant virions displayed a reduced sensitivity to penciclovir triphosphate [9]. Of interest is the clinical observation that patients with HBV containing these mutations still respond to lamivudine [293]. In a recent study, the L526M variation as well as a number of novel substitutions in other conserved domains of the HBV polymerase appeared in patients treated with famciclovir [259a].

Transient transfection studies, using replication competent cDNAs, confirmed that resistance to lamivudine is conferred by amino acid substitutions in the YMDD motif of the polymerase [4a]. In the case of HBV variants containing both the L526M and M550V substitutions in the polymerase, the EC_{50} for lamivudine was > 3000-fold higher for the mutant virus than for the wild-type virus [307a]. In addition, HBV polymerase containing M550V, M550I, or M550V and L526M displays reduced sensitivity to inhibition by lamivudine-triphosphate [322a].

HBV resistance to lamivudine has also been seen in immunocompetent patients with chronic HBV infection who were treated for a minimum of 6 months. As seen in viruses isolated from immunocompromised OLT patients, these viruses contained the M550V or M550I alterations in the YMDD motif [124]. In this study, resistant virus was found to recur gradually following incomplete suppression, or suddenly following complete suppression.

The appearance of drug-resistant HBV in patients treated long-term with lamivudine is now well documented (reviewed in [139a]). In a recent report, drug-resistance HBV was observed after 8 months in 52% of patients treated with lamivudine for two to four years [162a]. Although emergence of lamivudine-resistant YMDD-motif variants of HBV is frequent, as determined by PCR detection, it does not always occur with the reappearance of detectable serum HBV DNA or elevations in ALT [73a].

The biology, including virulence, pathogenicity, and replication competency, of drug resistant HBV variants requires further study. In recent experiments the replication capacity of lamivudine-resistant mutants was found to be lower than that of wild-type HBV [201a]. In addition, due to the fact that the open reading frame (ORF) for HBsAg is entirely contained within the

---

Fig. 2
Schematic representation of the linear sequence of reverse transcriptase (RT) from human immunodeficiency virus type 1 (HIV-1) and hepatitis B virus (HBV). The location of the terminal protein (TP) and spacer domains of HBV RT and the sub-domains of RT, as described by Kohlstaedt et al. [148], are indicated. The "thumb" and "connection" sub-domains of HBV RT are approximations since there is no significant homology between HIV-1 and HBV in these regions. The coordinates of the three asp residues which comprise the carboxylate triad of the active site are shown above each diagram. Shown below the diagrams are the coordinates of the wild-type sequence of HBV RT. The corresponding amino acids of HIV-1 RT are also indicated. Amino acids which are invariant between HIV-1 and HBV are shown in bold and the conserved YMDD motif is boxed. Amino acid sequence alterations found in the RT domain of reported drug-resistant variants of HBV are indicated. Numbering of the RT of HBV is according to Bartholomeusz and Locarnini [15].

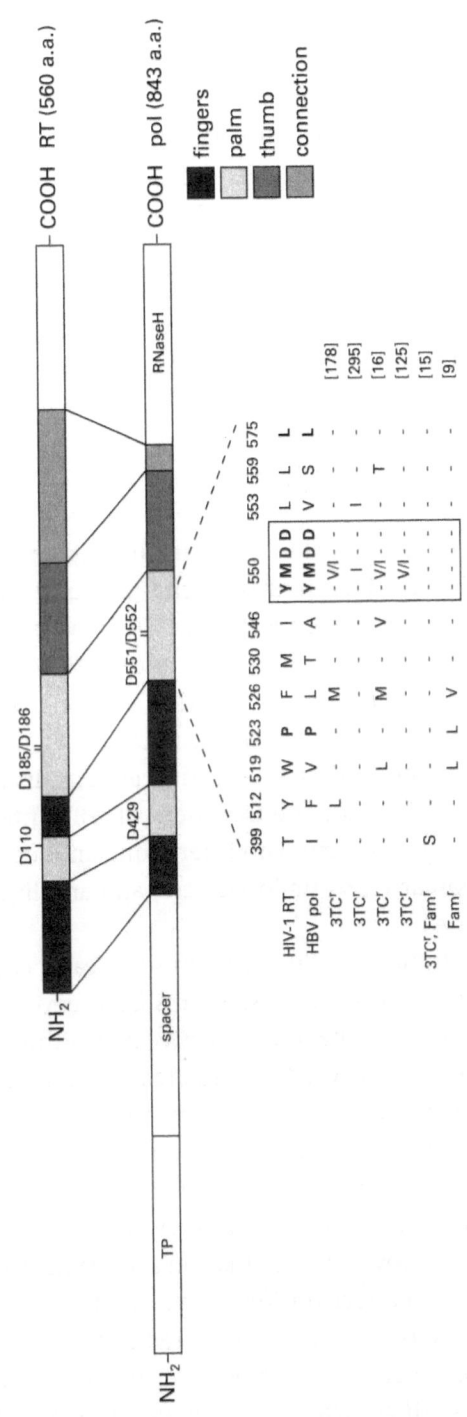

polymerase ORF, the mutations in the polymerase of drug-resistant viruses will lead also to changes in this envelope protein. Thus the issue of altered antigenicity among drug-resistant HBV variants possibly leading to altered sensitivity to neutralizing antibodies needs to be fully addressed. Indeed, in a recent study an HBsAg variant (G130D) along with the M550V substitution in the polymerase protein emerged in a patient treated with lamivudine [216a]. Moreover, several new famciclovir treatment-induced substitutions in the polymerase, which are predicted to lead to amino acid substitutions in or near the "a" determinant of HbsAg, have been described [259a].

9   Combination therapies

The emergence of clinical resistance to lamivudine, famciclovir, and possibly to other nucleoside analogs points to the difficulty in suppressing completely and permanently the replication of HBV *in vivo*. It is unlikely that the use of a single agent will result in the clearance of HBV infection. *In vitro* systems and animal models of HBV infection can be used for evaluation of potentially useful drug combinations including relevant nucleoside analogs, immunomodulators, and other treatment regimens. In this review, a number of drug combinations for the treatment of HBV infection have already been discussed such as ribavirin with interferon, lamivudine with interferon, ganciclovir with foscarnet or nalidixic acid, and ampligen with ganciclovir and coumermycin A1.

Earlier clinical studies indicated that in some cases combination therapy is more effective than monotherapy. For instance, acyclovir in combination with interferon appeared to be more effective than either alone and was well-tolerated in chronically infected patients [247]. Another study, using prednisolone withdrawal therapy followed by treatment with ara-A, demonstrated that the combination of an immunomodulatory agent with an antiviral is more efficacious than is monotherapy [216]. A recent study using hepatocytes derived from congenitally infected ducklings showed that lamivudine and famciclovir in combination acted synergistically over a range of clinically relevant concentrations. Importantly, this combination was more effective than either agent alone in reducing levels of CCC DNA [60]. This important observation indicates that the combination of these two drugs, both in Phase III clinical trials, may be effective in humans.

A number of issues concerning combination therapy needs to be resolved as discussed by Fontana and Lok [92]. These include whether the combination therapy will have additive or synergistic antiviral effects in humans, whether the prolonged use of combination therapy will result in greater toxicity, whether combination therapy will, as is hoped, delay or prevent the emergence of resistant variants, and finally, whether these variants will be cross-resistant to either agent alone. Although final resolution of these issues will require evaluation in animal models and, ultimately in the clinical setting, we can begin to address these questions using cell culture systems and animal models. For instance, using HBV-producing HepG2.2.15 cells, it has been shown that the combination of lamivudine with either interferon alpha or famciclovir increased the antiviral potency of these agents [149]. Building on these studies, it was shown very recently that a combination of lamivudine and IFNα was more effective than either alone in treating woodchucks chronically infected with WHV [153a].

10   Future directions

Since the discovery of the Dane particle as the etiologic agent of hepatitis type B infection, much has been learned concerning the molecular biology of the hepadnavirus genome and its replication. The in-depth knowledge of the replication of viral DNA has provided targets for the chemotherapeutic intervention of this process. Most notably, nucleoside analogs have been identified and developed which inhibit viral DNA replication and which have clinical utility. However, notwithstanding the rapid gains in our understanding of hepadnaviruses, there are still a number of areas in which the development of antiviral approaches has not been fully explored.

The difficulty in expressing functional hepadnaviral reverse transcriptases disassociated from the virion has limited our ability to identify novel and non-nucleoside inhibitors of this enzyme as has been accomplished for HIV reverse transcriptase [70]. The establishment of a cell-free *in vitro* translation system for DHBV reverse transcriptase [308], the expression of DHBV reverse transcriptase in yeast [285], and the expression of HBV reverse transcriptase in frog oocytes [259] or in a baculovirus system [161] are encouraging steps towards the development of assays which may uncover novel inhibitors of virus DNA replication.

Although hepadnaviruses appear to have a strict tropism for hepatocytes, the host cell receptor(s) for these viruses has not been unequivocally identified and characterized. Once the receptor is known, identification of inhibitors of virus attachment and entry into the cell may be facilitated. Additionally, the development of cell culture infection systems for hepadnaviruses may become feasible. This would enable the development of assays which can examine all stages of the virus infection cycle in detail.

As we learn more regarding the immunopathogenesis of HBV infection, it is hoped that new ways to modulate the host immune system in order to clear virus infection will be developed. For instance, the CTL response appears to play an important role in the clearance of HBV infection (reviewed in [47]) and recently Theradigm-HBV, a lipopeptide-based therapeutic vaccine designed to elicit an HBV-specific CTL response, has been described [45, 179]. In one clinical study, CY-1899, a therapeutic vaccine comprised of the hepatitis B core CTL epitope linked to a T helper epitope was shown to induce an HBV-specific CTL response but further studies are needed to determine the clinical efficacy of this approach [116].

Gene therapy has not been fully exploited and may offer novel approaches for the treatment of HBV infection. Gene therapy can be used for the intracellular expression of peptides or proteins which interfere with the virus replication cycle, an approach referred to as "intracellular immunization" [12]. Along these lines, it has been demonstrated that when expressed intracellulary, incompletely processed and non-secretory forms of the hepatitis B pre-Core protein [112, 159, 246] and dominant negative mutants of the core protein are inhibitors of HBV DNA replication [243, 245, 307]. In novel studies in which the C-terminal basic domain of the core protein of HBV was replaced with *Staphylococcus aureus* nuclease and co-expressed with wild-type core protein, chimeric virus particles were formed that contained enzymatically active nuclease [22a]. These results indicate that foreign proteins which can be used to inhibit virus replication can be incorporated into the virus capsid, thus comprising a "Trojan Horse" approach to anti-HBV therapy.

In the future it is expected that a more thorough understanding of the natural history of HBV disease will allow the successful implementation of existing approaches such as nucleoside analogs and their use in combination with other nucleoside analogs, with interferon, or with other immune modulators. A greater understanding of the disease process will also enable investigators to evaluate more fully the novel and untested approaches discussed in this review.

Acknowledgment

The authors thank Dr. Raymond F. Schinazi and Dr. Beverly Heinz for helpful comments and a critical review of the manuscript.

References

1   Abbruzzese, J.L., Schmidt, S., Raber, M.N., Levy, J.K., Castellanos, A.M., Legha, S.S. and Kroakoff I.H.: Invest. New Drugs 7, 195–201 (1989).

2   Acs, G., Sells, M.A., Purcell, R.H., Price, P., Engle, R., Shapiro, M. and Popper, H.: Proc. Natl. Acad. Sci. USA 84, 4641–4644 (1987).

2a Aguesse-Germon, S., Liu, S.H., Chevallier, M., Pichoud, C., Jamard, C., Borel, C., Chu, C.K., Trepo, C., Cheng, Y.C. and Zoulim, F.: Antimicrob. Agents Chemother. 42, 369–376 (1998).

3   Aldrich, C.E., Coates, L., Wu, T.T., Newbold, J., Tennant, B.C., Summers, J., Seeger, C. and Mason, W.S.: Virology 172, 247–252 (1989).

4   Alexander, G.J., Fagan, E.A., Hegarty, J.E., Yeo, J., Eddleston, A.L. and Williams, R.: J. Med. Virol. 21, 81–87 (1987).

4a Allen, M.I., Deslauriers, M., Andrews, C.W., Tipples, G.A., Walters, K.A., Tyrrell, D.L., Brown, N. (for the Lamivudine Clinical Investigation Group) and Condreay, L.D.: Hepatology 27, 1670–1677 (1998).

5   Anand, B.S., Yoffe, B. and Young, J.B.: J. Clin. Gastroenterology 22, 144–146 (1996).

6   Araki, K., Miyazaki, J., Hino, O., Tomita, N., Chisaka, O., Matsubara, K. and Yamamura, K.: Proc. Natl. Acad. Sci. USA 86, 207–211 (1989).

7   Ashwell, G. and Hartford, J.: Annu. Rev. Biochem. 51, 531–534 (1982).

8   Aye, T.T., Bartholomeuz, A., Shaw, T., Breschkin, A., Groenen, L., Bowden, S., McMillan, J., Angus, P., McCaughan, G.W. and Locarnini, S.: Hepatology 24, 285A (1996).

9   Aye, T.T., Bartholomeuz, A., Shaw, T., Bowden, S., Breschkin, A., McMillan, J., Angus, P. and Locarnini, S.: J. Hepatology 26, 1148–1153 (1997).

10 Bain, V.G., Daniels, H.M., Chanas, A., Alexander, G.J.M. and Williams, R.: J. Med. Virol. 29, 152–155 (1989).

11 Bain, V.G., Kneteman, N.M., Ma, M.M., Gutfreund, K., Shapiro, J.A., Fischer, K., Tipples, G., Lee, H., Jewell, L.D. and Tyrrell, D.L.: Transplantation 62, 1456–1462 (1996).

12 Baltimore, D.: Nature 325, 395–396 (1988).

13 Balzarini, .J, Kruining, J., Wedgwood, O., Pannecouque, C., Aquaro, S., Perno, C.F., Naesens, L., Witvrouw, M., Heijtink, R., De Clercq, E. and McGuigan, C.: FEBS Lett. 410, 324–328 (1997).

14 Barditch-Crovo, P., Toole, J., Hendrix, C.W., Cundy, K.C., Ebeling, D., Jaffe, H.S. and Lietman, P.S.: J. Inf. Dis. 176, 406–413 (1997).

15 Bartholomeusz, A. and Locarnini, S.: Intl. Antiviral News 5, 123–124 (1997).

15a Bartholomeusz, A., Groenen, L.C. and Locarnini, S.A.: Intervirology 40, 337–342 (1997).

16 Bartholomew, M.M., Jansen, R.W., Jeffers, L.J., Reddy, K.R., Johnson, L.C., Bunzendahl, H., Condreay, L.D., Tzakis, A.G., Schiff, E.R. and Brown, N.A.: Lancet 349, 20–22 (1997).

17 Bassendine, M.P., Chadwick, R.G., Salmeron, J., Shipton, U., Thomas, H.C. and Sherlock, S.: Gastroenterology 80, 1016–1022 (1981).

18 Bean, B.: Clin. Microbiol. Rev. 5, 146–182 (1992).

19 Beck, J. and Nassal, M.: Nucleic Acids Res. 23, 4954–4962 (1995).

20 Benhamou, Y., Katlama, C., Lunel, F., Coutellier, A., Dohin, E., Hamm, N., Tubiana, R., Herson, S., Poynard, T. and Opolom, P.: Ann. Int. Med. 125, 705–712 (1996).

21 Berk, L., Schalm, S.W. and Heijtink, R.A.: Antiviral Res. 19, 111–118 (1992).

22 Berk, L., Schalm, S.W., de Man, R.A., Heijtink, R.A., Berthelot, P., Brechot, C., Boboc, B., Degos et al.: J. Hepatology 14, 305–309 (1992).

22a Beterams, G., Bottcher, B. and Nassal, M.: FEBS Lett. 481, 169–176 (2000).

23 Bisacchi, G.S., Chao, S.T., Bachard, C., Daris, J.P., Innaimo, S., Jacobs, G.A., Kocy, O., Lapointe, P., Martel, A., Merchant, Z., Slusarchyk, W.A., Sundeen, J.I., Young, M.G., Colonno, R. and Zahler, R.: Bioorg. Med. Chem. Lett. 7, 127–132 (1997).

23a Block, T.M., Lu, X., Mehta, A.S., Blumberg, B.S., Tennant, B., Ebling, M., Korba, B., Lansky, D.M., Jacob, G.S. and Dwek, R.A.: Nat. Med. 4, 610–614 (1998).

24 Block, T.M., Lu, X., Platt, F.M., Foster, G.R., Gerlich, W.H., Blumberg, B.S. and Dwek, R.A.: Proc. Natl. Acad. Sci. USA 91, 2235–2239 (1994).

25 Blum, H.E., Zhang, Z.S., Galun, E., von Weizsacker, F., Garner, B., Liang, T.J. and Wands, J.R.: J Virol. 66, 1223–1227 (1992).

26 Boker, K.H.W., Ringe, B., Kruger, M., Pichlmayer, R. and Manns, M.P.: Transplantation 57, 1706–1708 (1994).

27 Boyd, M.R., Bacon, T.H., Sutton, D. and Cole, M.: Antimicrob. Agents Chemother. 31, 1238–1242 (1987).

28 Brook, M.G., Petrovic, L., McDonald, J.A., Scheuer, P.J. and Thomas, H.C.: J. Hepatol. 8, 218–225 (1989).

29 Bruss, V. and Ganem, D.: Proc. Natl. Acad. Sci. USA 88, 1059–1063 (1991).

30 Bunnell, B.A., Askari, F.K. and Wilson, J.M.: Cell Mol. Genet. 18, 559–569 (1992).

31 Burgess, J.B., Baenziger, J.U. and Brown, W.R.: Hepatology 15, 702–706 (1992).

32 Catapano, C.V., Perrino, F.W. and Fernandes, D.J.: J. Biol. Chem. 268, 7179–7185 (1993).

33 Catterall, A.P., Moyle, G.J., Hopes, E.A., Harrison, T.J., Gazzard, B.G. and Murray-Lyon, I.M.: J. Med. Virol. 37, 307–309 (1992).

34 Cerenzia, M.T., Fiume, L., Venon, W.D.B., Lavezzo, B., Brunetto, M.R., Ponzetto, M., Di Stefano, G., Busi, C., Mattioli, A., Gervasi, G.B., Bonino, F. and Verme, G.: Hepatology 23, 657–661 (1996).

35 Chachoua, A., Dieterich, D., Krasinski, K., Greene, J., Laubenstein, L., Wernz, J., Buhles, W. and Koretz, S.: Ann. Int. Med. 107, 133–137 (1987).

36 Chang, .IM.: Phytotherapy Res. 11, 189–192 (1997).

37 Chang, C.M., Jeng, K.S., Hu, C.P., Lo, S.J., Su, T.S., Ting, L.P., Chou, C.K., Han, S.H., Pfaff, E., Salfeld, J., et al.: EMBO J. 6, 675–680 (1987).

38 Chang, C.N., Doong, S.L., Zhou, J.H., Beach, J.W., Jeong, L.S., Chu, C.K., Tsai, C.H., Cheng, Y.C., Liotta, D. and Schinazi, R.: J. Biol. Chem. 267, 13938–13942 (1992).

39 Chang, L.J., Pryciak, P., Ganem, D. and Varmus, H.E.: Nature 337, 364–368 (1989).

40 Charvet, A.S., Turin, F., Faury, P., Hantz, O., Camplo, M., Mourier, N., Berthillon, P., Graciet, J.C., Chermann, J.C., Trepo, C. and Kraus, J.L.: Antiviral Res. 25, 161–168 (1994).

41 Chen, C.H. and Cheng, Y.C.: J. Biol. Chem. 264, 11934–11937 (1989).

42 Chen, C.H. and Cheng, Y.C.: J. Biol. Chem. 267, 2856–2859 (1992).

43 Chen, H.C., Chou, C.K., Sun, C.M. and Yeh, S.F.: Antiviral Res. 34, 137–144 (1997).

43a   Chen, H., Schinazi, R.F., Rajagopalan, P., Gao, Z., Chu, C.K., McClure, H.M. and Boudinot, F.D.: AIDS Res. Hum. Retroviruses 15, 1625–1630 (1999).

44   Chen, M.S., Van Nostrand, M. and Oshana, S.C.: Anal. Biochem. 156, 300–304 (1986).

45   Chesnut, R.W., Sette, A., Celis, E., Wentworth, P., Kubo, R.T., Alexander, J., Ishioka, G., Vitiello, A. and Grey, H.M.: Pharmaceutical Biotechnology 6, 847–874 (1995).

46   Chiou, J.F. and Cheng, Y.C.: Agents Chemother. 27, 416–418 (1985).

47   Chisari, F.V. and Ferrari, C.: Annu. Rev. Immunol. 13, 29–60 (1995).

48   Chisari, F.V., Ferrari, C. and Mondelli, M.U.: Microbial Pathogenesis 6, 311–325 (1989).

48a   Cho, G., Park, S.G. and Jung, G.: Biochem. Biophys. Res. Commun. 269, 191–196 (2000a).

48b   Cho, G., Suh, S.W. and Jung, G.: Biochem. Biophys. Res. Commun. 274, 203–211 (2000b).

49   Chou, T.C., Kong, X.B., Fanucchi, M.P., Cheng, Y.C., Takahashi, K., Watanabe, K.A. and Fox, J.J.: Antimicrob Agents Chemother. 31, 1355–1358 (1987).

49a   Chu, C.K., Boudinot, F.D., Peek, S.F., Hong, J.A., Choi, Y., Korba, B.E., Gerin, J.L., Cote, P.J., Tennant, B.C. and Cheng, Y.C.: Antivir. Ther. 3, 113–121 (1998).

50   Chu, C.K., Ma, T., Shanmuganathan, K., Wang, C., Xiang, Y., Pai, S.B., Yao, G.Q., Sommadossi, J.P. and Cheng, Y.C.: Antimicrob. Agents Chemother. 39, 979–981 (1995).

51   Civitico, G.M. and Locarnini, S.A.: Virology 203, 81–89 (1994).

52   Civitico, G., Shaw, T. and Locarnini, S.: Antimicrob. Agents Chemother. 40, 1180–1185 (1996).

53   Civitico, G., Wang, Y.Y., Luscombe, C., Bishop, N., Tachedjian, G., Gust, I. and Locarnini, S.: J. Med. Virol. 31, 90–97 (1990).

54   Coates, J.A., Cammack, N, and Jenkinson, H.J.: Antimicrob. Agents Chemother. 36, 202–205 (1992).

55   Colacino, J.M.: Antiviral Res. 29, 125–139 (1996).

56   Colacino, J. and Lopez, C.: Antimicrob. Agents Chemother. 25, 505–508 (1983).

57   Colacino, J., Brownridge, E., Greenberg, N. and Lopez, C.: Antimicrob. Agents Chemother. 29, 877–892 (1986).

58   Colacino, J.M., Malcolm, S.K. and Jaskunas, S.R.: Antimicrob. Agents Chemother. 38, 1997–2002 (1994).

59   Colacino, J.M., Horn, J.W., Horn D,M. and Richardson, F.C.: Tox. In Vitro 10, 297–303 (1996).

59a   Colacino, J.M. and Staschke, K.A.: Prog. Drug Res. 50, 259–322 (1998).

60   Colledge, D., Locarnini, S. and Shaw, T.: Hepatology 26, 216–225 (1997).

61   Colonno, R.J., Innaimo, S.F., Seifer, M., Genovesi, E., Clark, J., Yamanaka, G., Hamatake, R., Terry, B., Standring, D., Bisacchi, G., Sundeen, J. and Zahler, R.: Antiviral Res. 34, A51 (1997).

61a   Colonno, R.J., Genovesi, E.V., Medina, I., Lamb, L., Durham, S., Corey, L., Locarnini, S., Tennant, B.C. and Clark, J.M.: 40th Interscience Conference on Antimicrobial Agents and Chemotherapy, Abst. 172 (2000).

62   Condreay, L.D., Jansen, R.W., Powdrill, T.F., Johnson, L.C., Selleseth, D.W., Paff, M.T., Daluge, S.M., Painter, G.R., Furman, P.A., Ellis, M.N. and Averett, D.R.: Antimicrob. Agents Chemother. 38, 616–619 (1994).

63   Condreay, L.D., Condreay, J.P., Jansen, R.W., Paff, M.T. and Averett, D.R.: Antimicrob. Agents Chemother. 40, 520–523 (1996).

64   Cui, L., Yoon, S., Schinazi, R.F. and Sommadossi, J.P.: J. Clin. Inv. 95, 555–563 (1995).

65   Cui L., Schinazi, R.F., Gosselin, G., Imbach, J.L., Chu, C.K., Rando, R.F., Revankar, G.R., Sommadossi, J.P.: Bioch. Pharm. *52*, 1577–1584 (1996).
66   Cullen, J.M., Smith, S.L., Davis, M.G., Dunn, S.E., Botteron, C., Cecchi, A., Linsey, D., Linzey, D., Frick, L., Paff, M.T., Goulding, A. and Biron, K. Antimicrob. Agents Chemother. *41*, 2076–2082 (1997).
67   Cundy, K.C., Fishback, J.A., Shaw, J.P., Lee, M.L., Soike, K.F, Visor, G.C. and Lee, W.A.: Pharm. Res. *11*, 839–843 (1994).
68   Dannaoui, E., Trepo, C. and Zoulim, F.: Antiviral Chem. Chemother. *8*, 38–46 (1997).
69   Davis, M.G., Wilson, J.E., Van Draanen, N.A., Miller, W.H., Freeman, G.A., Daluge, S.M., Boyd, F.L., Aulabaugh, A.E., Painter, F.R. and Boone, L.R.: Antiviral Res. *30*, 133–145 (1996).
70   De Clercq, E.: AIDS Res. Human Retroviruses *8*, 119–134 (1992).
70a   de Man, R.A., Marcellin, P., Habgal, F., Desmond, P., Wright, T., Rose, T., Jurewicz, R. and Young, C.: Hepatology *32*, 413–417 (2000).
71   Denes A.E., Ebert, J.W., Berquist, K.R, Murphy, B.L. and Maynard, J.E.: Antimicrob. Agents Chemother. *10*, 571–572 (1976).
72   DeNoon, D.J.: Hepatitis Weekly, October 21, 1996.
73   Dienstag, J.L., Perrillo, R.P., Schiff, E.R, Bartholomew, M., Vicary, C., Rubin, M.: J. Hepatology *20*, 199A (1994).
73a   Dienstag, J.L., Schiff, E.R., Mitchell, M., Casey, D.E. Jr., Gitlin, N., Lissoos, T., Gelb, L.D., Condreay, L., Crowther, L., Rubin, M. and Brown, N.: Hepatology *30*, 1082–1087 (1999).
74   Doong, S.L., Tsai, C.H., Schinazi R.F., Liotta, D.C. and Cheng Y.C.: Proc. Natl. Acad. Sci. USA *88*, 8495–8499 (1991).
75   El Alaoui, A.M., Faraj, A., Pierra, C., Boudou, V., Johnson, R., Mathe, C., Gosselin G., Korba, B.E., Imbach, J.L., Schinazi R.F. and Sommadossi, J.P.: Antiviral Chem. Chemother. *7*, 276–280 (1996).
76   Elion, G.B.: J. Med. Virol. Suppl. *1*, S2–S6 (1993).
77   Enriquez, P.M., Jung, C., Josephson, L. and Tennant, B.C.: Bioconjugate Chem. *6*, 195–202 (1995).
78   Eriksson, B. and Oberg, B., in: Becker, Y. (ed.): Antiviral Drugs and Interferon, Martinus Nijhoff Publishing, Boston 1984, pp. 127–142.
79   Etta, L.V., Brown, J., Mastri, A. and Wilson, T.: J. Am. Med. Assoc. *246*, 1073–1075 (1981).
80   Fanucchi, M.P., Leyland-Jones, B., Young, C.W., Burchenal, J.H., Watanabe, K.A., Fox, J.J.: Cancer Treat. Rpts. *69*, 55–59 (1985).
81   Farquhar, D., Kahn, S., Srivastva, D.N., Saunders, P.P.: J. Med. Chem. *37*, 3902–3909 (1994).
82   Farza, H., Hadchouel, M., Scotto, J., Tiollais, P., Babinet, C. and Pourcel, C.: J. Virol. *62*, 4144–4152 (1988).
83   Feitelson, M.A., Millman, I., Halbherr, T., Simmons, H. and Blumberg, B.S.: Proc. Natl. Acad. Sci. USA *83*, 2233–2237 (1986).
84   Feitelson, M.A., Millman, I. and Blumberg, B.S.: Proc. Natl. Acad. Sci. USA. *83*, 2994–2997 (1986).
85   Field, A.K. and Goodchild, J.: Exp. Opin. Invest. Drugs *4*, 799–821 (1995).
86   Field, A.K., Davies, M.E., DeWitt, C., Perry, H.C., Liou, R., Germershausen, J., Karkas, J.D., Ashton, W.T., Johnston, D.B.R. and Tolman, R.L.: Proc. Natl. Acad. Sci. USA *80*, 4139–4143 (1983).
87   Fischer, K.P. and Tyrrell, D.L.J.: Antimicrob. Agents Chemother. *40*, 1957–1960 (1996).

88   Fiume, L., Busi, C., Mattioli, A., Balboni, P.G., Barbanti-Brodano, G.: FEBS Lett. *129*, 261–264 (1981).

89   Fiume, L., Bassi, B., Busi, C., Mattioli, A. and Spinosa, G.: Biochem. Pharmacol. 35, 967–972 (1986).

90   Fiume, L., Bassi, B., Busi, C., Mattioli, A., Sinosa, G. and Faulstich, H.: FEBS Lett. *203*, 203–206 (1986).

91   Fleet, G.W., Karpas, A., Dwek, R.A., Fellows, L.E., Tyms, A.S., Petursson, S., Namgoong, S.K., Ramsden, N.G., Smith, P.W., Son, J.C., Wilson, F., Witty, D.R., Jacob, G.S. and Radenmacher, T.W.: FEBS Lett. 237, 128–132 (1988).

92   Fontana, R.J. and Lok, A.S.F.: Hepatology *26*, 234–237 (1997).

93   Fourel, I., Hantz, O., Cova, L., Allaudeen, H.S. and Trepo, C.: Antimicrob. Agents Chemother. *34*, 473–475 (1990).

94   Fourel, I., Li, J., Hantz, O., Jacquet, C., Fox, J.J. and Trepo, C.: J. Med. Virol. *37*, 122–126 (1992).

95   Fourel, I., Saputelli, J., Schaffer, P.A. and Mason, W.S.: J. Virol. *68*, 1059–1065 (1994).

96   Fox, J.J., Watanabe, K.A., Chou, T.C., Schinazi R.F., Soike, K.F., Fourel, I., Hantz, O. and Trepo, C., in: Taylor, F.N. (ed.): Fluorinated Carbohydrates, Chemical and Biochemical Aspects, American Chemical Society, Washington, D.C. 1988, pp. 176–190.

97   Fried, M.W., Di Bisceglie, A.M., Straus, S.E., Savarese, B., Beames, M.P. and Hoofnagle, J.H.: Hepatology *16*, 127a (1992).

98   Fried, M.W., Fong, T.L., Swain, M.G., Beames, P.Y., Banks, S.M., Hoofnagle, J.H., Di Bisceglie, A.M.: J. Hepatology *21*, 145–150 (1994).

98a   Fu, L., Liu, S.H. and Cheng, Y.C.: Biochem. Pharmacol. *57*, 1351–1359 (1999).

99   Furman, P.A., Davis, M., Liotta, D.C., Paff, M., Frick, L.W., Nelson, D.J., Dornsife, R.E., Wurster, J.A., Wilson, L.J., Fyfe, J.A., Tuttle, J.V., Miller, W.H., Condreay, L., Averett, D.R., Schinazi, R.F. and Painter, G.R.: Antimicrob. Agents Chemother. *36*, 2686–2692 (1992).

100   Furman, P.A., Wilson, J.E., Reardon, J.E. and Painter, G.R.: Antiviral Chem. Chemother. *6*, 345–355 (1995).

101   Galle, P.R., Schlicht, H.J., F.ischer, M., Schaller H.: 1988. Production of infectious duck hepatitis B virus in a human hepatoma cell line. J. Virol. 62, 1736–1740 ().

102   Galle, P.R., Schlicht H.J., Kuhn, C., Schaller, H.: Hepatology *10*, 459–465 (1989).

102a   Galun, E., Nahor, O., Eid, A., Jurim, O., Rose-John, S., Blum, H.E., Nussbaum, O., Ilan, E., Daudi, N., Shouval, D. et al.: Virology *270*, 299–309 (2000).

103   Ganem, D., in: Fields, B.N., Knipe, D.M., Howley, P.M. (eds.): Virology, Lippincott-Raven Publishers, Philadelphia 1996, pp. 2703–2737.

104   Ganem, D. and Varmus, H.E.: Annu. Rev. Biochem. *56*, 651–693 (1987).

104a   Gao, H.Q., Boyer, P.L., Sarafianos, S.G., Arnold, E. and Hughes, S.H.: J. Mol. Biol. *300*, 403–418 (2000).

104b   Genovesi, E.V., Lamb, L., Medina, I., Taylor, D., Seifer, M., Innaimo, S., Colonno, R.J., Standring, D.N. and Clark, J.M.: Antimicrob. Agents Chemother. *42*, 3209–3217 (1998).

104c   Gilson, R.J.C., Chopra, K.B., Newell, A.M., Murray-Lyon, I.M., Nelson, M.R., Rice, S.J., Tedder, R.S., Toole, J., Jaffe, H.S. and Weller, I.V.: J. Viral Hep. *6*, 387–395 (1999).

105   Gish, R.G., Lau, J.Y., Brooks, L., Fang, J.W., Steady, S.L., Imperial, J.C., Garcia-Kennedy R., Esquivel, C.O. and Keeffe, E.B.: Hepatology. *23*, 1–7 (1996).

106   Gojobori, T. and Yokoyama, S.: Proc. Natl. Acad. Sci. USA *82*, 4198–4201 (1985).

107   Gojobori, T., Moriyama, E.N. and Kimura, M.: Proc. Natl. Acad. Sci. USA *87*, 10015–10018 (1990).

108   Goodarzi G., Gross, S.C., Tewari, A. and Watabe, K.: J. Gen. Virol. *71*, 3021–3025 (1990).

109   Grant, A.J., Feinberg, A., Chou, T.C., Watanabe, K.A., Fox, J.J. and Philips, F.S.: Bioch. Pharmacol. *31*, 1103–1108 (1982).

110   Grellier, L., Mutimer, D., Ahmed, M., Brown, D., Burroughs, A.K., Rolles, K., McMaster, P., Beranek, P., Kennedy, F., Kibbler, H., McPhillips, P., Elias, E. and Dushieko, G.: Lancet *348*, 1212–1215 (1996).

111   Gripon, P., Diot, C., Theze, N., Fourel, I., Loreal, O., Brechot, C., Guguen-Guillouzo, C.: J. Virol. *62*, 4136–4143 (1988).

112   Guidotti, L.G., Matzke, B., Pasquinelli, C., Schoenberger, J.M., Rogler, C.E., Chisari, F.V.: J. Virol. *70*, 7056–7061 (1996).

113   Hagelstein, J., Fathinejad, F., Stemmel, W. and Galle, P.R.: Virology *229*, 292–294 (1997).

113a   Hagmeyer, K.O. and Pan, Y.Y.: Annals Pharmacother. *33*, 1104–1112 (1999).

114   Hantz, O., Allaudeen, H.S., Ooka, T., De Clercq, E. and Trepo, C.: Antiviral Res. *4*, 187–199 (1984).

115   Harrell, A.W., Wheeler, S.M., Pennick, M., Clarke, S.E., Chenery, R.J.: Drug Met. Disp. *21*, 18–23 (1993).

116   Heathcote, J., McHutchison, J., Benner, K., Wright, T., Minuk, G., Sacks, S., Sherman, M., Rustgi, V., Perrillo, R., King, P., Redeker, A., Davis, G., Lok, A. and Chesnut, R.: Hepatology *24*, 283A (1996).

117   Heijtink, R.A., De Wilde, G.A., Kruining, J., Berk, L., Balzarini, J., De Clercq, E., Holy, A. and Schalm, S.W.: Antiviral Res. *21*, 141–153 (1993).

118   Helgstrand, E., Eriksson, B., Johansson, N.G., Lannero, B., Larsson, A., Misiorny, A., Noren, J.O., Sjoberg, B., Stenberg, K., Stening, G., Stridh, S. and Oberg, B.: Science *201*, 819–821 (1978).

119   Hess, G., Arnold, W. and Meyer zum Buschenfelde, K.H.: J. of Med. Virol. 5, 309–316 (1980).

120   Hino, O., Nomura, K., Ohtake, K., Saito, I., Abe, K., Rogler, C.E., Sugano, H. and Kitagawa, T.: Gastroenterologia Japonica *25*, (Suppl. 2), 53–56 (1990).

121   Hirota, K., Sherker, A.H., Omata, M., Yokosuka, O., Okuda, K.: Hepatology 7, 24–28 (1987).

122   Honkoop, P., de Man, R.A., Zondervan, P.E. and Schalm, S.W.: Liver *17*, 103–106 (1997).

123   Honkoop, P., de Man, R.A., Scholte, H.R., Zondervan, P.I., van den Berg, J.W.O., Rademakers, L.H.P.M. and Schalm, S.W.: Hepatology *26*, 211–215 (1997).

124   Honkoop, P., Niesters, H.G.M., De Man, R.A., Osterhaus, A.D.M.E. and Schalm, S.W.: c. J. Hepatology 26, 1393–1395 (1997).

125   Honkoop, P., Scholte, H.R., de Man, R.A. and Schalm, S.W.: Drug Safety 17, 1–7 (1997).

126   Hoofnagle, J.H., Di Bisceglie, A.M.: N. Engl. J. Med. *336*, 347–356 (1997).

127   Hoofnagle, J.H., Lau, D.: N. Engl J. Med. *334*, 1470–1471 (1996).

128   Hoofnagle, J.H., Dushieko, G.M., Seeff, L.B., Jones, E.A., Waggoner, J.G., Bales, Z.B.: Ann. Intern. Med. *94*, 744–748 (1981).

129   Hoofnagle, J.H., Minuk, G.Y., Dusheiko, G.M., Schafer, D.F., Johnson, R., Straus, S., Jones, E.A., Gerin, J.L. and Ishak, K.: Hepatology *2*, 784–788 (1982).

130   Hoofnagle, J.H., Hanson, R.G., Minuk, G.Y., Pappas, S.C., Schafer, D.F., Dusheiko, G.M., Straus, S.E., Popper, H. and Jones, E.: Gastroenterology *86*, 150–157 (1984).

131   Hoofnagle, J.H., Davis, G.L., Hanson, R.G., Pappas, S.C, Peters, M.G., Avigan, M.I., Waggoner J.G., Howard, R., Jones, E.A. and Straus, S.E.: J. Med. Virol. *15*, 121–128 (1985).

131a   Hostetler, K.Y., Beadle, J.R., Hornbuckle, W.E., Bellezza, C.A., Tochkov, I.A., Cote, P.J.,

Gerin, J.L., Korba, B.E. and Tennant, B.C.: Antimicrob. Agents Chemother. *44*, 1964–1969 (2000).

132 Hostetler, K.Y, Beadle, J.R., Kini, G.D., Gardner, M.F., Wright, K.N, Wu, T.H. and Korba, B.A.: Biochem. Pharmacol. *53*, 1815–1822 (1997).

133 Howe, A.Y.M., Elliott, J.F. and Tyrrell, D.L.J.: Bioch. Biophys. Res. Comm. *189*, 1170–1176 (1992).

134 Hu, J. and Seeger, C.: Proc. Natl. Acad. Sci. USA *93*, 1060–1064 (1996).

135 Hu, J., Toft, D.O. and Seeger, C.: EMBO J. *16*, 59–68 (1997).

136 Hudson, J.B., Lopez-Bazzocchi, I. and Towers, G.H.N.: Antiviral Res. *15*, 101–112 (1991).

137 Ikeda, N., Kaneko, S., Shimoda, A., Inagaki, Y., Unoura, M., Yonekawa, Y., Takahasi, K. and Kobayashi, K.: J. Animicrob. Chemother. *33*, 83–89 (1994).

137a Innaimo, S.F., Seifer, M., Bisacchi, G.S., Standring, D.N., Zahler, R. and Colonno, R.J.: Antimicrob. Agents. Chemother. *41*, 1444–1448 (1997).

138 Innaimo, S.F., Seifer, M., Bisacchi, G.S., Standring, D.N., Zahler, R., Colonno, R.J.: Antimicrob. Agents. Chemother. *41*, 1444–1448 (1997).

139 Jacyna, M.R. and Thomas, H.C.: British Med. Bull. *46*, 368–382 (1990).

139a Jarvis, B. and Faulds, D.: Drugs *58*, 101–141 (1999).

140 Jilg, W., Schmidt, M., Deinhardt, F., Zachoval, R.: Lancet *2*, 458 (1989).

140a Josefson, D.: BMJ *317*, 1034 (1998).

141 Kakumu, S., Yoshioka, K., Wakita, T., Ishikawa, T., Takayanagi, M. and Higashi, Y.: Hepatology *18*, 258–263 (1993).

142 Karpas, A., Fleet, G.W., Dwek, R.A., Petursson, S., Namgoong, S.K., Ramsden, N.G., Jacob, G.S. and Rademacher, T.W.: Proc. Natl. Acad. Sci. USA *85*, 9229–9233 (1988).

143 Kassianides, C., Hoofnagle, J.H., Miller, R.H., Doo, E., Ford, H., Broder, S. and Mitsuya, H.: Gastroenterology *97*, 1275–1280 (1989).

144 Khudyakov, Y.E. and Makhov, A.M.: FEBS Lett. *243*, 115–118 (1989).

145 Klecker, R.W., Katki, A.G., Collins, J.M.: Mol. Pharmac. *46*, 1204–1209 (1994).

145a Klein, N.P., Bouchard, M.J., Wang, L.H., Kobarg, C. and Schneider, R.J.: EMBO *18*, 5019–5027 (1999).

146 Klein, M., Geoghegan, J., Schmidt, K., Bockler, D., Korn, K., Wittekind, C., Scheele, J.: . Transplantation *64*, 162–163 (1997).

146a Knaus, E.E., Parang, K., Wiebe, L.I., Huang, J.S. and Tyrrell, D.L.: J. Pharm Pharm. Sci. *1*, 108–114 (1998).

147 Kock, J., Borst, E.M. and Schlicht, H.J.: J. Virol. *70*, 5827–5831 (1996).

148 Kohlstaedt, L.A., Wang, J., Friedman, J.M., Rice, P.A. and Steitz, T.A.: Science *256*, 1783–1790 (1992).

148a Korba, B.E., Cote, P., Hornbuckle, W., Schinazi, R., Gangemi, J.D., Tennant, B.C. and Gerin, J.L.: Antiviral Ther. *5*, 95–104 (2000).

149 Korba, B.E.: Antiviral Res. *29*, 49–51 (1996).

150 Korba, B.E. and Milman, G.: Antiviral Res. *15*, 217–228 (1991).

151 Korba, B.E. and Gerin, J.L.: Antiviral Res. *17*, 1–16 (1992).

152 Korba, B.E. and Gerin, J.L.: Antiviral Res. *28*, 225–242 (1995).

153 Korba, B.E., Cote, P.J., Tennant, B.C. and Gerin, J.L., in: Hollinger, F.B., Lemon, S.M. and Margolis, H.S. (eds.): Viral Hepatitis and Liver Disease, Williams & Williams, Baltimore 1991, pp. 663–665.

153a Korba, B.E., Schinazi, R.F., Cote, P., Tennant, B.C. and Gerin, J.L.: Antimicrob. Agents Chemother. *44*, 1757–1760 (2000).

154 Kreis, W., Damin, L., Colacino, J., Lopez, C.: Biochem. Pharm. *31*, 767–773 (1982).

155 Kufe, D.W., Major, P.P., Egan, E.M. and Beardsley, G.P.: J. Biol. Chem. *255*, 8997–9000 (1980).

155a Kukhanova, M., Lin, Z.Y., Yas'co, M. and Cheng, Y.C.: Biochem. Pharmacol. *55*, 1181–1187 (1998).

156 Kukhanova, M., Liu, S.H., Mozzherin, D., Lin, T.S., Chu, C.K. and Cheng, Y.C.: J. Biol. Chem. *270*, 23055–23059 (1995).

156a Kuroki, K., Cheung, R., Marion, P.L. and Ganem, D.: J. Virol. *68*, 2091–2096 (1994).

156b Kuroki, K., Eng, F., Ishikawa, T., Turck, C., Harada, F. and Ganem, D.: J. Biol. Chem. 270, 15022–15028 (1995).

156c Ladner, S.K., Miller, T.J., Otto, M.J. and King, R.W.: Antiviral Chem Chemother. 9, 65–72 (1998).

157 Ladner, S.K., Otto, M.J., Marker, C.S., Zaifert, K., Wang, G.H., Guo, J.T., Seeger, C. and King, R.W.: Antimicrob. Agents Chemother. *41*, 1715–1720 (1997).

158 Lai, C.L., Ching, C.K., Tung, A.K.M., Li, E., Young, J., Hill, A., Wong, B.C.Y., Dent, J. and Wu, P.C.: Hepatology *25*, 241–244 (1997).

159 Lamberts, C., Nassal, M., Velhagen, I., Zentgraf, H., Schroeder, C.H.: J. Virol. *67*, 3756–3762 (1993).

160 Lampertico, P., Malter, J.S. and Gerber, M.A.: Hepatology *13*, 422–426 (1991).

160a Lanford, R.E., Chavez, D., Brasky, K.M., Burns, R.B. III. and Rico-Hesse, R.: Proc. Natl. Acad. Sci USA 95, 5757–5761 (1998).

160b Lanford, R.E., Chavez, D., Rico-Hesse, R. and Mootnick, A.: J. Virol. *74*, 2955–2959 (2000).

161 Lanford, R.E., Notvall, L. and Beames, B.: J. Virol. *69*, 4431–4439 (1995).

162 Lanford, R.E., Michaels, M.G., Chavez, D., Brasky, K., Fung, J. and Starzl, T.E.: J. Med. Virol. *46*, 207–212 (1995).

162a Lau, D.T., Farooq Khokhar, M., Doo, E., Ghany, M.G., Herion, D., Park, Y., Kleiner, D., Schmid, P., Condreay, L.D., Gaulthier, J. et al.: Hepatology *32*, 828–834 (2000).

163 Lavie, G., Mazur, Y., Lavie, D., Prince, A.M., Pascual, D., Liebes, L., Levin, B. and Meruelo, D.: Transfusion *35*, 392–400 (1995).

164 Lee, B., Luo, W.X., Suzuki, S., Robins, M.J. and Tyrrell, D.L.: Antimicrob. Agents Chemother. *33*, 336–339 (1989).

165 Lee, C.D., Ott, M., Thyagarajan, S.P., Shafritz, D.A., Burk, R.D. and Gupta, S.: Eur. J. Clin. Invest. *26*, 1069–1076 (1996).

166 Lee, Y.I., Hong, Y.B., Kim, Y., Rho, H.M. and Jung, G.: Biochem. Biophys. Res. Comm. *233*, 401–407 (1997).

167 Leinbach, S.S., Reno, J.M., Lee, L.F., Isbell, A.F. and Boezi, J.A.: Biochem. *15*, 426–430 (1976).

168 Levine, A.J.: Viruses. The hepatitis B virus, Scientific American Library, New York, New York 1992, pp. 177–193.

169 Lewis, W., Meyer, R.R., Simpson, J.F., Colacino, J.M., Perrino, F.W.: Biochemistry 33, 14620–14624 (1994).

170 Lewis, W., Levine, E.S, Griniuviene, B., Tankersley, K.O, Colacino, J.M., Sommadossi, J.P., Watanabe, K.A. and Perrino, F.W.: Proc. Natl. Acad. Sci. USA 93, 3592–3597 (1996).

170a Li, J., Tong, S. and Wands, J.R.: J. Virol. *70*, 6029–6035 (1996).

170b Li, J., Tong, S. and Wands, J.R.: J. Biol. Chem. *274*, 27658–27665 (1999).

171   Liaw, Y.F., Chu, C.M., Su, I.J., Huang, M.J., Lin, D.Y. and Chang-Chien, C.S.: Gastroenterology 84, 216–219 (1983).

172   Lieberman, K.C. and Heidelberger, C.: J. Biol. Chem. 316, 823–830 (1955).

173   Lin, E., Luscombe, C., Wang, Y.Y., Shaw, T. and Locarnini, S.: Antimicrob. Agents Chemother. 40, 413–418 (1996).

174   Lin, J.C., Smith, M.C. and Cheng, Y.C.: Science 221, 578–579 (1983).

175   Lin, T.S., Luo, M.Z., Liu, M.C., Pai, S.B., Dutschman, G.E. and Cheng, Y.C.: Biochem. Pharm. 47, 171–174 (1994).

176   Lin, T.S., Luo MZ, Zhu J.L., Liu MC, Zhu YL., Dutschman GE, Cheng YC.: 1995. Synthesis of a series of purine 2′,3′–dideoxy–L–nucleoside analogues as potential antiviral agents. Nucleosides Nucleotides 14, 1759–1783 ().

177   Lin, T.S., Luo, M.A., Liu, M.C., Zhu, Y.L., Gullen, E., Dutschman, G.E. and Cheng, Y.C.: J. Med. Chem. 39, 1757–1759 (1996).

178   Ling, R., Mutimer, D., Ahmend, M., Boxall, E.H., Elias, E., Dushieko, G.M. and Harrison, T.J.: Hepatology 24, 711–713 (1996).

178a   Liu, S.H., Grove, K.L. and Cheng, Y.C.: Antimicrob. Agents Chemother. 42, 833–839 (1998).

179   Livingston, B.D., Crimi, C., Grey, H., Ishioka, G., Chisari, F.V., Fikes, J., Grey, H., Chesnut, R.W. and Sette, A.: J. Immunol. 159, 1383–1392 (1997).

180   Lofgren, B., Vickery, K., Zhang, Y.Y. and Nordenfelt, E.: J. Viral Hep. 3, 61–65 (1996).

181   Lofgren, B., Habteyesus, A., Nordenfelt, E., Eriksson, S. and Oberg, B.: Antiviral Chem. Chemother. 1, 361–366 (1990).

182   Lofgren, B., Nordenfelt, E. and Oberg, B.: Antiviral Res. 12, 301–310 (1989).

182a   Lok, A.S.: Gastroenterol. 119, 263–266 (2000).

183   Lopez, C., Watanabe, K.A. and Fox, J.J.: Antimicrob. Agents Chemother. 17, 803–806 (1980).

184   Lopez-Bazzochi, I., Hudson, J.B. and Towers, G.H.N.: Photochem. Photobiol. 54, 95–98 (1991).

185   Lu, X., Block, T.M. and Gerlach, W.H.: J. Virol. 70, 2277–2285 (1996).

186   Lu, X., Mehta, A., Dadmarz, M., Dwek, R., Blumberg, B.S. and Block, T.M.: Proc. Natl. Acad. Sci. USA 94, 2380–2385 (1997).

187   Luscombe, C., Pedersen, J., Uren, E. and Locarnini, S.: Hepatology. 24, 766–773 (1996).

188   Ma, T., Pai, S.B., Zhu, Y.L., Lin, J.S., Shanmuganathan, K., Du, J., Wang, C., Kim, H., Newton, M.G., Cheng, Y.C. and Chu, C.K.: J. Med. Chem. 39, 2835–2843 (1996).

189   Macrae, D.R., Bruss, V. and Ganem, D.: Virology 181, 359–63 (1991).

190   Main, J., Brown, J.L., Howells, C., Galassini, R., Crossey, M., Karayiannis, P., Gerogiou, P., Atkinson, G. and Thomas, H.C.: J. Viral. Hepatitis 3, 211–215 (1996).

190a   Malik, A.H. and Lee, W.M.: Annals Intern. Med. 132, 723–731 (2000).

191   Mansour, T.S., Tse, A. and Charron, M.: Med. Chem. Res. 5, 417–425 (1995).

192   Mansour, T.S. and Storer, R.: Curr. Pharm. Design 3, 227–264 (1997).

193   Mao, J.C. and Robishaw, E.E.: Biochem. 14, 5475–5479 (1975).

194   Margolis, H.S., Alter, M.J. and Halder, S.C.: Semin. Liv. Dis. 11, 84–92 (1991).

195   Marshall, J.S., Williams, S. and Jones, P.: J. Lab. Clin. Med. 92, 30–37 (1978).

196   Mason, W.S., Cullen, J., Saputelli, J., Wu, T.T., Liu, C., London, W.T., Lustbader, E., Schaffer, P., O'Connell, A.P., Fourel, I., Aldrich, C.E. and Jilbert, A.R.: Hepatology.: 19, 398–411 (1994).

197 Matthes, E., Langen, P., von Janta-Lipinski, M., Will, H., Schroeder, H.C., Merz, H., Weiler, B.E. and Muller, W.E.G.: Antimicrob. Agents Chemother. *34*, 1986–1990 (1990).

198 McKenzie, R., Fried, M.W., Sallie, R., Conjeevaram, H., Di Bisceglie, A.M., Park, Y., Savarese, B., Kleiner, D., Tsokos, M., Luciano, C., Pruett, T., Stotka, J.L., Straus, S.E. and Hoofnagle, J.H.: N. Engl. J. Med. *333*, 1099–1105 (1995).

199 Mehrotra, R.and Srivastava, S.: Ind. J. Med. Res. *85*, 113–119 (1987).

200 Mehta, A., Lu, X., Block, T.M., Blumberg, B.S. and Dwek, R.A.: Proc. Natl. Acad. Sci. USA *94*, 1822–1827 (1997).

201 Meijer, D.K.F. and Molema, G.: Semin. Liver. Dis. *15*, 202–256 (1995).

201a Melegari, M., Scaglioni, P.P. and Wands, J.R.: Hepatology *27*, 628–633 (1998).

202 Meruelo, D., Lavie G. and Lavie D.: Proc. Natl. Acad. Sci. USA 85, 5230–5234 (1988).

203 Moraleda, G., Wu, T.T., Jilbert, A.R., Aldrich, C.E., Condreay, L.D., Larsen, S.H., Tang, J.C., Colacino, J.M. and Mason, W.S.: Antiviral Res. *20*, 235–247 (1993).

204 Muller, W.E.G., Maidhof, A., Taschner, H. and Zahn, R.K.: Biochem. Pharmacol. *26*, 1071–1075 (1977).

204a Mutchnick, M.G., Appelman, H.D., Chung, H.T., Aragona, E., Guota, T.P., Cummings, G.D., Waggoner, J.G., Hoofnagle, J.H. and Shafritz, D.A.: Hepatology *14*, 409–415 (1991).

204b Mutchnick, M.G., Lindsay, K., Schiff, E., Cummings, G. and Appelman, H.D.: Gastroenterology *108*, A1127 (1995).

204c Mutchnick, G.M., Lindsay, K.L., Schiff, E.R., Cummings, G.D., Appelman, H.D., Peleman, R.R., Silva, M., Roach, K.C., Simmons, F., Milstein, S. et al.:J. Viral Hepat. 6, 397–403 (1999).

205 Naessens, L., Snoeck, R., Andrei, G., Balzarini, J., Neyts, J. and De Clercq, E.: Antiviral Chem. Chemother. *8*, 1–23 (1997).

206 Nagahata, T., Araki, K., Yamamura, K. and Matsubara, K.: Antimicrob. Agents Chemother. *36*, 2042–2045 (1992).

207 Nagahata, T., Kitagawa, M. and Matsubara, K.:Antimicrob. Agents Chemother. *38*, 707–712 (1994).

208 Nakazono, K., Ito, Y., Wu, C.H. and Wu, G.Y.: Hepatology. *23*, 1297–303 (1996).

209 Newbold, J.E., Xin, H., Tencza, M., Sherman G., Dean, J., Bowden, S. and Locarnini, S.: J. Virol. *69*, 3350–3357 (1995).

210 Nishiyama, Y., Yamamoto, N., Yamada, Y., Fujioka, H., Shimada, N. and Takahashi, Y.: J. Antibiotics *42*, 1308–1311 (1989).

211 Niu, J., Wang, Y., Dixon, R., Bowden, S., Qiao, M., Einck, L. and Locarnini, S.: Antiviral Res. *21*, 155–171 (1993).

212 Niu, J., Wang, Y., Qiao, M., Gowans, E., Edwards, P., Thyagarajan, S.P., Gust, I. and Locarnini, S.: J. Med. Virol. *32*, 212–218 (1990).

213 Nommensen, F.E., Go, S.T. and Maclaren, D.M.: Lancet *2*, 847–849 (1989).

214 Nordenfelt, E., Oberg, B., Helgstrand, E. and Miller, E.: Acta Path. Microbiol. Scand. Sect. B. *88*, 169–175 (1980).

215 Offensperger, W.B., Offensperger, S., Walter, E., Teubner, K., Igloi, G., Blum, H. and Gerok, W.: EMBO J. *12*, 1257–1262 (1993).

216 Omata, M. and Uchiumi, K.: J. Hepatology 3 (Suppl. 2), S65–69 (1986).

216a Oon, C.J., Chen, W.N., Lim, N., Koh, S., Lim, G.K., Leong, A.L., Tan, G.S.: Antiviral Res. *41*, 113–118 (1999).

217 Orito, E., Mizokami, M., Ina, Y., Moriyama, N.E., Kameshima, N., Yamamoto, M. and Gojobori, T.: Proc. Natl. Acad. Sci. USA *86*, 7059–7062 (1989).

218   Ozer, A., Khaoustov, V.I., Mearns, M., Lewis, D.E., Genta, R.M., Darlington, G.J. and Yoffe, B.: Gastroenterology *110*, 1519–1528 (1996).

219   Pai, S.B., Liu, S.H., Zhu, Y.L., Chu, C.K. and Cheng, Y.C.: Antimicrob. Agents Chemother. *40*, 380–386 (1996).

220   Parang, K., Wiebe, L.I., Knaus, E.E., Huang, J.S., Tyrrell, D.L. and Csizmadia, F.: Antiviral Res. *34*, 75–90 (1997).

220a   Parkin, D.M., Pisani, P., Munoz, N. and Ferlay, J.: Cancer Surv. *33*, 5–33 (1999).

221   Perri, S. and Ganem, D.: J. Virol. *70*, 6803–6809 (1996).

221a   Perrillo, R., Schiff, E., Yoshida, E., Statler, A., Hirsch, K., Wright, T., Gutfreund, K., Lamy, P. and Murray, A.: Hepatology *32*, 29–34 (2000).

222   Persing, D.H., Varmus, H.E. and Ganem, D.: J. Virol. *61*, 1672–1677 (1987).

223   Petcu, D.J., Aldrich, C.J., Coates, L., Taylor, J.M. and Mason, W.S.: Virology *167*, 385–392 (1988).

223a   Petry, W., Erhardt, A., Heintges, T. and Haussinger, D.: Z. Gastroenterol. *38*, 77–87 (2000).

224   Poch, O., Sauvaget, I., Delarue, M. and Tordo, N.: EMBO J. *8*, 3867–3874 (1989).

225   Pollard, R.B., Smith, J.L., Neal, A., Gregory, P.B., Merigan, T.C. and Robinson, W.S.: J. Am. Med. Assoc. *239*, 1648–1650 (1978).

226   Ponzetto, A., Fiume, L., Forzani, B., Song, S.Y., Busi, C., Mattioli, A., Spinelli, C., Marinelli, M., Smedile, A., Chiaberge, E.F., Gervasi, G.B., Rapicetta, M. and Verme, G.: Hepatology *14*, 16–24 (1991).

227   Preiksaitis, J.K., Lan, K.B., Ng, P.K., Brox, L., LePage, G.A. and Tyrrell, D.L.J.: J. Inf. Dis. *144*, 358–364 (1981).

228   Price, P.M., Banerjee, R., Acs, G.: Proc. Natl. Acad. Sci. USA *86*, 8541–8544 (1989).

229   Price, P.M., Banerjee, R., Jeffrey, A.M. and Acs, G.: Hepatology *16*, 8–12 (1992).

230   Pugh, J.C. and Summers, J.W.: Virology *172*, 564–572 (1989).

230a   Qadri, I. and Siddiqui, A.: J. Biol. Chem. *274*, 31359–31365 (1999).

231   Radziwill, G., Tucker, W. and Schaller, H.: J. Virol. *64*, 613–620 (1990).

232   Rajagopalan, P., Boudinot, F.D., Chu, C.K., Tennant, B.C., Baldwin, B.H. and Schinazi, R.F.: Antiviral Chem. Chemother. *7*, 65–70 (1996).

233   Realdi G., Alberti, A., Rugge, M., Bortolotti, F., Rigoli, A.M., Tremolada, F. and Ruol, A.: Gastroenterology *79*, 195–199 (1980).

234   Reardon, J.E.: J. Biol. Chem. *264*, 19039–19044 (1989).

235   Rensen, P.C.N., de Vrueh, L.A., van Berkel, T.J.C.: Drug Delivery Systems *31*, 131–155 (1996).

236   Richardson, F.C., Engelhardt, J.A. and Bowsher, R.R.: Proc. Natl. Acad. Sci. USA *91*, 12003–12007 (1994).

237   Rijintjes, P.J., Moshage, H.J. and Yap, S.H.: Virus. Res. *10*, 95–110 (1988).

238   Roll, P.M., Weinfeld, H., Carroll, E. and Brown, G.B.: J. Biol. Chem. *220*, 439–454 (1956).

239   Roome, A.J., Walsh, S.J., Cartter, M.L. and Hadler, J.L.: J. Am. Med. Assoc. *270*, 2931–2934 (1993).

240   Rosowsky, A., Saha, J., Fazely, F., Koch, J. and Ruprecht, R.: Biochem. Biophys. Res. Comm. *172*, 288–293 (1990).

240a   Ryu, C.J., Cho, D.Y., Gripon, P., Kim, H.S., Guguen-Guillouzo, C. and Hong, H.J.: J. Virol. *74*, 110–116 (2000).

241   Sacks, S.L., Smith, J.L., Pollard, R.B., Sawhney, V., Mahol, A.S., Gregory, P., Merigan, T.C. and Robinson, W.S.: J. Am. Med. Assoc. *241*, 28–29 (1979).

242   Sawamura, T., Nakada, H., Hazama, H., Shiozaki, Y., Sameshima, T. and Tashiro, Y.: Gastroenterology 87, 1217–1221 (1984).

243   Scaglioni, P.P., Melegari, M. and Wands, J.R.: Virology 205, 112–120 (1994).

244   Scaglioni, P.P., Melegari, M. and Wands, J.R.: Bailliere's Clinical Gastroenterology 10, 207–225 (1996).

245   Scaglioni, P.P., Melegari, M., Takahashi, M., Chowdhury, J.R. and Wands, J.R.: Hepatology 24, 1010–1017 (1996).

246   Scaglioni, P.P., Melegari, M. and Wands, J.R.: J. Virol. 71, 345–353 (1997).

247   Schalm, S.W., Heijtink, R.A., Van Buuren, H.R. and de Man, R.A.: .J. Hepatology 3 (Suppl. 2), S189–192 (1986).

248   Schalm, S.W., de Man, R.A., Heijtink, R.A. and Niesters, H.G.M.: J. Hepatology 22 (Suppl. 1), 52–56 (1995).

249   Schat, K.A., Schinazi, R.F. and Calnek, B.W.: Antiviral Res. 4, 259–270 (1984).

250   Schilke, A.J., Staschke, K.A. and Colacino, J.M.: Antiviral Res. 23 (Suppl. 1), 80 (1994).

251   Schinazi, R.F., Fox, J.J., Watanabe, K.A. and Nahmias, A.J.: Antimicrob Agents Chemother. 29, 77–84 (1986).

252   Schinazi, R.F., Chu, C.K., Babu, J.R., Oswald, B.J., Saalman, V., Cannon, D.L., Eriksson, B.F.H. and Nasr, M.: Antiviral Res. 13, 265–272 (1990).

253   Schinazi, R.F., Lloyd, R.M. Jr., Nguyen, M.H., Canon, D.L., McMillan, A., Ilksoy, N., Chu, C.K., Liotta, D.C., Bazmi, H.Z. and Mellors, J.W.: Antimicrob. Agents Chemother. 37, 875–881 (1993).

254   Schinazi, R.F., McClure, H.M., Boudinot, F.D., Jxiang, Y. and Chu, C.K.: Antiviral Res. 23 (Suppl), 81 (1994).

255   Schinazi, R.F., Gosselin, G., Faraj, A., Korba, B.E., Liotta, D.C., Chu, C.K., Mathe, C., Imbach, J.L. and Sommadossi, J.P.: Antimicrob. Agents Chemother. 38, 2172–2174 (1994).

256   Schlicht, H.J., Radziwill, G. and Schaller, H.: Cell. 56, 85–92 (1989).

257   Schreiber, G.B., Busch, M.P., Kleinman, S.H. and Korelitz, J.J. and The Retrovirus Epidemiology Donor Study: N. Engl. J. Med. 334, 1685–1690 (1996).

258   Scullard, G.B., Pollard, R.B., Smith, J.L., Sacks, S.L., Gregor, P.B., Robinson, W.S. and Merigan, T.C.: J. Inf. Dis. 143, 772–783 (1981).

258a   Seeger, C. and Mason, W.S.: Micro. and Mol. Biol. Rev. 64, 51–68 (2000).

258b   Seifer, M., Hamatake, R.K., Colonno, R.J. and Standring, D.N.: Antimicrob. Agents Chemother. 42, 3200–3208 (1998).

258c   Seifer, M., Hamatake, R., Bifano, M. and Standring, D.N.: J. Virol. 72, 2765–2776 (1998).

259   Seifer, M. and Standring, D.N.: J. Virol. 67, 4513–4520 (1993).

259a   Seigneres, B., Pichoud, C., Ahmed, S.S., Hantz, O., Trepo, C. and Zoulim, F.: J. Inf. Dis. 181, 1221–1233 (2000).

260   Sells, M.A., Chen, M.L. and Acs, G.: Proc. Natl. Acad. Sci. USA 84, 1005–1009 (1987).

260a   Semino-Mora, C., Leon-Monzon, M. and Dalakas, M.C.: Lab. Invest. 76, 487–495 (1997).

261   Severini, A., Liu, X.Y., Wilson, J.S. and Tyrrell, D.L.: Antimicrob. Agents Chemother. 39, 1430–1435 (1995).

262   Shaw, T., Amor, P., Civitico, G., Boyd, M. and Locarnini, S.: Antimicrob. Agents Chemother. 38, 719–723 (1994).

263   Shaw, T., Mok, S.S. and Locarnini, S.A.: Hepatology 24, 996–1002 (1996).

264   Shepp, D.H., Dandliker, P.S., DeMiranda, P., Burnette, T.C., Cederberg, D.M., Kirk, L.E. and Meyers, J.D.: Ann. Int. Med. 103, 368–373 (1985).

265 Sherker, A.H., Hirota, K., Omata, M. and Okuda, K.: Gastroenterology *91*, 818–824 (1986).

266 Sherman, M., Chan, R., Kwan, S., Bloomer, J., Bechtold, C., Ingraham, P., Dehertogh, D., and 008 Study Group: Abstracts of the 37th International Conference on Antimicrobial Agents and Chemotherapy, September 28–October 1, 1997. H-32 (1997).

267 Shimada, N., Hasegawa, S., Harada, T., Tomisawa, T., Fujii, A. and Takita, T.: J. Antibiotics *39*, 1623–1625 (1986).

268 Shimada, N., Hasegawa, S., Saito, S., Nishikiori, T., Fujii, A. and Takita, T.: J. Antibiotics *40*, 1788–1790 (1987).

269 Sidwell, R.W., Huffman, J.H., Khare, G.P., Allen, L.B., Witkowski, J.T. and Robins, R.K.: . Science *177*, 705–706 (1972).

270 Singh, N. and Gayowski, T.: Transplantation. *59*, 1629–30 (1995).

271 Smilkstein, M.J., Gary, M.D., Knapp, M.S., Kenneth, W., Kulig, M.D. and Rumack, M.D.: J. Med. *24*, 1557–1562 (1988).

272 Staschke, K.A. and Colacino, J.M.: J. Virol. *68*, 8265–8269 (1994).

273 Staschke, K.A., Colacino, J.M., Mabry, T.E. and Jones, C.D.: Antiviral Res. *23*, 45–61 (1994).

274 Staschke, K.A., Richardson, K.K, Mabry, T.E., Baxter, A.J., Scheuring, J.C., Huffman, D.M., Smith, W.C., Richardson, F.C. and Colacino, J.M.: Nucl. Acids Res. *24*, 4111–4116 (1996).

275 Stephenson, M.L. and Zamecnik, P.C.: Proc. Natl. Acad. Sci. USA *75*, 285–288 (1978).

276 Stevenson, W., Gaffey, M., Ishitani, M., McCullough, C., Dickson, R., Caldwell, S., Lobo, P. and Pruett, T.: Transpl. Proc. *27*, 1219–1221 (1995).

277 Streeter, D.G., Witkowski, J.T., Khare, G.P., Sidwell, R.W., Bauer, R.J., Robins, R.K. and Simon, L.N.: Proc. Natl. Acad. Sci. USA *70*, 1174–1178 (1973).

278 Streeter, D.G., Miller, J.P., Robins, R.K. and Simon, L.N.: Ann. NY. Acad. Sci. *284*, 201–210 (1977).

279 Sudo, K., Konno, K., Shigeta, S. and Yokota, T.: Microbiol. Immunol. *40*, 153–159 (1996).

280 Summers, J. and Mason, W.S.: Cell *29*, 403–415 (1983).

281 Sureau, C., Romet-Lemonne, J.L., Mullins, J.I. and Essex, M.: Cell *47*, 37–47 (1986).

282 Syamasundar, K.V, Singh, B., Thakur, R.S., Husain, A., Kiso, Y. and Hikino, H.: J. Ethnopharmacol. *14*, 41–44 (1985).

283 Sydiskis, R.J., Owen, D.G., Lohr, J.L., Rosler, K.H.A. and Blomster, R.N.: Antimicrob. Agents Chemother. *35*, 2463–2466 (1991).

283a Tam, R.C., Pai, B., Bard, J., Lim, C., Averett, D.R., Phan, U.T. and Milovanovic, T.: J. Hepatol. *30*, 376–382 (1999).

284 Tang, J., Colacino, J.M., Larsen, S.H. and Spitzer, W.: Antiviral Res. *13*, 313–326 (1990).

285 Tavis, J.E. and Ganem, D.: Proc. Natl. Acad. Sci. USA *90*, 4107–4111 (1993).

286 Tavis, J.E. and Ganem, D.: J. Virol. *70*, 5741–5750 (1996).

287 Tencza, M.G. and Newbold, J.E.: J. Med. Virol. *51*, 6–16 (1997).

287a Tennant, B.C.: Clinics Liver Dis. 3, 241–266 (1999).

288 Tennant, B., Jacob, J., Graham, L.A., Peek, S., Korba, B., Gerin, J.L., Witcher, J.W., Boudinot, F.D., Du, J. and Chu, C.K.: Antiviral Res. *34*, A52 (1997).

289 Tennant, B.C., Baldwin, B.H., Graham, L.A., Ascenzi, M.A., Hornbuckle, W.E., Rowland, P.H., Tochkov, I.A., Yeager, A.E., Erb, H.N., Colacino, J.M. et al.: Hepatol. *28*, 179–191 (1998).

290   Thomas, D.L., Factor, S.H., Kelen, G.D., Washington, A.S., Taylor, E. Jr. and Quinn, T.C.: Arch. Int. Med. *153*, 1705–1712 (1993).

291   Thyagarajan, S.P., Thiruneelakantan, K., Subramanian, S. and Sundaravelu, T.: Ind. J. Med. Res. Supplement *76*, 124–130 (1982).

292   Thyagarajan, S.P., Subramanian, S., Thirunalasundari, T., Venkateswaran, P.S., Blumberg, B.S.: Lancet *2*, 764–766 (1988).

293   Tillman, H.L., Troutwein, C., Kruger, M., Boker, K., Schlitt H.J., Condreay, L., Deslauri-ars, M., Bruns, I., Pichlmayr, R. and Manns, M.P.: J. Hepatology *26* (Suppl. 1), 153 (1997).

294   Tiollais, P., Pourcel, C. and Dejean, A.: Nature *317*, 489–495 (1985).

295   Tipples, G.A., Ma, M.M., Fischer, K.P, Bain, V.G., Kneteman, N.M. and Tyrrell, D.L.: Hepa-tology *24*, 714–717 (1996).

296   Toh, H., Hayashida, H. and Miyata, T.: Nature *305*, 827–829 (1983).

296a   Tong, S., Li, J. and Wands, J.R.: J. Virol. *73*, 8696–8702 (1999).

296b   Torresi, J. and Locarnini, S.: Gastroenterol. 118, S83–S103 (2000).

297   Tsiquaye, K.N, Collins, P. and Zuckerman, A.J.: J. Antimicrob. Chemother. *18*, 223–228 (1986).

298   Tsiquaye, K.N, Slomka, M.J. and Maung, M.: J. Med. Virol. *42*, 306–310 (1994).

299   Tsurimoto, T., Fujiyama, A. and Matsubara, K.: Proc. Natl. Acad. Sci. USA *84*, 444–448 (1987).

300   Tuttleman, J.S., Pugh, J.C. and Summers, J.W.: J. Virol. *58*, 17–25 (1986).

301   Tyrrell, D.L., Fischer, K., Savani, K., Tan, W. and Jewell, L.: Clin. Invest. Med. *16* (Suppl. 4), B77 (1993).

302   Tyrrell, D.L.J., Mitchell, M.C., de Man, R.A., Schalm, S.W., Main, J., Thomas, H.C. et al.: J. Hepatology *18*, 112A (1993).

303   Ueda, K., Tsurimoto, T., Nagahata, T., Chisaka, O. and Matsubara, K.: Virology *169*, 213–316 (1989).

304   Van Draanen, N.A., Tisdale, M., Parry, N.R, Jansen, R., Dornsife, R.E., Tuttle, J.V., Averett, D.R. and Koszalka, G.W.: Antimicrob. Agents Chemother. *38*, 868–871 (1994).

305   Venkateswaran, P.S., Millman, I. and Blumberg, B.S.: Proc. Natl. Acad. Sci. USA *84*, 274–278 (1987).

306   von Weizsacker, F., Blum, H.E. and Wands, J.R.: Biophys. Res. Commun. *189*, 743–748 (1992).

307   von Weizsacker, F., Wieland, S. and Blum, H.E.: Hepatology *24*, 294–299 (1996).

307a   Walters, K., Tipples, G., Allen, M.I. et al.: Hepatology 28 (4 Pt 2), 589A, Abst. No. 1706 (1998).

308   Wang, G.H. and Seeger, C.: Cell *71*, 663–670 (1992).

309   Wang, G.H. and Seeger, C.: J. Virol. 67, 6507–6512 (1993).

310   Wang, Y., Bowden, S., Shaw, T., Civitico, G., Chan, Y., Qiao, M. and Locarnini, S.: Antivi-ral Chem. Chemother. *2*, 107–114 (1991).

311   Wang, Y., Luscombe, C., Bowden, S., Shaw, T. and Locarnini, S.: Antimicrob. Agents Chemother. *39*, 556–558 (1995).

312   Weber, M., Bronsema, V., Bartos, H., Bosserhoff, A., Bartenschlager, R., and Schaller, H.: J. Virol. *68*, 2994–2999 (1994).

313   Weiss, L., Hildt, E., Hofschneider, P.H.: Antiviral Res. *32*, 43–53 (1996).

314   Welch, P.J., Tritz, R., Yei, S., Barber, J. and Yu, M.: Gene Ther. *4*, 736–743 (1997).

315   Weller, I.V.D., Bassendine, M.F., Craxi, A., Fowler, M.J.F., Monjardino, J., Thomas, H.C. and Sherlock, S.: Gut *23*, 717–723 (1982).

316 Willis, R.C., Carson, D.A. and Seegmiller, J.E.: Proc. Natl. Acad. Sci. USA *75*, 3042–3044 (1978).

317 Witcher, J.W., Boudinot, F.D., Baldwin, B.H., Ascenzi, M.A., Tennant, B.C., Du, J.F. and Chu, C.K.: Antimicrob. Agents Chemother. *41*, 2184–2187 (1997).

317a Wolters, L.M., Honkoop, P., Niesters, H.G. and de Man, R.A.: J. Hepatol. *28*, 909–910 (1998).

318 Woo, M.H. and Burnakis, T.G.: Ann. Pharmacother. *31*, 330–337 (1997).

319 Wood, R.C., MacDonald, K.L., White, K.E., Hedberg, C.W., Hanson, M. and Osterholm, M.T.: J. Am. Med. Assoc. *270*, 2935–2939 (1993).

320 Wright, J.D., Ma, T., Chu, C.K. and Boudinot, F.D.: Pharm. Res. *12*, 1350–1353 (1995).

321 Wright, J.D., Ma, T., Chu, C.K. and Boudinot, F.D.: Drug. Disp. *17*, 197–207 (1996).

322 Wu, G.Y. and Wu, C.H.: J. Biol. Chem. *267*, 12436–12439 (1992).

322a Xiong, X., Flores, C., Yang, H., Toole, J.J. and Gibbs, C.S.: Hepatology *28*, 1669–1673 (1998).

323 Yaginuma, K., Shirakata, Y., Kobayashi, M. and Koike, K.: Proc. Natl. Acad. Sci. USA *84*, 2678–2682 (1987).

323a Yamanaka, G., Wilson, T., Innaimo, S., Bisacchi, G.S., Egli, P., Rinehart, J.K., Zahler, R. and Colonno, R.J.: Antimicrob. Agents Chemother. *43*, 190–193 (1999).

323b Yao, F. and Gish, R.G.: Curr. Gastroenterol. Rep. *1*, 20–26 (1999).

324 Yao, G.Q., Liu, S.H., Chou, E., Kukhanova, M., Chu, C.K. and Cheng, Y.C.: Biochem. Pharm. *51*, 941–947 (1996).

324a Ying, C., De Clercq, E., Nicholson, W., Furman, P. and Neyts, J.: J. Viral Hepat. *7*, 161–165 (2000).

325 Yokota, T., Mochizuki, S., Konno, K., Mori, S., Shigeta, S. and De Clercq, E.: Antimicrob. Agents Chemother. *35*, 394–397 (1991).

326 Yu, W., Hongsong, C., Fengshui, W., Qianhong, L., Guanghui, C. and Baifang, F.: Chinese Med. J. *109*, 674–679 (1996).

327 Yuen, G.J., Morris, D.M., Mydlow, P.K., Haidar, S., Hal,l S.T. and Hussey, E.K.: J. Clin. Pharm. *35*, 1174–1180 (1995).

328 Zahm, F.E., d'Urso, N., Bonino, F. and Ponzetto, A.: Liver *16*, 88–93 (1996).

329 Zamecnik, P.C. and Stephenson, M.L.: Proc. Natl. Acad. Sci. USA *75*, 280–284 (1978).

330 Zhu, Y.L., Pai, S.B., Liu, S.H., Grove, K.L., Jones, B.C.N.M., Simmons, C., Zemlicka, J. and Cheng, Y.C.: Antimicrob. Agents Chemother. *41*, 1755–1760 (1997).

331 Zoulim, F. and Seeger, C.: J. Virol. *68*, 6–13 (1994).

332 Zoulim, F., Saputelli, J. and Seeger, C.: J. Virol. *68*, 2026–2030 (1994).

333 Zoulim, F., Dannaoui, E., Borel, C., Hantz, O., Lin, T.S., Liu, S.H., Trepo, C. and Cheng, Y.C.: Antimicrob. Agents Chemother. *40*, 448–453 (1996).

334 Zuckerman, A.J.: J. Virol. Methods *17*, 119–126 (1987).

335 zu Putlitz, J., Yu, Q., Burke, J.M. and Wands, J.R.: J. Virol. *73*, 5381–5387 (1999).

Antiviral Agents – Advances and Problems (E. Jucker, Ed.)
©2001 Birkhäuser Verlag, Basel (Switzerland)

Current and potential therapies for the treatment of herpes-virus infections

By Elcira C. Villarreal

Eli Lilly and Company
Infectious Diseases Research
Drop Code 0438
Lilly Research Laboratories
Indianapolis, IN 46285, USA
<villarreal_elcira_c@lilly.com>

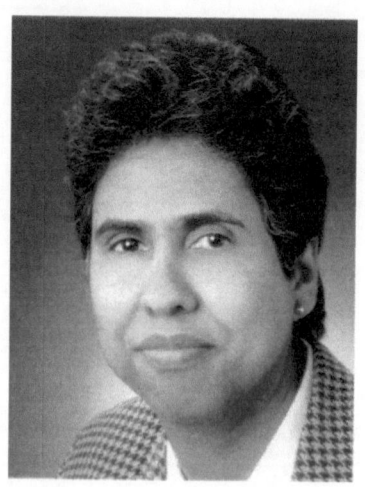

Elcira C. Villarreal

was born and raised in Colon, Republic of Panama. She received a BA degree in biology and a MS degree in microbiology from Incarnate Word College in San Antonio, Texas. She earned her doctoral degree at Oregon State University in Corvallis, Oregon, for her work on host cell nuclear involvement in vaccinia virus replication. After a post-doctoral fellowship at Harvard Medical School in Boston, she obtained a position in 1990 as Senior Virologist at Eli Lilly and Company, advancing to Research Scientist in 1995 and to Chairperson of the Virology Action Group in 1996.

Summary

Human herpesviruses are found worldwide and are among the most frequent causes of viral infections in immunocompetent as well as in immunocompromised patients. During the past decade and a half a better understanding of the replication and disease causing state of herpes simplex virus types 1 and 2 (HSV-1 and HSV-2), varicella-zoster virus (VZV), and human cytomegalovirus (HCMV) has been achieved due in part to the development of potent antiviral compounds that target these viruses. While some of these antiviral therapies are considered safe and efficacious (acyclovir, penciclovir), some have toxicities associated with them (ganciclovir and foscarnet). In addition, the increased and prolonged use of these compounds in the clinical setting, especially for the treatment of immunocompromised patients, has led to the emergence of viral resistance against most of these drugs. While resistance is not a serious issue for immunocompetent individuals, it is a real concern for immunocompromised patients, especially those with AIDS and the ones that have undergone organ transplantation. All the currently approved treatments target the viral DNA polymerase. It is clear that new drugs that are more efficacious than the present ones, are not toxic, and target a different viral function would be of great use especially for immunocompromised patients. Here, we provide an overview of the diseases caused by the herpesviruses as well as the replication strategy of the better studied members of this family for which treatments are available. We also discuss the various drugs that have been approved for the treatment of some herpesviruses in terms of structure, mechanism of action, and development of resistance. Finally, we present a discussion of viral targets other than the DNA polymerase, for which new antiviral compounds are being considered.

Contents

Elcira C. Villarreal

Key words

Acyclovir, antiviral agents, antisense, cytomegalovirus, DNA polymerase, Epstein-Barr virus, famciclovir, fomivirsen, foscarnet, ganciclovir, herpesviruses, herpes simplex viruses, nucleoside analogs, penciclovir, prodrugs, thymidine kinase, resistance, valaciclovir, varicella zoster virus, virus replication.

Glossary of abbreviations

ACV, 9-(2-hydroxyethoxymethyl)guanine (acyclovir); ACV^r, acyclovir-resistant; BDCRB, 5,6-dichloro-2-bromo-1β-D-ribofuranosyl-1H-benzimidazole; BMT, bone marrow transplant; CDV, (S)-1-(3-hydroxy-2-phosphonylmethoxypropyl)cytosine (cidofovir); CMV, cytomegalovirus; EBV, Epstein-Barr virus; FCV, famciclovir; FCV^r, famciclovir-resistant; GCV, ganciclovir; GCV^r, ganciclovir-resistant; HCMV, human cytomegalovirus; HPMPC, (S)-1-(3-hydroxy-2-phosphonylmethoxypropyl)cytosine (cidofovir); HSV-1, herpes simplex virus type 1; HSV-2, herpes simplex virus type 2; IC$_{50}$, inhibitory concentration, 50%; kbp, kilobase pair; L-FMAU, the L enantiomer of 2'-deoxy-2'-fluoro-1-β-D-arabinofuranosyl-5-methyluracil; MP, monophosphate; PCV, penciclovir; PCV^r, penciclovir-resistant; PFA, phosphonoformic acid (foscarnet); PFA^r, foscarnet-resistant; SI, selective index; TCRB, 2,5,6-trichloro-1-(β-D-ribofuranosyl)benzimidazole; TK, thymidine kinase; tk, thymidine kinase gene; TP, triphosphate; VZV, varicella zoster virus.

1   Introduction

Human herpesviruses are found worldwide and are among the most frequent causes of viral infections in immunocompetent as well as in immunocompromised patients. To date, eight herpesviruses have been isolated from humans and these include herpes simplex virus type 1 (HSV-1), herpes simplex virus type 2 (HSV-2), varicella-zoster virus (VZV), human cytomegalovirus (HCMV), Epstein-Barr virus (EBV), and human herpesviruses 6, 7 and 8 (HHV-6, 7 and 8). The fact that potent antiviral drugs are available for the treatment of HSV-1, HSV-2, VZV, and HCMV, has contributed in part to a better understanding of these members of the herpesvirus family [1–8].

A common feature of all herpesviruses is that following primary infection, they establish long-term latency and reactivate intermittently, particularly during periods of serious immunosuppression [8–10]. Among immunocompetent patients, herpesvirus infections can be troublesome but in most cases are self-limited and usually do not require antiviral therapy. In contrast, immunocompromised individuals may develop severe viral disease which can be life-threatening and needs prompt treatment with antiviral agents [7,

11–24]. During the last decade and a half, the number of immunocompromised patients has increased as a result of an expansion in organ transplantation, more aggressive chemotherapy regimens and the higher incidence of individuals with acquired immunodeficiency syndrome (AIDS) [16]. Immunocompromised patients are extremely susceptible to a number of herpesvirus infections. The rise in the number of immunocompromised patients has led to an increase in the use of anti-herpetic drugs in the clinical setting. This in turn has resulted in the rapid emergence of resistance to most of these antiviral drugs [12–24]. It is clear that new medications are needed to be able to continue the efficient treatment of herpes infections especially in the immunocompromised patients [16]. To date, the approved drugs for the treatment of herpesvirus infections all target the viral DNA polymerase. However, there are numerous efforts underway to try to find new anti-herpes drugs that target other viral functions. The focus of these efforts is to try to find compounds that will (a) exhibit improved oral bioavailability and pharmacokinetics which will allow less frequent oral or topical dosing, will (b) target different viral functions such that they are effective against resistant HSV infections, and will (c) have improved efficacy [16].

This review will focus on the current therapies for HSV-1, HSV-2, VZV, and HCMV, will discuss viral resistance to these therapies, and will end with a discussion of additional viral targets, other than the viral DNA polymerase, that are currently being considered as alternatives for the development of new antiherpes drugs.

2 Diseases caused by herpesviruses

Infection with HSV-1 is universal, regardless of geography and race. Approximately 70% of people older than 40 years have antibodies against HSV-1 [25]. The most common manifestation is gingivostomatitis [26–28]. It is estimated that HSV-1 causes approximately 70% of orolabial infections [29]. HSV-2 is the most common cause of genital ulcer disease worldwide [25]. It is estimated that HSV-2 is responsible for approximately 70% of genital infections. In the U.S. alone there are between 40 to 60 million people infected with HSV-2 [21, 30–31]. Reactivation of acyclovir-resistant (ACV^r) HSV is particularly problematic in AIDS patients and recipients of bone marrow transplants (BMT). In immunocompetent individuals, the vast majority of primary infections or infections due to reactivation of HCMV, are assymptomatic. However, HCMV is a serious opportunistic pathogen in immunocompromised patients. In AIDS patients, HCMV infections can lead to retinitis that can cause blindness [32] and in bone marrow and solid organ transplant recipients can produce life-threatening infections such as pneumonitis and hepatitis [17, 18, 33] and gastrointestinal hemorrhage [34]. HCMV retinitis accounts for over 70% of cases of CMV disease in AIDS patients [35]. If left untreated, CMV retinitis is progressive and generally leads to blindness within 6 months [36, 37]. VZV is responsible for the primarily childhood disease known as varicella (chickenpox) and in adults herpes zoster (shingles). Reactivation of VZV in immunocompromised patients that are resistant to acyclovir, can be devastating as reported by Leport et al. [38].

3 Replication of herpesviruses

In order to consider new approaches to treat herpesvirus infections, an understanding of the viral replication process is necessary. A brief consideration of this topic is provided in this section. For a more thorough discussion of basic herpesvirus virology, excellent review articles by Matthews et al. [39], Haarr and Skulstad [28], Homa and Brown [40], Subak-Sharpe and Dargan [41], and Miller et al. [42], among others, are available.

All human herpesviruses studied to date share three common characteristics: First, the typical particle morphology; second, a large double-stranded DNA genome that ranges in size from 120–250 kilobase pairs (kbp); and third, the ability to undergo disease producing productive replication followed by a period of latency and given the proper stimulus, reactivation. The replication cycle of HSV, the best studied of the herpesviruses, is illustrated schematically in Figure 1.

HSV is a large enveloped virus that contains a genome of approximately 150 kbp. Following entry of the virus into the cell, and the localization of the viral DNA into the nucleus, the expression of viral genes occurs in a highly regulated manner. Three classes of genes have been identified and they are classified as immediate-early or alpha genes, early or beta genes and late or gamma genes. The alpha genes are responsible for the regulated expression of the viral genome while the beta genes encode for all the proteins involved in viral DNA replication. Examples of early gene products include viral DNA

HSV Infection

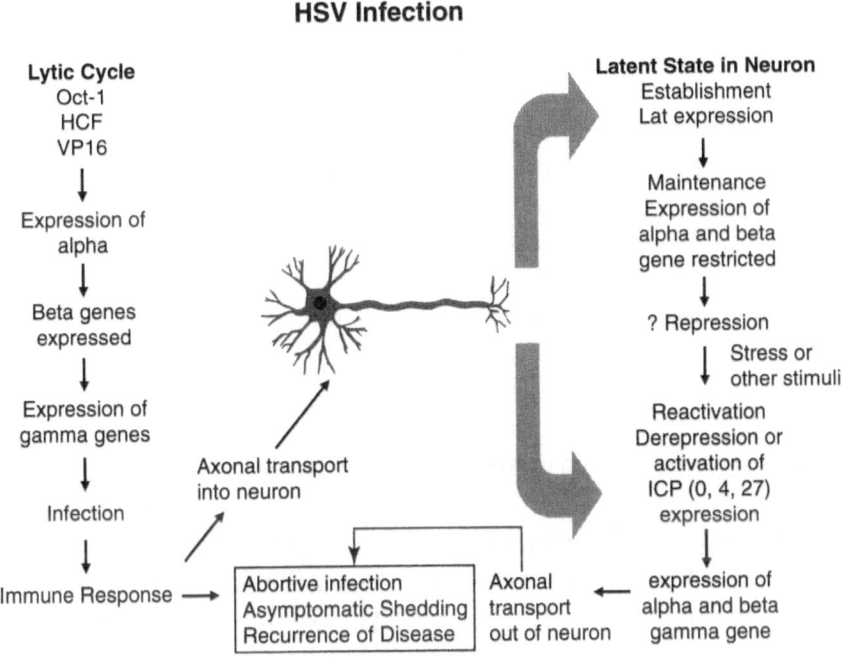

Lytic Cycle
Oct-1
HCF
VP16
↓
Expression of
alpha
↓
Beta genes
expressed
↓
Expression of
gamma genes
↓
Infection
↓
Immune Response →

Axonal transport
into neuron

Abortive infection	Axonal
Asymptomatic Shedding	transport
Recurrence of Disease	out of neuron

Latent State in Neuron
Establishment
Lat expression
↓
Maintenance
Expression of
alpha and beta
gene restricted
↓
? Repression
↓ Stress or
other stimuli
Reactivation
Derepression or
activation of
ICP (0, 4, 27)
expression
↓
expression of
alpha and beta
gamma gene

Fig. 1
Replication cycle of herpes simplex virus type 1.

polymerase and thymidine kinase (TK). The gamma, or late genes, are mainly involved in assembly of the virus particle and egress from the cell. The VZV genome is somewhat smaller (~ 125 kbp) and even though this virus has not been as well studied as the HSV virus has, there is evidence to show that VZV has the same classes of genes with similar functions as those of HSV. It has now been clearly established that VZV encodes homologs of most HSV proteins, including the DNA polymerase and TK [18, 28, 39–43].

HCMV has the largest genome of any of the herpesviruses (~ 230 kbp). Approximately 33 of the 208 ORFs of HCMV show a high level of amino acid similarity to ORFs in HSV-1 and VZV [44]. HCMV shares with other herpesviruses the ability to establish latency following primary infection, and to reactivate subsequently as host cell-mediated immunity diminishes [44]. However, HCMV has evolved unique strategies for intracellular replication, pathogenesis and persistence in the host. The regulatory mechanisms and biological sites for viral persistence and reactivation of CMV are not well understood, but what is clear is that they are different from those neurotropic pathways employed by HSV and VZV [44].

After the occurrence of the lytic cycle which generally leads to productive infection, all herpesviruses enter a latent state in which the viral genome is present in a non-replicating state in the infected cell and from which, given the proper stimulus, the virus can intermittently reactivate [42, 45, 46]. What is known about the three different stages of HSV-1 latency (i.e., establishment, maintenance, and reactivation) has been reviewed recently by Miller et al. [42].

4   Approved treatments for herpesvirus infections

The various points in the replication cycle of herpesviruses (Fig. 1), such as viral attachment, entry, uncoating, protein synthesis, DNA replication, assembly, and egress from the infected cell represent potential targets for the development of antiviral drugs. However, despite intensive efforts on the part of numerous pharmaceutical and academic laboratories to examine other herpesvirus targets and develop antivirals against them, all the approved treatments are directed at the viral DNA polymerase. Currently, there are approved therapies for HSV-1, HSV-2, VZV, and HCMV. The therapeutic efficacy of these approved drugs, in controlled clinical trials, has not been determined for the rest of the herpesviruses namely EBV and HHV-6–8 [47–49].

4.1   Acyclic nucleoside analogs

4.1.1 Acyclovir and valaciclovir

Acyclovir (1; ACV; 9-(2-hydroxyethoxymethyl)guanine) is a synthetic analog of the nucleoside guanosine and in its triphosphate form has marked inhibitory activity against HSV types 1 and 2, and VZV [2]. In HSV-1, HSV-2 and VZV-infected cells, the viral thymidine kinase (TK) is responsible for phosphorylating ACV to its monophosphate (MP) [50, 51]. Host cellular kinases then convert ACV-MP to its triphosphate (TP) form, which then selectively inhibits the viral DNA polymerase activity [50, 52]. Incorporation of the ACV-MP into the nascent viral DNA chain results in premature chain termination [52, 53].

Valaciclovir (VCV) is the valine ester prodrug of ACV and it is rapidly and almost completely converted to ACV after oral administration [54]. Plasma ACV levels that are comparable to those achieved by intravenous administration of ACV are found after VCV administration [55]. The advantage of VCV over ACV is its high oral bioavailability, which allows less frequent dosing in the treatment of HSV and VZV disease [4, 56–60]. It is currently approved for the treatment of genital herpes and VZV infections. However, recent data shows that VCV has good activity both as a preemptive and a prophylactic agent against HCMV-associated disease in AIDS patients [61, 62]. Work still needs to be done in determining the ideal doses of VCV for treatment of HCMV disease [61]. Currently, ACV and VCV are used in high doses to prevent CMV infection following allogeneic stem cell and renal transplantation [49].

An important question is by what mechanism do VCV and ACV get phosphorylated by HCMV. A very interesting report published recently by Talarico et al. [63] in which they examined the role of HCMV UL97 in both the intracellular and extracellular activation of ACV showed that purified UL97 protein can phosphorylate ACV as well as GCV. This is the first report indicating that purified UL97 directly phosphorylates either GCV or ACV. This work showed a direct role of the HCMV UL97 protein in the phosphorylation of ACV in HCMV-infected cells. The observation of phosphorylation of ACV by the HCMV UL97 protein provides a rationale for the efficacy of ACV and VCV therapy in preventing HCMV infection and disease in the immunocompromised patients.

4.1.2 Ganciclovir

Ganciclovir (2; GCV; 9-(1,3-dihydroxy-2-propoxymethyl)guanine) is an acyclic guanosine nucleoside analog with potent activity against members of the herpesvirus family, especially, HCMV [64]. In HCMV-infected cells, the product of the UL97 open reading frame (ORF) is responsible for phosphorylating GCV to its MP form [65]. Like is the case with ACV, cellular kinases then convert GCV-MP to its TP form and this leads to selective inhibition of CMV DNA polymerase activity [66]. Structurally, GCV is very similar to ACV but differs from ACV in that is has the functional equivalent of a 3'-OH group. This structural difference allows GCV-MP to incorporate into the growing viral DNA chain without being an absolute chain terminator like ACV [67, 68]. GCV has been shown to be very effective for the treatment of CMV retinitis in AIDS patients [69], and HCMV-associated disease in bone marrow, heart and renal transplant patients [70–72] and is currently marketed for these indications. Despite the fact that GCV can act as a good substrate for HSV-1 TK and as a result of this is an excellent inhibitor of HSV replication, it is not used to treat HSV infections. Due to its poor oral bioavailability (< 10%) intravenous administration is usually necessary for most indications [73].

4.1.3 Penciclovir and famciclovir

Penciclovir (3; PCV (9-4-hydroxy-3-hydroxymethylbut-1-yl)guanine) is an acyclic nucleoside analog which differs slightly from ganciclovir in that it has a methylene bridge instead of the ether oxygen in the acyclic side chain [74]. Like ACV, it inhibits the viral DNA polymerase following conversion to triphosphates by the virus encoded TK and cellular enzymes. Unlike ACV, the PCV-TP suppresses viral replication through competitive inhibition of the viral DNA polymerase, rather than DNA chain termination [75]. Penciclovir has demonstrated antiviral activity against hepatitis B virus, HSV-1, HSV-2 and VZV [76]. The intracellular triphosphate of PCV is considerably more stable than ACV-TP (*in vitro* half-life of 10–20 h in HSV-infected cells compared to 0.7 to 1 h for ACV) which gives PCV a potential pharmacological advantage [77]. Also of importance is the fact that PCV has been shown to be effective against a small percentage of ACV[r] HSV strains *in vitro* [76]. This could present a benefit for some immunocompromised patients.

PCV is currently marketed, as a topical formulation, for the treatment of recurrent herpes labialis in immunocompromised patients. An open, dose-escalation study where PCV was administered intravenously to immunocompromised patients with mucocutaneous HSV infections showed that the drug was effective for the treatment of mucocutaneous HSV infection. The optimum intravenous dose of PCV for the treatment of HSV disease in this group of patients was 5 mg/kg q8h or q12h. This study was followed by a randomized, double-blind, multicenter study comparing these two doses of PCV with ACV (5 mg/kg q8h for 7 days) [78]. The results of this study showed

(1) Acyclovir

(2) Ganciclovir

(3) Penciclovir

(4) Famciclovir

(5) Cidofovir

(6) Foscarnet

that PCV given either q8h or q12h is safe and as effective as ACV for the treatment of mucocutaneous HSV infection in immunocompromised patients [78]. The success of the PCV q12h regimen is important because the reduced frequency of administration translates into possible patient convenience.

Famciclovir (4; FCV), the orally bioavailable prodrug of PCV, is approved in the United States and other countries for the treatment of acute herpeszoster virus infection and the treatment and suppression of genital herpes

[56, 57, 79]. The major metabolic pathway of FCV involves the deacetylation at the 3 and 4 positions of the acyclic side chain followed by oxidation at the 6 position of the purine ring to yield the active metabolite, PCV [80, 81]. A major advantage of FCV over ACV is its high oral bioavailability which permits less frequent dosing in the treatment of HSV and VZV disease [4, 56–60].

4.2 Phosphonate analogs

4.2.1 Cidofovir

Cidofovir (5; CDV, HPMPC) is an acyclic phosphonate analog of CMP with potent *in vitro* and *in vivo* activity against a broad spectrum of herpesviruses [82–84]. CDV differs from other nucleoside analogs in that it does not contain a sugar ring and, because of the phosphonate group, it only needs to undergo two additional phosphorylations in order to be metabolically equivalent to the nucleoside triphosphates. CDV is phosphorylated by cellular enzymes [85] and as a result of this, its metabolism is not affected by HSV infection [86]. In its diphosphate form, CDV inhibits herpesvirus DNA polymerase [86]. Consequently, CDV is active against ACV[r] TK[−] and TK[a] HSV mutants *in vitro* and in animal models [87, 88]. This is an important point given the fact that TK[−] and TK[a] mutants make up the vast majority of ACV[r] HSV strains. More recently, CDV has been used successfully to treat ACV[r], PCV[r] and GCV[r] herpesvirus infections [89, 90]. One of the advantages of CDV is its prolonged antiviral effect which requires less frequent administration [88, 91]. CDV was originally approved for the treatment of CMV retinitis. The ability to use CDV topically for localized lesions, or as an infrequent intravenous administration for disseminated disease, combined with the increased susceptibility of TK-deficient HSV mutants to this agent, has made CDV an attractive potential therapy for the treatment of infections caused by wild-type and ACV[r] HSV strains. CDV is currently approved in its intravenous form for the treatment of disseminated disease. A CDV gel product (Forvade) is currently being reviewed by the FDA for the treatment of refractory HSV. Currently, Forvade is in phase II clinical trials. In addition, cidofovir as a topical ophthalmic drug is in phase II clinical trials for HSV and VZV infections.

4.3   Pyrophosphate analogs

4.3.1 Foscarnet

Foscarnet (6; phosphonoformic acid, PFA) is a pyrophosphate analog that does not require activation by either cell or viral enzymes, but rather inhibits the polymerase directly [3]. The drug inhibits the viral DNA polymerase of herpesviruses, including CMV. PFA binds close to the pyrophosphate binding site on the viral DNA polymerase, and in this manner prevents cleavage of pyrophosphate from the deoxynucleoside triphosphates, which terminates elongation of the viral DNA chain [3]. Or, in this manner prevents normal pyrophosphate release so that the polymerase cannot complete the catalytic cycle [12, 93]. The selectivity for this compound arises from the viral polymerase being more sensitive than cellular enzymes [94]. PFA was originally approved for the treatment of CMV infection, especially for rescue therapy in patients who show no response to GCV treatment. More recently it has also been approved for the treatment of patients with ACV^r HSV and VZV infection [95, 96]. At the present time, PFA is the only drug approved for the treatment of ACV^r HSV infection [21].

4.4   Antisense

4.4.1 Fomivirsen

Fomivirsen (ISIS 2922 or Vitravene; 5'-GCGTTTGCTCTTCTTCTTGCG-3') is a 21-base antisense phosphorothioate oligonucleotide that is complementary to the human CMV immediate early 2 (IE2) mRNA [97, 98]. In 1998, the FDA approved Fomivirsen for the local treatment of CMV retinitis in patients with AIDS. It is specifically intended for patients who cannot tolerate, who have a contraindication to, or who do not sufficiently respond to other treatments [99]. Because it specifically targets the viral RNA, it avoids some of the toxicity of other drugs used to treat CMV retinitis [99]. Fomivirsen is the first antisense drug to have demonstrated safety and efficacy in the clinic and is the first antisense product approved as a therapeutic agent [100]. Administration consists of an intravitreal injection. Advantages of the new agent in the management of CMV retinitis include avoidance of intravenous lines and the systemic toxicities of intravenous therapies, and decreased frequency of injections compared with other antiviral compounds [99].

5 Resistance to herpesvirus drugs

Infections due to HSV-1, HSV-2, CMV and VZV have been well-studied, in part because potent antiviral drugs against these viruses have been introduced into clinical use during the past ten years [1–7]. Following the widespread use of antiviral agents against herpesviruses, the isolation of resistant virus strains has been reported with increasing frequency. A number of excellent review articles have been written on this topic [3, 8–10, 18, 21, 101–107]. This chapter will attempt to update and expand upon certain aspects covered in earlier reviews.

5.1 Acyclovir

Four mechanisms of acyclovir resistance in the treatment of HSV-1 and 2 and VZV have been described to date. Three of these mechanisms involve the *tk* gene and one the *pol* gene. The two most common causes of resistance are mutations in the *tk* gene, which result in absent or decreased production of enzyme [101, 108, 109]. This impaired production leads to an inability to phosphorylate acyclovir to the monophosphate form, leading to a deficiency in the active acyclovir-triphosphate form. These isolates are called thymidine kinase-deficient mutants (TK⁻). This mechanism of resistance has proven to be important in the clinical use of acyclovir [110]. These mutants are cross-resistant to ganciclovir and famciclovir, which also require thymidine kinase for their initial phosphorylation, but are sensitive to CDV and foscarnet which do not require viral-specific TK phosphorylation for their antiviral activity [101, 111, 112].

The third mechanism of resistance identified is a mutation of the *tk* gene that results in an altered enzyme (TKᵃ) with decreased affinity for acyclovir [113, 114]. This mutation results in a TK that retains the ability to phosphorylate thymidine but is unable to phosphorylate acyclovir [101, 115]. These isolates are susceptible to CDV and foscarnet. In the case of the TKᵃ mutants, cross-resistance to other nucleosides is variable; these isolates are generally resistant to ganciclovir but sensitive to famciclovir. The fourth mechanism of resistance affects the viral DNA polymerase, and this results in decreased affinity of DNA polymerase for ACV-TP. These isolates are cross-resistant to foscarnet and CDV but retain sensitivity to ganciclovir [101, 108, 114, 116, 117].

A number of large surveys of viral isolates taken from patients receiving acyclovir have shown that in immunocompetent patients, the prevalence of acyclovir-resistance has been ~ 3% in both pre- and postacyclovir therapy isolates. These studies also indicate that the prevalence of acyclovir-resistant HSV in immunocompetent individuals has remained essentially unchanged over the past 15 years, and even following prolonged administration of the drug, there does not appear to be an increased incidence of the emergence of resistance [21].

Unlike the situation in immunocompetent patients, *in vitro* acyclovir resistance has been reported with increasing frequency in immunocompromised patients [reviewed in references 8, 21]. HSV resistance to acyclovir in immunocompromised hosts was first described by Crumpacker et al. [118] in 1982, and since that time, resistance to antivirals has become recognized as a clinically significant problem in patients with acquired immunodeficiency syndrome (AIDS) and other immunosuppressive conditions [119]. Factors that appear to play a role in the development of resistance are the degree of immunosuppression and length of acyclovir therapy [120]. Sub-therapeutic levels of acyclovir in patients receiving prolonged prophylactic therapy may also be an important issue. As the number of immunocompromised patients increases, particularly those with advanced HIV disease, in whom the prevalence of HSV and the use of acyclovir is high, the incidence of acyclovir-resistant disease should be expected to increase [8, 21, 101–107].

The resistance to acyclovir observed in most clinical HSV strains examined to date in immunocompromised hosts has been caused by TK- mutants [8, 21, 101–107]. Results from a number of studies reports the level of resistance to be as high as 5% [120, 121] in AIDS patients and up to 9% in bone marrow transplant patients [122]. In the case of VZV, an analysis of ACV^r strains in immunocompromised patients shows that the resistance is associated with altered or deficient TK function [8, 21]. A few strains have been isolated that are resistant to both acyclovir and foscarnet [122], suggesting mutations in the viral DNA polymerase gene.

A major question and concern regarding acyclovir-resistant isolates is whether they are transmissible. Approximately 95–96% of isolates in surveys of patients with acyclovir resistance are TK⁻. The remaining 4–5% are usually TKᵃ mutants [21]. DNA polymerase mutants have for the most part been described in single case reports [21]. The few HSV isolates resistant to both acyclovir and foscarnet [123, 124] suggested alterations of the viral DNA polymerase. At present, there are no reports documenting person-to-person transmission of a TK⁻ mutant. Acyclovir-resistant isolates with TKᵃ or DNA polᵃ have been able to induce latency and cause reactivation illness in animal models [125]. Theoretically, these isolates can be transmitted from person to person. Fortunately, they constitute only a small proportion of acyclovir-resistant mutants, and as yet there have been no reported cases of person-to-person transmission with these phenotypes [21].

Of concern is the appearance of resistance to non-thymidine kinase dependent therapy in patients undergoing bone marrow transplantation [126]. Up to the time of the study by Darville et al. [126], failure of clinical response to foscarnet had only been seen with HIV-infected individuals.

Another area worth discussing is that of the appearance of acyclovir-resistant HSV isolates that have been identified in immunocompetent patients and their correlation with clinical disease [127]. Prior to 1998, acyclovir-resistant HSV isolates had been identified in immunocompetent patients, but drug resistance for the most part had not correlated with clinical disease [128]. The paper by Swetter et al. [127] describes the first case of a clinically significant acyclovir-resistant disease caused by a TK-deficient HSV isolate from an otherwise healthy HIV-negative woman.

Recently, a very interesting study by Sasadeusz et al. [129] showed that the majority of HSV-2 ACVʳ clinical isolates studied contained frameshift mutations within two long homopolymer nucleotide stretches which the authors postulated functioned as hot spots within the HSV *tk* gene and produced nonfunctional, truncated TK proteins. The study consisted of taking plaque isolates from eight ACVʳ clinical isolates from AIDS patients and sequencing them to determine the genetic lesion within the *tk* gene conferring resistance. What they found was that the mutations were clustered within two homopolymer nucleotide stretches. Three of the mutants had insertions within a 7 guanosine stretch and two of the mutants had frameshift mutations within a 6 cytosine stretch. To demonstrate that the mutation was responsible for the loss of TK activity, one of the homopolymer frameshift mutations was corrected and this resulted in the restoration of activity. Prior to this work, two other reports of clinical isolates had described frameshift mutations in the 7 guanosine homopolymer stretch, but in each case only one mutant was analyzed [130, 131]. Previously, it had been observed that laboratory-derived isolates occurred more frequently at G-C homopolymer stretches [132]. The Sasadeusz et al. study [129] contained the largest collection of HSV-1 ACV^r clinical isolates sequenced to date. Their data solidify the evidence that frameshift mutations at homopolymer sites are a major mechanism responsible for ACV resistance.

Until the appearance of a paper in 1999 by Saijo et al. [133], the consensus was that TK$^-$ ACV^r HSV mutants can establish latency in mouse trigeminal ganglia but cannot reactivate [134–136]. This would suggest that these mutants should be unable to reactivate in patients. In recent years there have been several reports of reactivated TK$^-$ clinical isolates [137–139]. A previous study [139] had shown the possibility of reactivation from latency of TK$^-$ ACV^r HSV-2 in immunocompromised patients. The present study showed very strongly that TK-associated ACV^r HSV-1 had the ability to reactivate from latency and to cause recurrent ACV^r herpes simplex virus infections in immunocompromised hosts [133]. The present work deals with the genetic characterization of seven sequential isolates recovered from 1993–1997 from a patient suffering from Wiskott-Aldrich Syndrome. Saijo et al. [133] showed, using thin-layer chromatography, that the HSV-1 TA2 mutant acquired resistance to ACV was a result of the loss of ACV phosphorylation activity by the viral TK. This indicated that the resistance to ACV was associated with mutations in the viral TK polypeptide. Nucleotide sequencing of the five ACV^r isolates was carried out and the data was compared with that of the two ACV^s isolates. This analysis showed that the nucleotide sequence of all the ACV^r isolates was identical, indicating that they all originated from the same strain. The only difference in nucleotide sequence between the five ACV^r mutants and the two ACV^s isolates was the deletion of a cytosine located within a homopolymer, at position 1064 of the ORF which gave rise to a frameshift mutation and a longer TK polypeptide. The data seems to indicate that the ACV^r HSV-1 isolate was derived from the ACV^s isolate during a long-term of prophylactic administration of ACV (March 1993–April 1994). This conclusion is supported by the fact that there is great diversity in HSV-1 TK nucleotide sequence among clinical isolates recovered from Japanese children. The DNA polymerase of the five mutants was intact as shown by their pattern of sensitivity to vidarabine and foscarnet. Prior to this study, the TK$^-$ mutants that have been reported have had either an amino acid substitution at the ATP-binding site in the TK polypeptide [140] or a frameshift mutation resulting in a the production of a truncated TK polypeptide [139, 141, 142]. This represents a different type of mutation and indicates that the carboxy terminus of the TK polypeptide plays an important role in acquisition of resistance to ACV.

5.2   Ganciclovir

Ganciclovir, one of the three approved treatments for CMV retinitis is a virustatic drug and hence has to be administered for prolonged periods of time. The use of repeated courses of GCV for treatment of CMV retinitis predisposes to the development of viral drug resistance. In addition, it has been shown that the prevalence of antiviral resistance increases with the duration of therapy [65, 143, 144]. In one study, 38% of patients treated for more than three months with GCV demonstrated resistance to the drug [144]. In another study, GCV^r isolates could be identified in 27% of AIDS patients that were treated for CMV retinitis with GCV for nine months [145]. Clinical reactivation of disease with CMV seldom occurs in the immunocompetent individuals but patients with AIDS, are at high risk of reactivation of latent infection or superinfection from a different strain of CMV [17, 146].

Two mechanisms of CMV resistance to ganciclovir have been identified. One deals with mutations in the UL97-encoded phosphotransferase which results in deficient phosphorylation of ganciclovir [8]. Loss of UL97 phosphotransferase activity as a result of mutation leads to decreased phosphorylation of GCV to GCV monophosphate and, subsequently, reduced GCV triphosphate levels. A reduction of intracellular phosphorylation of GCV may render the drug ineffective [147]. This has been demonstrated with mutants isolated in the laboratory as well as in the clinical setting [148]. Mutations in the UL97 gene are the most common types of mutations isolated in clinical patients [17]. It is estimated that mutations in the HCMV UL97 gene account for 70% of clinical resistant isolates [17]. Until 1997, usually the resistance in clinical isolates was caused by a single amino acid change in the UL97 gene product and the most commonly affected amino acids were M460, H520, A594, K595 [17]. Following a number of very comprehensive reviews of GCV resistance [17, 149, 150], there have been two reports of new mutations in clinical isolates that cause GCV resistance [151, 152]. Baldanti et al. [151], reported on the isolation of a GCV[r] mutant with a single amino acid change at residue 598 (G598S) from an AIDS patient. This mutation falls within a UL97 phosphotransferase region (residues 590–607) that is involved in GCV recognition and binding [151]. Even though the role of this mutation in conferring GCV resistance was not confirmed by marker transfer experiments, there are several pieces of data that point in this direction. The G598S mutant was detected *in vivo* when treatment failure was observed and was not seen in 50 GCV-sensitive isolates that were examined; there were no other amino acid changes in the UL97 and UL54 genes of this mutant; GCV phosphorylation was impaired; the G598S mutation is adjacent to other mutations that confer GCV resistance [151].

A second report by Baldanti et al. [152] described the isolation of two GCV[r] mutants recovered from an AIDS patient and a heart transplant patient. In both cases, the resistance was conferred by a single amino acid change at position 607 (Cys607Tyr). Sequencing of these mutants showed no amino acid substitutions in the viral polymerase gene. Marker transfer experiments restored the sensitive phenotype to the mutants. The identification of this new mutation extends the region of the carboxy-terminal domain of the UL97 phosphotransferase involved in GCV substrate recognition [152].

Ganciclovir resistance can also be caused by alterations of the viral DNA polymerase [8, 149] even though these mutations are less frequent. Polymerase mutations usually occur in addition to UL97 mutations and may increase the level of drug resistance [149]. It has been demonstrated that some GCV resistant strains with DNA polymerase mutations exhibit cross-resistance to cidofovir but usually not to foscarnet [17, 149]. However, there have been some reports of patients with AIDS where viral isolates resistant to both GCV and foscarnet have been seen [149].

A recent study by Erice et al. [153] has looked at the rapid emergence of GCV[r] mutants in bone marrow transplant recipients who are treated with GCV after receiving prophylaxis with ACV. Because ACV shares the same mechanism of activation and action as GCV against CMV, it is theoretically possible for UL97 mutations causing resistance to GCV to occur under selective pressure during exposure to ACV. To test this hypothesis, they looked at GCV susceptibilities and UL97 sequences of CMV isolates recovered from bone marrow transplant recipients who developed active CMV infection after receiving prophylaxis with ACV. The study was able to show that CMV isolates containing GCV resistance UL97 mutations may emerge rapidly in bone marrow transplant recipients treated with GCV. Therefore, active CMV infections that occur in this setting should be considered as potentially caused by GCV^r viruses. The question of whether these resistant isolates are selected for during prior prophylaxis with ACV remains to be answered.

Of interest in the area of understanding the function of the UL97 ORF is a recent study that addresses this issue [154]. Little is known about the role of UL97 in CMV replication. Biochemical studies have demonstrated protein kinase activity from UL97 that can result in both autophosphorylation [155, 156] and transphosphorylation [154]. However, at this time it is not known what the natural substrate for UL97 is. To address the question of whether UL97 is essential for viral replication, Prichard et al. [154], constructed recombinant HCMV viruses with a large deletion in UL97 and then examined these viruses for their ability to replicate in tissue culture. What this study showed was that the mutants were severely impaired in their ability to replicate in primary fibroblasts as demonstrated by the formation of small, slowly growing plaques. This would indicate that the UL97 gene is not absolutely required for replication in cell culture. The replication deficit was corrected when UL97 was provided in *trans* in a UL97 complementing cell line, confirming that the phenotype observed was due to a deficiency in UL97. What this work shows is that even though the product of the *UL97* gene may not be absolutely essential for viral replication in tissue culture, it still plays an important role and may be a good target for antiviral chemotherapy.

5.3 Penciclovir and famciclovir

The mechanisms of herpesvirus resistance to penciclovir remain to be elucidated, but are likely to be similar to those described for acyclovir. For most isolates that are resistant to acyclovir but not foscarnet, there is cross-resistance with penciclovir [8]. However, this is not always the case [8]. No laboratory or clinical penciclovir resistant isolates have been obtained to date for HSV or VZV.

5.4   Cidofovir (HPMPC)

Cidofovir might prove to be an important treatment alternative when herpesvirus resistance to nucleoside analogs is associated with deficient production or altered substrate specificity of the enzymes responsible for conversion to the monophosphate form during drug activation [8]. It has been observed that HSV TK⁻ and TKᵃ mutants are more susceptible to CDV in tissue culture than are the parental strains [157]. The difference in susceptibility to CDV of mutant viruses and wild-type is not due to viral effects on CDV metabolism, as is the case for ACV. During infection of cells, the elevation of the dCTP pool by the TK mutant viruses is less than that induced by the wild-type virus. CDV diphosphate is a competitive inhibitor with respect to dCTP for HSV DNA polymerase [157]. The competition between CDV diphosphate and dCTP at the viral polymerase is therefore changed in favor of CDV diphosphate, enhancing its activity.

Alternating ACV and CDV regimens appears to be a rational approach for dealing with immunocompromised patients. Several studies have shown that ACV resistance can be overcome, as ACVʳ strains became sensitive after CDV therapy [158]. This may happen because TK⁺ viruses can establish latency more readily than do TK⁻ viruses [158]. This would suggest that alternating between ACV and CDV therapies may be a good strategy for managing the emergence of alternatively ACV-sensitive and -resistant infections [158]. This treatment may prolong the usefulness of both agents by delaying the development of an isolate that is resistant to both drugs. Topical CDV seems to be effective and safe in the treatment of immunocompromised patients with HSV infections that are refractory to treatment with other antiviral agents [159].

An interesting study designed to look at the incidence of clinical resistance to intraocular CDV injection for treatment of AIDS-related CMV retinitis has shown that clinical failure of intravitreal CDV occurs infrequently but may be associated with CDVʳ CMV selected by prior GCV or CDV treatment [160]. To date, all polymerase alterations in HCMV known to confer GCV resistance also confer CDV resistance [160]. A look at polymerase mutations that confer resistance to GCV and CDV has shown that there is an association between polymerase residue 513 alterations and *in vitro* GCV and CDV resistance [160]. Smith et al.'s work [160] reports a new polymerase G678S alteration that is responsible for causing antiviral resistance. The fact that this residue does not lie within one of the conserved polymerase regions does not detrack from its importance in resistance due to the fact that alteration of residue S676, which also lies outside of the conserved polymerase regions, has been associated with resistance [160].

Jabs et al. [161], as part of a study for the Cytomegalovirus Retinitis and Viral Resistance Study Group, looked at the development of resistance in AIDS patients treated for CMV retinitis. The frequencies of a CDV^r isolate at the time of diagnosis of CMV retinitis are low [161]. However, with prolonged therapy use, 29% of patients treated with CDV for three months had a CDV^r isolate. This study also showed that CDV resistance is not less likely to occur than GCV resistance is when patients are treated for comparable time periods.

5.5 Foscarnet

Because of the difference in mechanism of action of foscarnet as compared to the nucleoside and nucletide analogs, herpesvirus resistance to foscarnet results exclusively from mutations in the viral DNA polymerase gene [8]. With the recommendation in 1996 to use foscarnet in patients suspected to have acyclovir-resistant HSV disease [8] foscarnet resistance has increased. Foscarnet has also been used for the treatment of acyclovir-resistant herpes zoster [8]. Analysis of clinical CMV isolates has shown that a few of the strains were resistant to foscarnet alone, or to both foscarnet and ganciclovir [8].

Most studies of VZV sensitivity to foscarnet have yielded conflicting results between clinical and *in vitro* resistance [95]. Safrin et al. [162] described a case of herpes zoster in a patient with AIDS, which responded to foscarnet despite altered *in vitro* sensitivity. In contrast, two patients with *in vitro*-susceptible strains failed to respond to foscarnet. One of these patients had AIDS [162] and one had received a bone marrow transplant [163]. The first case of a correlation between *in vitro* resistance and clinical resistance came from an AIDS patient [122]. More recently, there has been a report of a VZV foscarnet resistant clinical isolate mutant in which a single amino acid change glutamic acid to lysine (E512K) in DNA polymerase was associated with resistance [95]. An analysis of foscarnet VZV resistant mutants generated in the laboratory indicates that a single mutation is sufficient for causing resistance to foscarnet and the mutations were mapped to domains II and III of the VZV DNA polymerase [164]. A similar study done with foscarnet resistant HSV-1 mutants isolated from 8 AIDS patients indicated that most of the mutations conferring resistance to the drug consisted of single base substitutions in conserved regions of domains II, III and VI of the DNA polymerase gene [96]. Foscarnet resistant clinical isolates from patients with CMV retinitis have a single amino acid change (Ala to Val at codon 809) in conserved region III of the DNA polymerase that is responsible for resistance to the drug [165].

As is the case with CDV, the frequencies of a foscarnet-resistant isolate at the time of diagnosis of CMV retinitis is low. However, with prolonged therapy 37% of patients treated with foscarnet for nine months had a foscarnet-resistant isolate [161]. Jabs et al. [161] concluded in their study that the probability of developing resistance to foscarnet is about the same as that of developing resistance to GCV when patients are treated for comparable time periods.

5.6 Fomivirsen

The drugs currently used to treat CMV retinitis such as ganciclovir, cidofovir and foscarnet are all virustatic rather than virucidal. As a result of their shared mechanism of action, inhibition of DNA polymerase, clinical resistance to one of these three drugs usually indicates reduced clinical utility of the others. Because fomivirsen has a different target than the other three approved drugs, it makes it a good alternative for the treatment of CMV retinitis. To date no clinical resistance has been seen with fomivirsen. However, Mulamba et al. [166] have published a very interesting study in which they isolated and studied a fomivirsen-resistant virus (2922^{r}A-32-1) obtained by passaging the parental strain AD169 in increasing concentrations of the drug. There is considerable evidence that phosphorothioate oligonucleotides can inhibit viral replication by both sequence-dependent and sequence-independent mechanisms [167]. The Mulamba et al. study showed that fomivirsen inhibits CMV in a sequence dependent manner [166]. The ability to isolate a mutant resistant to fomivirsen implies that this compound acts at least in part via a virus-specific mechanism [166]. This would agree with previous mechanism of action studies for this compound [97, 98]. This work represents the first published report of a sequence-dependent viral mutant resistant to an antisense drug. Because such nonantisense mechanisms as inhibition of virus adsorption may also contribute to the antiviral activity of this type of compound, the isolation of the fomivirsen-resistant mutant shows that at least in part fomivirsen is working through an antisense mechanism [168]. The isolation of this mutant raises the possibility that resistant mutants could arise during administration of fomivirsen to patients. What remains to be seen is whether the degree of resistance observed by Mulamba et al. [166] is clinically significant and whether such mutants would retain sufficient pathogenicity to cause CMV disease.

6 Inhibitors for other viral targets

Potentially, the areas of viral attachment, entry, uncoating, protein synthesis, DNA replication, assembly and egress represent targets for therapeutic intervention. However, to date, all the anti-herpes drugs in the market target the viral DNA polymerase and hence viral DNA replication. During the last decade, the increase in the number of immunocompromised patients and the resulting emergence of resistance to the existing therapies has made the need for new medications obvious. To circumvent the rise of resistance in immunocompromised patients, medications that target new processes in the replication of the virus are needed. The following section will address ongoing work in these other viral targets.

6.1 Protease inhibitors

Herpesviruses encode a unique protease that is essential for viral replication [169, 170]. The protease is encoded by the UL26 gene in HSV-1 [169] and by the homologous UL80 gene in CMV [170]. The protease plays an essential role in virus capsid maturation by cleaving a scaffold protein which is encoded in-frame with the C-terminal part of the gene product [171]. There is a varying degree of sequence homology across the members of the herpesvirus family with a highly conserved P_4–P_1' cleavage motif, in which proteolysis occurs between alanine and serine residues. These proteases do not show homology with any known proteases outside of the herpes virus family and the recent determination of the crystal structures of HCMV, HSV-1 and VZV proteases indicates that they belong to an entirely new family of serine proteases with a novel Ser-His-His catalytic triad [172]. Recently, it has also been shown that dimerization is required for activity of the CMV and HSV proteases [172].

Previous reports of herpes protease inhibitors with drug-like qualities include the spiro-oxazolones, imidazolones, oxazinones and β-lactams (reviewed in [172]). To date, one of the most promising series of herpes protease inhibitors include the N-acyl analogues of 5-methylthieno [2,3-d]oxazinone based inhibitors (7, 8). The compounds in this series were tested for antiviral activity against HSV-2, VZV and HCMV and the IC_{50} values for the best compounds were in the submicromolar range for HSV-2 and HCMV and in the nanomolar range for VZV. Testing of the most potent compounds in this series in a MRC-5 cell culture assay (XTT) for cytotoxicity showed low to moderate cytotoxity [173]. Furthermore, selectivity testing of the most potent compounds against elastase and trypsin demonstrated no significant inhibition up to 100 μM [173]. These compounds were also tested for their effect on protease processing in HSV-2 virus infected cells using a pulse chase assay, and cytotoxicity data under the assay conditions was also obtained. The best compounds (7, 8) demonstrated inhibition of viral protease processing at the micromolar range and a > 30-fold separation from cytotoxicity. This series of compounds is still in preclinical development.

Another interesting series is the enedione-thieno[2,3-d]oxazinones (9) [174]. The aryl ketones in this series showed an order of magnitude improvement in IC_{50} for CMV protease compared to the most potent cinnamide thieno[2,3-d]oxazinones [173]. This series of compounds acts by not only acylating the catalytic serine, but also by alkylating cysteine 161 of the protease [174]. Unfortunately, when they tested the best compounds in this series for cytotoxicity severe toxicity was uncovered. Based on the high level of cytotoxicity of these compounds, the decision was made to not further evaluate them as CMV antiviral agents.

6.2   Helicase inhibitors

The 5'-3' helicase activity of herpes simplex virus is encompassed within a heterotrimeric protein complex that includes helicase, primase, and ATPase activities encoded by the UL5, UL8, and UL52 genes [175, 176]. Several lines of evidence seem to indicate that the UL5 gene encodes the helicase activity

(7) Cinnamide derivative of
5-methylthieno[2,3-d]oxazinone

(8) 5-bromo substituted derivative of
5-methylthieno[2,3-d]oxazinone

(9) Phenyl enedione-thieno
[2,3-d]oxazinone

of the complex. The UL5 gene contains six conserved motifs found in a number of RNA and DNA helicases [177–181]. Furthermore, site-directed mutagenesis of amino acids within each of the six motifs showed that all six are critical for the function of the UL5 protein as a helicase in transient replication assays [181, 182].

The compound T157602 (10), a 2-amino thiazole, was identified as an inhibitor of the UL5/8/52 helicase-primase complex from HSV [183, 184]. Three lines of evidence indicated that T157602 is an inhibitor of the product of the UL5 gene. First, T157602-resistant mutants were isolated and analyzed and it was shown that single point mutations within the UL5 gene were suf-

(10) 2-amino thiazole

ficient to confer resistance to T157602 to wild-type viruses. The molecular target of T157602 is the UL5 component of the HSV helicase-primase complex [184]. Second, Marker rescue experiments demonstrated that the UL5 gene from T157602-resistant viruses conferred resistance to T157602-sensitive wild-type viruses. Third, recombinant UL5/8/52 helicase-primase complex purified from baculoviruses expressing mutant UL5 protein, showed complete resistance to T157602 in an *in vitro* helicase assay. T157602 inhibited reversibly the helicase activity of the HSV UL5/8/52 helicase-primase complex with an IC_{50} of 5 μM. Testing of this compound against a number of other helicases showed that the inhibition is specific for the HSV-1 UL5/8/52 helicase. The primase activity of the Ul5/8/52 complex was also inhibited by T157602 with an IC_{50} of 20 μM. This compound was tested for cytotoxicity and shown to be non-cytotoxic at a concentration exceeding 100 μM which gave a therapeutic index of approximately 33. Of importance is the fact that T157602 showed good inhibitory activity against ACV^r laboratory strains and clinical isolates of HSV (as good as that of wild-type) [184]. Testing of this compound against VZV, CMV, and EBV showed the three viruses to be resistant.

6.3   Ribonucleotide reductase inhibitors

Herpes simplex virus encodes a ribonucleotide reductase enzyme that catalyzes the formation of deoxyribonucleotides from ribonucleotides [185, 186]. The enzyme consists of a large R1 subunit which contains redox-active thiols that provide the hydrogen for nucleotide reduction [187–190] and a small R2 subunit that contains a binuclear μ-oxo bridged iron center associ-

(11) BILD 1633 SE

ated with a tyrosyl free radical [190–193]. It has been shown that the carboxy terminus of the R2 subunit is essential for subunit association and for the catalytic activity of the enzyme [194, 195]. Although HSV ribonucleotide reductase is not essential for virus replication in exponentially growing cells, it is necessary in nondividing cells [196] and is necessary for the full expression of pathogenicity of HSV in animal models of primary infection [194, 197–199]. In addition, the RR has also been shown to be required for reactivation from latency [197–198]. As a result of this, the HSV RR represents a potential target for therapeutic intervention [194, 195, 198].

Early efforts to create peptidomimetic ribonucleotide reductase inhibitors have met with mixed results [16]. The results of these initials efforts were compounds that either had good antiviral activity *in vitro* but were too toxic in animal studies, or were not too toxic but did not have sufficient antiviral activity when tested in humans [16]. Recently, there have been reports of a new class of selective HSV RR subunit association inhibitors that act as mimics of the carboxy terminus of the small subunit [200]. The most promising compound in this series is BILD 1633 SE (11) [200]. Examination of this compound against cutaneous ACV[r] HSV-1 infections in the athymic nude mouse model either alone or in combination therapy with acyclovir showed that this compound is very effective. BILD 1633 SE was effective against both TK and polymerase mutants. Given the rise in ACV[r] HSV infections, this type of compound may be considered as an alternative to or used in combination with ACV. While the activity and toxicity profiles of BILD 1633 SE are much better than its predecessors in the series, this compound, like other peptidomimetic compounds, does not have good systemic absorption. There-

(12) 6-(4-acylanilino)-uracil

fore, the therapeutic potential with this class of inhibitors may be limited to topical treatment only [200]. Of note is the fact that HSV-1 isolates resistant to peptidomimetic RR inhibitors are more sensitive to ACV [201]. As a result of this, combination therapy with ACV and RR inhibitors could be beneficial.

6.4 Uracil-DNA glycosylase inhibitors

The HSV-1 uracil-DNA glycosylase (UDG) is involved in postreplicative DNA repair by the removal of uracil residues from DNA, resulting from either cytosine deamination or dUTP incorporation, by cleavage of the N-glycosidic bond linking the base to the deoxyribose phosphate backbone. Recent evidence suggests that the viral UDG is required both for virus reactivation from latency and for efficient replication in nerve tissue [202]. To date, the best UDG inhibitors that have been identified are the 6-anilinouracils which contain large n-alkyl groups in the para position of the anilino ring [203]. These compounds exhibited potent activity against the HSV-1 enzyme and retained a high degree of selectivity for the viral enzyme [203]. The most potent compound, 6-(4-octylanilino)-uracil (12), had an IC_{50} of 8 µM against the viral enzyme and a > 300 µM IC_{50} against the human enzyme. One problem with this series of compounds is their low solubility. Recently, the x-ray structure of the HSV-1 UDG complexed with uracil was solved [204]. This information has been used to design and improve UDG inhibitors [205]. The model derived from the x-ray structure data predicts that a 1-substitution may enhance activity as well as solubility of these compounds. The 1-(hydroxyalkyl) derivative was as potent as 6-(4-octylanilino)-uracil and more water soluble [205].

6.5 DNA processing inhibitors

Currently, GCV, foscarnet and CDV are the only FDA-approved drugs for the treatment of HCMV disease. These drugs all have low oral bioavailability and/or dose-related toxicities [206, 207] which limit their usefulness, particularly in AIDS patients on antiretroviral therapies. Furthermore, resistance to GCV and foscarnet in this patient group has been correlated with clinical failure [106]. There is a clear need for an orally bioavailable, effective, nontoxic anti-HCMV agent to treat the immunocompromised patient population. A series of compounds that may fit these criteria are the ribobenzimidazoles [208]. The best compounds in this series were 2-bromo-5,6-dichloro-1-β-D-ribofuranosyl benzimidazole (BDCRB) (14) and its 2-chloro analog (TCRB) (13) [208]. TCRB had an IC_{50} of 2.9 μM and BDCRB an IC_{50} of 0.7 μM against HCMV. Both compounds were only weakly active against HSV-1 and VZV [209]. Little to no cytotoxicity was observed at concentrations of up to 100 μM for these compounds [208]. The activity and selectivity of these two compounds are better than that observed with either GCV or foscarnet.

It has been demonstrated that the mechanism of action by which BDCRB and TCRB inhibit HCMV is by preventing concatemer processing which is an essential step in DNA maturation. BDCRB and TCRB inhibit the cleavage of concatemers to monomeric genomes without inhibiting the synthesis of viral DNA, mRNA, or proteins [209]. Marker rescue experiments and sequence comparison studies have shown that resistance to BDCRB maps to the U_L89 ORF. Based on motif analysis as well as homology analysis with the T4 gp17 protein and the blockage of concatemer cleavage resulting from its inhibition by BDCRB, it has been postulated that the U_L89 of HCMV encodes a DNA terminase [209]. An analysis of strains resistant to TCRB has mapped the mutations responsible for conferring resistance to the U_L89 and U_L56 ORFs [210]. The HCMV U_L56 ORF has a homolog U_L28 in HSV-1 which is involved in concatemer cleavage and packaging [211–214]. This further supports the notion that the benzimidazole ribonucleosides inhibit viral DNA processing [210].

In 1998, the compound BDCRB (GW-275175) was in phase I chinical trials in the UK in HIV-infected patients as a potential treatment for CMV infection. In 1999, Glaxo Wellcome discontinued development of GW-275175 and is in the process of out-licensing this compound.

While initial data on TCRB was exciting, pharmacokinetic studies in rats and monkeys revealed the instability of this compound *in vivo*. The phar-

(13) TCRB   (14) BDCRB   (15) 1263 W94

macokinetic data indicated that the instability was due to a cleavage of the glycosidic bond *in vivo* which released the heterocycle (2,5,6-trichlorobenzimidazole) into the bloodstream [215]. Attempts to increase the stability of TCRB and its antiviral activity against HCMV have included the synthesis of TCRB analogs with a fluoro group on the carbohydrate moiety, replacement of a C-N glycosidic bond with a C-C bond, and adding a benzene spacer between the imidazole ring and the dichlorobenzene ring. Synthesis of TCRB analogs with a fluoro group on the carbohydrate moiety resulted in compounds that exhibited a marked decrease in activity against HCMV as compared to TCRB. In addition, there was an increase in cytotoxicity which resulted in a dramatic decrease in the selectivity index of these analogs. Synthesis of TCRB analogs containing a C-N glycosidic bond in place of the C-C bond gave unexpected results. The simple transposition of the N-1 and C-7a atoms of TCRB [215] resulted in a complete lack of activity and cytotoxicity. Addition of the benzene spacer resulted in a compound that retained the same activity as TCRB against HCMV, but the activity was accompanied by a large increase in cytotoxicity yielding essentially no selectivity. Studies using other spacers are currently underway.

6.6   DNA synthesis inhibitors

In an effort to improve the metabolic stability of BDCRB, L-riboside benzimidazole analogs of this compound were synthesized [216]. The best of these analogs, 1263W94 (**15**), showed selective activity against HCMV and EBV. It is not active against HSV-1 and 2 or VZV as measured in a plaque reduction assay. The IC_{50} value of this compound against the AD169 laboratory strain of HCMV is 0.04 to 0.1 μM and has a similar range of 0.03 to 0.132 μM against

HCMV clinical isolates. This compound has shown > 50% oral bioavailability in monkeys and rats and no toxic effects in monkeys dosed at 180 mg/kg for 30 days [216]. In addition, it has shown oral bioavailability in humans of 30–40% and is three- to 20-fold more potent than GCV against CMV. It has been shown that 1263W64 inhibits HCMV replication by a novel mechanism which involves inhibition of viral DNA synthesis, but not of the viral DNA polymerase (pap 5, ref. [6]). More recently, HCMV resistance to 1263W94 has been mapped to the viral kinase UL97 [216]. The fact that 1263W94 has a novel mechanism of action against HCMV is very important because it would predict that this compound should be active against strains resistant to current therapies.

An interesting observation was made when the compound 1263W94 was tested against EBV in a latently infected Burkitt lymphoma (BL) cell line in which viral reactivation and lytic replication can be efficiently induced [217, 218]. The IC_{50} value against EBV was 0.15 to 1.1 μM. This activity was at least ten-fold higher than that seen for ACV in identical assays. The TC_{50} value for 1263W94 was determined for several lymphocyte lines and it varied from 55 to 90 μM giving an *in vitro* therapeutic index of 50 to 100. Phase I clinical trials in asymptomatic HIV positive volunteers showed that 1263W94 was well tolerated at these levels, with no adverse side effects [216].

There is evidence that shows that 1263W94 acts against the EBV essential replication factor EA-D. In the presence of this compound both the accumulation and phosphorylation of EA-D are decreased [216]. It has been proposed that EA-D may be a substrate for a viral kinase encoded by the EBV BGLF4 ORF.

Studies of 1263W94 (maribavir) in volunteers have indicated good oral bioavailability and acceptable tolerance and the compound appears not to interfere with the anti-HIV activity of antiretroviral drugs. Glaxo Wellcome was conducting phase I/II clinical studies in the European Union and the US but decided that the compound should be out-licensed. Currently 1263W94 is in a suspended phase II stage.

6.7 Thymidine kinase inhibitors

HSV-1 encodes a thymidine kinase enzyme that is not required for the efficient replication of virus in dividing cells [219], but may be important in reac-

(16) HBPG

tivation of virus from latency [220]. A strategy for preventing the recurrence of herpes infections would be to interfere with the reactivation process by targeting inhibitors against the virus-encoded TK. To address this issue, the N^2-phenylguanine series was synthesized [221–224]. The original compounds in this series showed selective inhibitory activity against the HSV-1 and HSV-2 TKs relative to the human enzyme *in vitro* and *in vivo*. The best inhibitors in this series were tested for their ability to inhibit the reactivation of HSV-1 from explant cultures of latently infected murine trigeminal ganglia. Both compounds greatly reduced the frequency of reactivation at 150 µM compared with that of untreated control ganglia [224]. Further examination of these compounds confirmed that they had poor water solubility which made the use of high concentrations very difficult. Efforts to increase potency, water solubility and maintain lipid solubility yielded the compound 9-(4-hydroxybutyl)-N^2-phenylguanine (HBPG) (16) [225]. The IC$_{50}$ value for this compound against thymidine phosphorylation of HSV-1 and HSV-2 TKs is 0.16 and 2.15 µM respectively. Biochemical analysis of HBPG showed that it is a competitive, nonsubstrate inhibitor of HSV-1 TK (K_I = 50 nM). Further analysis of this compound demonstrated that it had a good pharmacokinetic profile and lacked acute toxicity in mice *via* the ip route. When tested for its capacity to suppress viral reactivation of HSV-1 following hyperthermic stress in latently infected mice, HBPG showed that it can inhibit viral reactivation and viral DNA synthesis in nervous system tissue, such as the trigeminal ganglia of mice.

More recently, another series of compounds, the 6-azapyrimidine-2'-deoxynucleosides, first synthesized in the 1960's, and which showed very little activity against herpesviruses [226], have come into the limelight again. The 6-azapyrimidine-2'-deoxynucleosides had received little attention due to their poor biological activity. This was the result of their testing in antiviral

(17) 5-(1-Thienyl)-6-aza-4'-thio-2'-deoxyuridine

assays *in vitro*, where the expression of the TK enzyme is not necessary for viral replication although it is an important enzyme for the pathogenicity of the virus [226]. However, recent data has shown that they are specific inhibitors of the herpesvirus TK. When tested for their effect on thymidine phosphorylation of the HSV-1 and human TK, the IC_{50} values for the best compound in this series were 0.40 and > 100 respectively [226]. Not only are these compounds good inhibitors of the enzyme but they are very poor substrates. Further evaluation of these compounds will determine if they are potential candidates for treating herpesvirus infections such as herpetic encephalitis which affects non-replicating cells such as neurons, or for suppressing reactivation of such infections in the clinic.

6.8   DNA polymerase inhibitors

Despite the fact that nucleoside analogs have played an important role in the treatment of viral infections, the toxicities associated with a number of these compounds [227, 228] as well as the emergence of resistant viral strains have led to the search for new classes of molecules. Among these new classes of nucleoside analogs are the L-nucleosides which exhibit either equal or more potent activities compared to their D-counterparts while exhibiting less toxicity [229]. L-nucleosides have less toxicity due to the fact that they are usually not recognized by normal mammalian enzymes but only by virus-encoded or bacterial enzymes [230].

L-nucleosides are the enantiomers of the natural nucleosides which have an inverted configuration at all chiral centers. Although L-nucleosides had been synthesized as early as 1964, this class of compounds did not gain seri-

(18) L-FMAU

ous attention until the appearance of 3TC which is now marketed for AIDS and HBV infection. To date, the L-nucleoside exhibiting the best antiherpesvirus activity is 2'-fluoro-5-methyl-β-L-arabinofuranosyluracil (L-FMAU) (18) [231]. This compound shows potent anti-EBV activity with a favorable toxicity profile [232]. D-FMAU also showed excellent anti-EBV activity, but the severe toxicity exhibited by the compound precluded it from being considered as a potential clinical candidate [231]. L-FMAU has no significant anti-HSV-1 or 2 activity [231].

Very recently, a new series of L-nucleoside analogs that has shown great promise as inhibitors of herpesviruses are the cyclohexene nucleoside analogs [233]. A concept that has become very important in the area of antiviral nucleosides is the difference in biological behavior of enantiomers. It has become clear until the synthesis of the cyclohexene nucleoside analogs that D- and L-nucleosides have a different activity and toxicity profile [233]. D-cyclohexenyl-G (19) and L-cyclohexenyl-G (20) are the first example of two enantiomeric nucleosides that show similar activity and toxicity profile against the whole series of classical herpesviruses. This is an unexpected finding for nucleosides that have three chiral centers. D-cyclohexenyl-G as well as L-cyclohexenyl-C showed potent and selective activity against HSV-1, HSV-2, CMV, and VZV. Their activity spectrum was comparable to that of ACV and GCV.

7   Conclusion

Herpesvirus infections and the emergence of resistance to the old and most of the newer treatments constitute a serious problem in the immunocompromised patient population. It is clear that the development of new drugs

(19) D-cyclohexenyl nucleoside   (20) L-cyclohexenyl nucleoside

against viral targets, other than the DNA polymerase, would be a useful addition to the armamentarium of already existing anti-herpes therapies. With the continued understanding of the viral replication process, it is not unrealistic to expect that future anti-herpes drugs could target such processes as viral attachment, entry, uncoating, protein synthesis, DNA replication and assembly.

Acknowledgments

I would like to thank Ms. Elizabeth Estansell for her technical support and my colleague Dr. Doreen Ma for helpful comments during the preparation of the manuscript.

References

1   D. Faulds and R.C. Heel: Drugs 39, 597–638 (1990).
2   R.J. Whitley and J.W. Gnann Jr.: N. Engl. J. Med. 327, 782–789 (1992).
3   A.J. Wagstaff and H.M. Bryson: Drugs 48, 199–226 (1994).
4   K.R. Beutner, D.J. Friedmann, C. Forszpaniak, P.L. Andersen and M.J. Wood: Antimicrob. Agents Chemother. 39, 1546–1553 (1995).
5   W.L. Drew, D. Ives and J.P. Lalezari: N. Engl. J. Med. 333, 615–620 (1995).
6   J.P. Lalezari, W.L. Drew, E. Glutzer, C. James, D. Miner, J. Flaherty, P.E. Fisher, K. Cundy, J. Hannigan, J.C. Martin et al.: J. Infect. Dis. 171, 788–796 (1995).
7   P. Reusser: Bailliere's Clin. Infect. Dis. 1, 523–544 (1994).
8   P. Reusser: J. Hosp. Infect. 33, 235–248 (1996).
9   P. Reusser, S.R. Riddell, J.D. Meyers and P.D. Greenberg: Blood 78, 1373–1380 (1991).
10   J.L. Meier and S.E. Straus: J. Infect. Dis. 166, S13–S23 (1992).
11   M.S. Hirsch, in: R.H. Rubin and L.S. Young (eds.): Clinical approach to infection in the

compromised host, Plenum Medical Book Company, New York and London 1994, 379–396.

12   P. Reusser: J. Suisse de Med. *130*, 101–112 (2000).

13   E. De Clercq: Clin. Microbiol. Rev. *10*, 674–693 (1997)

14   D.W. Kimberlin, D.M. Coen, K.K. Biron, J.I. Cohen, R.A. Lamb, M. McKinlay, E.A. Emini and R.J. Whitley: Antiviral Res. *26*, 369–401 (1995).

15   K.K. Biron: Antiviral Chemother. *4*, 135–143 (1996).

16   K.A. Cassady and R.J. Whitley: J. Antimicrob. Chemother. *39*, 119–128 (1997).

17   J.L. Perez: Microbiol. Sem. *13*, 343–352 (1997).

18   D.M. Coen, in: D.D. Richman (ed.): Nucleosides and foscarnet – mechanisms, John Wiley & Sons, Chichester, New York, Brisbane, Toronto and Singapore 1996, 81–102.

19   J. Balzarini, L. Naesens and E. De Clercq: Curr. Opinion Microbiol. *1*, 535–546 (1998).

20   D. Pillay: Comm. Dis. Pub. Health *1*, 5–13 (1998).

21   J.C. Pottage, Jr. and H.A. Kessler: Infect. Agents and Dis. *4*, 115–125 (1995).

22   D.M. Coen: Antiviral Chemother. *4*, 49–57 (1996).

23   F.A. Alrabiah and S.L. Sacks: Drugs *52*, 17–32 (1996).

24   C.M. Perry and A.J. Wagstaff: Drugs *50*, 396–415 (1995).

25   W.E. Rawls and J. Campione-Piccardo, in: A. Nahmias, W. Dowdle and R. Schinazi (eds.): The human herpes viruses: an interdisciplinary perspective, Elsevier, Amsterdam 1981, 137–152.

26   F.M. Burnet and S.W. Williams: Med. J. Aust. *1*, 637–642 (1939).

27   K. Dodd, L.M. Johnston and G.J. Buddingh: J. Pediatr. *12*, 95–102 (1938).

28   L. Haarr and S. Skulstad: APMIS *102*, 321–346 (1994).

29   J.J. Gibson, C.A. Hornung, G.R. Alexander, F.K. Lee, W.A. Potts and A.J. Nahmias: J. Infect. Dis. *162*, 306–312 (1990).

30   L.S. Magder, A.J. Nahmias, R.E. Johnson, F.K. Lee, C. Brooks and C. Snowden: N. Engl. J. Med. *321*, 7–12 (1989).

31   J.C. Overall, Jr., in: G.J. Galasso, T.C. Merigan and R.A. Buchanan (eds.): Antiviral agents and viral diseases of man, Raven Press, New York 1984, 251–252.

32   W.L. Drew, W. Buhles and K.S. Erlich: Infect. Dis. Clin. N. Am. *2*, 495–509 (1988).

33   P.K. Peterson, H.H. Balfour, S.C. Marker, D.S. Fryd, R.J. Howard and R.L. Simmons: Medicine *59*, 283–300 (1980).

34   J. Glenn: Rev. Infect. Dis. *3*, 1151–1178 (1981).

35   B.D. Kuppermann: J. Acquired Imm. Def. Syn. Human Retrovirol. *14*, S13–S21 (1997).

36   D.A. Jabs, C. Enger and J.G. Bartlett: Arch. Ophthalmol. *107*, 75–80 (1989).

37   M.A. Polis and H. Masur: JAMA *273*, 1457–1459 (1995).

38   C. Leport, S. Puget and J.M. Pepin: J. Infect. Dis. *168*, 1330–1331 (1993).

39   J.T. Matthews, B.J. Terry and A.K. Field: Antiviral Res. *20*, 89–114 (1993).

40   F.L. Homa and J.C. Brown: Rev. Med. Virol. *7*, 107–122 (1997).

41   J.H. Subak-Sharpe and D.J. Dargan: Virus Genes *16*, 239–251 (1998).

42   C.S. Miller, R.J. Danaher and R.J. Jacob: Crit. Rev. Oral Biol. Med. *9*, 541–562 (1998).

43   A.J. Davison and J.E. Scott: J. Gen. Virol. *67*, 1759–1816 (1986).

44   E.S. Mocarski, Jr., in: B.N. Fields, D.M. Knipe and P.M. Howley (eds.): Cytomegaloviruses and their replication, Lippincott-Raven Publishers, Philadelphia 1996, 2447–2492.

45   B. Roizman and A.E. Sears: Annu. Rev. Microbiol. *41*, 543–571 (1987).

46   J.G. Stevens: Microbiol. Rev. *53*, 318–332 (1989).

47   S.E. Straus, J.L. Cohen, G. Tosato and J. Meier: Ann. Intern. Med. *118*, 45–58 (1993).

48   N. Singh and D.R. Carrigan: Ann. Intern. Med. *124*, 1065–1071 (1996).

49   P. Reusser, in: J. Klastersky, S.C. Schimpff and H.J. Senn (eds.): Supportive care in cancer: A handbook for oncologists, Marcel Dekker, Inc., New York 1999, 87–112.

50   G.B. Elion, P.A. Furman, J.A. Fyfe, P. de Miranda, L. Beauchamp and H.J. Schaeffer: Proc. Natl. Acad. Sci. USA *74*, 5716–5720 (1977).

51   J.A. Fyfe, P.M. Keller, P.A. Furman, R.L. Miller and G.B. Elion: J. Biol. Chem. *253*, 8721–8727 (1978).

52   Y.C. Cheng, S.P. Grill, G.E. Dutschman, K. Nakayama and K.F. Bastow: J. Biol. Chem. *258*, 12460–12464 (1983).

53   P.V. McQuirt and P.A. Furman: Am. J. Med. *73*, 67–71 (1982).

54   S. Weller, M.R. Blum, M. Doucette, T. Burnette, D.M. Cederberg, P. de Miranda et al.: Clin. Pharmacol. Ther. *54*, 595–605 (1993).

55   M.A. Jacobson, J. Gallant, L.H. Wang, D. Coakley, S. Weller, D. Gary, L. Squires, M.L. Smiley, M.R. Blum and J. Feinberg: Antimicrob. Agents Chemother. *38*, 1534–1540 (1994).

56   S.L. Sacks, F.Y. Aoki, F. Diaz-Mitoma, J. Sellors, S.D. Shafran: JAMA *276*, 44–49 (1996).

57   S. Tyring, R.A. Barbarash, J.E. Nahlik, A. Cunningham, J. Marley, M. Heng et al.: Ann. Intern. Med. *123*, 89–96 (1995).

58   R. Patel, N.J. Bodsworth, P. Woolley, B. Peters, G. Vejlsgaard, S. Saari et al.: Genitourin. Med. *73*, 105–109 (1997).

59   M. Reitano, S. Tyring, W. Lang, C. Thoming, A.-M. Worm, S. Borelli et al.: J. Infect. Dis. *178*, 603–610 (1998).

60   T. Schacker, H-L. Hu, D.M. Koelle, J. Zeh, R. Saltzman, R. Boon et al.: Ann. Intern. Med. *128*, 21–28 (1998).

61   J.E. Feinberg, S. Hurwitz, D. Cooper, F.R. Sattler, R.R. MacGregor, W. Powderly, G.N. Holland, P.D. Griffiths, R.B. Pollard, M. Youle et al.: J. Infect. Dis. *177*, 48–56 (1998).

62   P.D. Griffiths, J.E. Feinberg, J. Fry, C. Sabin, L. Dix, D. Gor, A. Ansari and V.C. Emery: J. Infect. Dis. *177*, 57–64 (1998).

63   C.L. Talarico, T.C. Burnette, W.H. Miller, S.L. Smith, M.G. Davis, S.C. Stanat, T.I. Ng, Z. He, D.M. Coen, B. Roizman et al.: Antimicrob. Agents Chemother. *43*, 1941–1946 (1999).

64   A.K. Field, M.E. Davies, C. DeWitt, H.C. Perry, R. Liou, J. Germershausen, J.D. Karkas, W.T. Ashton, D.B.R. Johnston and R.L. Tolman: Proc. Natl. Acad. Sci. USA *80*, 4139–4143 (1983).

65   V. Sullivan, C.L. Talarico, S.C. Stanat, M. Davis, D.M. Coen and K.K. Biron: Nature *358*, 162–164 (1992).

66   T. Matthews and R. Boehme: Rev. Infect. Dis. *10*, S490–S494 (1988).

67   J.E. Reardon: J. Biol. Chem. *264*, 19039–19044 (1989).

68   F.M. Hamzeh, P.S. Lietman, W. Gibson and G.S. Hayward: J. Virol. *64*, 6184–6195 (1990).

69   B.E. Sha, C.A. Benson, T.A. Deutsch, P.A. Urbanski, J.P. Phair and H.A. Kessler: J. Infect. Dis. *164*, 777–780 (1991).

70   H.H. Balfour, Jr., B.A. Chace, J.T. Stapleton, R.L. Simmons and D.S. Fryd: N. Engl. J. Med. *320*, 1381–1387 (1989).

71   C.C. Elkins, W.H. Frist, J.S. Dummer, J.R. Stewart, W.H. Merrill, K.A. Carden and H.W. Bender: Ann. Thorac. Surg. *56*, 1267–1273 (1993).

72   T.O. Nunan, M. King, P. Bull, J.E. Banatvala, N.F. Jones and P.J. Hilton: Clin. Nephrol. *22*, 28–31 (1984).

73   C.S. Crumpacker: N. Engl. J. Med. *335*, 721–729 (1996).

74 M.R. Boyd, T.H. Bacon, D. Sutton and M. Cole: Antimicrob. Agents Chemother. *31*, 1238–1242 (1987).

75 R.A. Vere Hodge and R.M. Perkins: Antimicrob. Agents Chemother. *33*, 223–229 (1989).

76 M.R. Boyd, S. Safrin and E.R. Kern: Antivir. Chem. Chemother. *4*, 3–11 (1993).

77 R.A. Vere Hodge: Antivir. Chem. Chemother. *4*, 67–84 (1993).

78 H.M. Lazarus, R. Belanger, A. Candoni, M. Aoun, R. Jurewicz, L. Marks: Antimicrob. Agents Chemother. *43*, 1192–1197 (1999).

79 S.L. Spruance, T.L. Rea, C. Thoming, R. Tucker, R. Saltzman and R. Boon: JAMA *277*, 1374–1379 (1997).

80 A.W. Harrell, S.M. Wheeler, M. Pennick, S.E. Clarke and R.J. Chenery: Drug Met. Disp. *21*, 18–23 (1993).

81 J.M. Colacino and K.A. Staschke: Prog. Drug Res. *50*, 261–322 (1998).

82 J.J. Bronson, I. Ghazzouli, M.J.M. Hitchcock, R.R. Webb II, E.R. Kern and J.C. Martin, in: J.C. Martin (ed.): Nucleotide analogues as antiviral agents, American Chemical Society, Washington, D.C. 1989, 88–102.

83 J.J. Bronson, I. Ghazzouli, M.J.M. Hitchcock, R.R. Webb II and J.C. Martin: J. Med. Chem. *32*, 1457–1463 (1989).

84 E. De Clercq, T. Sakuma, M. Baba, R. Pauwels, J. Balzarini, I. Rosenberg and A. Holy: Antiviral Res. *8*, 261–272 (1987).

85 T. Cihlar, I. Votruba, K. Horska, R. Liboska, I. Rosenberg and A. Holy: Collect. Czech. Chem. Commun. *57*, 661–672 (1992).

86 H.-T. Ho, K.L. Woods, J.J. Bronson, H. De Boeck, J.C. Martin and M.J.M. Hitchcock: Mol. Pharmacol. *41*, 197–202 (1992).

87 G. Andrei, R. Snoeck, P. Goubau, J. Desmyter and E. De Clercq: Eur. J. Clin. Microbiol. Infect. Dis. *11*, 143–151 (1992).

88 P.C. Maudgal and E. De Clercq: Invest. Ophthalmol. Visual Sci. *32*, 1816–1820 (1991).

89 J.P. Lalezari, W.L. Drew, E. Glutzer, D. Miner, S. Safrin, W.F. Owen, Jr., J.M. Davidson, P.E. Fisher and H.S. Jaffe: J. Infect. Dis. *170*, 570–572 (1994).

90 R. Snoeck, G. Andrei, E. De Clercq, M. Gerard, N. Clumeck and C. Sadzot-Delvaux: N. Engl. J. Med. *329*, 968–969 (1993).

91 K. Soike, J.-L. Huang, J.E. Zhang, R. Boem, M.J.M. Hitchcock and J.C. Martin: Antiviral Res. *16*, 17–28 (1991).

92 B. Erickson, A. Larsson, E. Helgstrand, N.-G. Johansson and B. Oberg: Biochim. Biophys. Acta *607*, 53–64 (1980).

93 M. Ostrander and Y.C. Cheng: Biochim. Biophys. Acta *609*, 232–245 (1980).

94 B. Erickson and B. Oberg: Antimicrob. Agents Chemother. *15*, 758–762 (1979).

95 B. Visse, B. Dumont, J.-M. Huraux and A.-M. Fillet: J. Infect. Dis. *178*, S55–S57 (1998).

96 I. Schmit and G. Boivin: J. Infect. Dis. *180*, 487–490 (1999).

97 R.F. Azad, V.B. Driver, K. Tanaka, R.M. Crooke and K.P. Anderson: Antimicrob. Agents Chemother. *37*, 1945–1954 (1993).

98 K.P. Anderson, M.C. Fox, V. Brown-Driver, M.J. Martin and R.F. Azad: Antimicrob. Agents Chemother. *40*, 2004–2011 (1996).

99 P. Piascik: J. Am. Pharm. Assoc. *39*, 84–85 (1999).

100 C. Marwick: JAMA *280*, 871 (1998).

101 B.A. Larder and G. Darby: Antiviral Res. *4*, 1–42 (1984).

102 D.M. Coen: J. Antimicrob. Chemother. *18B*, 1–10 (1986).

103 D.M. Coen: Antiviral Res. *15*, 287–300 (1991).

104 P.A. Chatis and C.S. Crumpacker: Antimicrob. Agents Chemother. *36*, 1589–1595 (1992).

105 D.M. Coen: Int. Antiviral News *1*, 98–99 (1993).

106 A.K. Field and K.K. Biron: Clin. Microbiol. Rev. *7*, 1–13 (1994).

107 D.M. Coen: Trends Microbiol. *2*, 481–485 (1994).

108 D.M. Coen and P.A. Schaffer: Proc. Natl. Acad. Sci. USA *77*, 2265–2269 (1980)

109 G. Palu, W.P. Summers, S. Valisena and M. Tognon: J. Med. Virol. *24*, 251–262 (1988).

110 H.J. Field: Br. Med. Bull. *41*, 345–350 (1985).

111 H.J. Field, G. Darby and P. Wildy: J. Gen. Virol. *49*, 115–124 (1980).

112 H.J. Field, B.A. Larder and G. Darby: Am. J. Med. *73*, 369–371 (1982).

113 G. Darby, H.J. Field and S.A. Salisbury: Nature *289*, 81–83 (1981).

114 B.A. Larder and G. Darby: Virology *146*, 262–271 (1985).

115 B.A. Larder, Y.C. Cheng and G. Darby: J. Gen. Virol. *64*, 523–532 (1983).

116 P. Collins, B.A. Larder, N.M. Oliver, S. Kemp, I.W. Smith and G. Darby: J. Gen. Virol. *70* 375–382 (1989).

117 C.B. Hwang, K.L. Ruffner and D.M. Coen: J. Virol. *66*, 1774–1776 (1992).

118 C.S. Crumpacker, L.E. Schnipper, S.I. Marlowe, P.N. Kowalsky, B.J. Hershey and M.J. Levin: N. Engl. J. Med. *306*, 343–346 (1982).

119 S. Safrin: J. Acquir. Immune Defic. Syndr. *5*, S29–S32 (1992).

120 J.A. Englund, M.E. Zimmerman, E.M. Swierkosz, J.L. Goodman, D.R. Scholl and H.H. Balfour: Ann. Intern. Med. *112*, 416–422 (1990).

121 F. Nugier, J.N. Colin, M. Aymard and M. Langlois: J. Med. Virol. *36*, 1–12 (1992).

122 A.M. Fillet, B. Visse, E. Caumes, B. Dumont, M. Gentilini and J.M. Huraux: Clin. Infect. Dis. *21*, 1348–1349 (1995).

123 C.J. Birch, G. Tachedjian, R.R. Doherty, K. Hayes and I.D. Gust: *162*, 731–734.

124 S.L. Sacks, R.J. Wanklin, D.E. Reece, K.A. Hicks, K.L. Tyler and D.M. Coen: Ann. Intern. Med. *111*, 893–899 (1989).

125 P.A. Chatis, C.H. Miller, L.E. Schrager and C.S. Crumpacker: N. Engl. J. Med. *320*, 297–300 (1989).

126 J.M. Darville, B.E. Ley, A.P.C.H. Roome and A.B.M. Foot: Bone Marrow Trans. *22*, 587–589 (1998).

127 S.M. Swetter, E.L. Hill, E.R. Kern, D.M. Koelle, C.M. Posavad, W. Lawrence and S. Safrin: J. Infect. Dis. *177*, 543–550 (1998).

128 S.N. Lehrman, E.L. Hill, J.F. Rooney, M.N. Ellis, D.W. Barry and S.E. Strauss: J. Antimicrob. Chemother. *18*, 85–94 (1986).

129 J.J. Sasadeusz, F. Tufaro, S. Safrin, K. Schubert, M.M. Hubinette, P.K. Cheung and S.L. Sacks: J. Virol. *71*, 3872–3878 (1997).

130 C.B.C. Hwang, B. Horsburgh, E. Pelosi, S. Roberts, P. Digard and D. Coen: Proc. Natl. Acad. Sci. USA *91*, 5461–5465 (1994).

131 S. Kit, M. Sheppard, H. Ichimura, S. Nusinoff-Lehrman, M.N. Ellis, J.A. Fyfe and H. Otsuka: Antimicrob. Agents Chemother. *31*, 1483–1490 (1987).

132 C.B.C. Hwang and H.J.H. Chen: Gene *152*, 191–193 (1995).

133 M. Saijo, T. Suzutani, K. Itoh, Y. Hirano, K. Murono, M, Nagamine, K. Mizuta, M. Niikura and S. Morikawa: J. Med. Virol. *58*, 387–393 (1999).

134 D.M. Coen, M. Kosz-Vnenchak, J.G. Jacobson, D.A. Leib, C.L. Bogard, P.A. Schaffer, K.L. Tyler and D.M. Knipe: Proc. Natl. Acad. Sci. USA *86*, 4736–4740 (1989).

135 S. Efsthaniou, S. Kemp, G. Darby and A.C. Minson: J. Gen. Virol. 70, 869–879 (1989).

136 R.B. Tenser, K.A. Hay and W.A. Edris: J. Virol. *63*, 2861–2865 (1989).

137 S. Safrin, C. Crumpacker, P. Chatis, R. Davis, R. Hafner, J. Rush, H.A. Kessler, B. Landry, J. Mills, et al.: N. Engl. J. Med. *325*, 551–555 (1991).

138 J.J. Sasadeusz and S.L. Sacks: J. Infect. Dis. *174*, 476–482 (1996).

139 G. Palu, G. Gerna, F. Bevilacqua and A. Marcello: Virus Res. *25*, 133–144 (1992).

140 Q.Y. Liu and W.C. Summers: Virology *163*, 638–642 (1988).

141 M.H. Sawyer, G. Inchauspe, K.K. Biron, D.J. Waters, S.E. Straus and J.M. Ostrove: J. Gen. Virol. *69*, 2585–2593 (1988).

142 D.M. Coen, A.F. Irmiere, J.G. Jacobson and K.M. Kerns: Virology 168, 221–231 (1989).

143 P. Chrisp and S.P. Clissold: Drugs *41*, 104–129 (1991).

144 W.L. Drew, R.C. Miner, D.F. Busch, S.E. Follansbee, J. Gullet, S.G. Mehalko et al.: J. Infect. Dis. *163*, 716–719 (1991).

145 D.A. Jabs, C. Enger, J.P. Dunn and M. Forman: J. Infect. Dis. *177*, 770–773 (1998).

146 M.S. Pasternack, D.N. Medearis, Jr. and R.H. Rubin: Rev. Infect. Dis. *12*, S720–S726 (1990).

147 S.C. Stanat, J.E. Reardon, A. Erice, E.C. Jordan, W.L. Drew and K.K. Biron: Antimicrob. Agents Chemother. *35*, 2191–2197 (1991).

148 A. Erice, S. Chou, K.K. Biron, S.C. Stanat, H.H. Balfour, Jr. and M.C. Jordan: N. Engl. J. Med. *320*, 289–293 (1989).

149 S. Noble and D. Faulds: Drugs *56*, 115–146 (1998).

150 W.L. Drew: Am. J. Health System. Pharm. *53*, S17–S23 (1996).

151 F. Baldanti, L. Simoncini, C.L. Talarico, A. Sarasini, K.K. Biron and G. Gerna: AIDS *12*, 816–818 (1998).

152 F. Baldanti, M.R. Underwood, C.L. Talarico, L. Simoncini, A. Sarasini, K.K. Biron and G. Gerna: Antimicrob. Agents Chemother. *42*, 444–446 (1998).

153 A. Erice, N. Borrell, W. Li, W.J. Miller and H.H. Balfour Jr.: J. Infect. Dis. *178*, 531–534 (1998).

154 M.N. Prichard, N. Gao, S. Jairath, G. Mulamba, P. Krosky, D.M. Coen, B.O. Parker and G.S. Pari: J. Virol. *73*, 5663–5670 (1999).

155 Z. He, Y.S. He, Y. Kim, L. Chu, C. Ohmstede, K.K. Biron and D.M. Coen: J. Virol. *71*, 405–411 (1997).

156 M. van Zeijl, J. Fairhurst, E.Z. Baum, L. Sun and T.R. Jones: Virology *231*, 72–80 (1997).

157 D.B. Mendel, D.B. Barkhimer and M.S. Chen: Antimicrob. Agents Chemother. *39*, 2120–2122 (1995).

158 C.M. Martinez and D.B. Luks-Golger: Ann. Pharmacotherapy *31*, 1519–1521 (1997).

159 L. Farooq, P.C. Don, M. Kaufmann, S.M. White and J.M. Weinberg: Arch. Dermatol. *134*, 1169–1170 (1998).

160 I.L. Smith, I. Taskintuna, F.M. Rahhal, H.C. Powell, E. Ai, A.J. Mueller, S.A. Spector and W.R. Freeman: Arch. Ophthalmol. *116*, 178–185 (1998).

161 D.A. Jabs, C. Enger. M. Forman and J.P. Dunn: Antimicrob. Agents Chemother. *42*, 2240–2244 (1998).

162 S. Safrin, T.G. Berger, I. Gilson, P.R. Wolfe, C.B. Wofsy, J. Mills and K.K. Biron: Ann. Intern. Med. *115*, 19–21 (1991).

163 A.E. Bendel, T.G. Gross, W.G. Woods, C.K. Edelman and H.H. Balfour Jr.: Lancet *341*, 1342 (1993).

164 B. Visse, J.M. Huraux and A.M. Fillet: J. Med. Virol. *59*, 84–90 (1999).

165 S. Chou, G. Marousek, D.M. Parenti, S.M. Gordon, A.G. LaVoy, J.G. Ross, R.C. Miner and W.L. Drew: J. Infect. Dis. *178*, 526–530 (1998).

166 G.B. Mulamba, A. Hu, R.F. Azad, K.P. Anderson and D.M. Coen: Antimicrob. Agents Chemother. 42, 971–973 (1998).

167 J.L. Tonkinson and C.A. Stein: Antiviral Chem. Chemother. 4, 193–200 (1993).

168 C.M. Perry and J.A. Barman Balfour: Drugs 57, 375–380 (1999).

169 F. Liu and B. Roizman: J. Virol. 65, 5149–5156 (1991).

170 A.R. Welch , A.S. Woods, L.M. McNally, R.J. Cotter and W. Gibson: Proc. Natl. Acad. Sci. USA 88, 10792–10796 (1991).

171 M. Gao, L. Matusick-Kumar, W. Hurlburt, S.F. DiTusa, W.W. Newcomb, J.C. Brown, P.J. McCann III, I. Deckman and R.J. Colonno: J. Virol. 68, 3702–3712 (1994).

172 L. Waxman and P.L. Darke: Antiviral Chem. Chemother. 11, 1–22 (2000).

173 R.L. Jarvest, I.L. Pinto, S.M. Ashman, C.E. Dabrowski, A.V. Fernandez, L.J. Jennings, P. Lavery and D.G. Tew: Bioorg. Med. Chem. Lett. 9, 443–448 (1999).

174 I.L. Pinto, R.L. Jarvest, B. Clarke, C.E. Dabrowski, A. Fenwick, M.M. Gorczyca, L.J. Jennings, P. Lavery, E.J. Sternberg, D.G. Tew et al.: Bioorg. Med. Chem. Lett. 9, 449–452 (1999).

175 J.J. Crute and I.R. Lehman: J. Biol. Chem. 266, 4484–4488 (1991).

176 J.J. Crute, L. Tsurumi, L. Zhu, S.K. Weller, P.D. Olivo, E.S. Mocarski, M.D. Challberg and I.R. Lehman: Proc. Natl. Acad. Sci. USA 86, 2186–2189 (1989).

177 A.E. Gorbalenya, E.V. Koonin, A.P. Donchenko and V.M. Blinov: FEBS Lett. 235, 16–24 (1988).

178 T.C. Hodgeman: Nature 333, 22–23 (1988).

179 D.J. McGeoch, M.A. Dalrymple, A. Dolan, D. McNab, L.J. Perry, P. Taylor and M.D. Challberg: J. Virol. 62, 444–453 (1988).

180 J.E. Walker, M. Saraste, M.J. Runswicke and N.J. Gay: EMBO J. 1, 945–951 (1982).

181 L. Zhu and S.K. Weller: J. Virol. 66, 469–479 (1992).

182 L. Zhu and S.K. Weller: Virology 166, 366–378 (1988).

183 M. Sivaraja, H. Giordano and M.G. Peterson: Anal. Biochem. 265, 22–27 (1998).

184 F.C. Spector, L. Liang, H. Giordano, M. Sivaraja and M.G. Peterson: J. Virol. 72, 6979–6987 (1998).

185 V.G. Preston, J.A.V. Coates and F.J. Rixon: J. Virol. 45, 1056–1064 (1983).

186 M. Ponce De Leon, R.J. Eisenberg and G.H. Cohen: J. Gen. Virol. 36, 163–173 (1977).

187 R.L. Krogsrud, E. Welchner, E. Scouten and M. Liuzzi: Anal. Biochem. 213, 386–394 (1993).

188 W. McClements, G. Yamanaka, V. Garsky, H. Perry, S. Bacchetti, R. Colonno and R.B. Stein: Virology 162, 270–273 (1988).

189 P. Nordlund, B.-M. Sjoberg and H. Eklund: Nature 345, 593–598 (1990).

190 P. Reichard: Annu. Rev. Biochem. 57, 349–374 (1988).

191 J.M. Bollinger Jr., D.E. Edmondson, B.H. Huynh, J. Filley, J.R. Norton and J. Stubbe: Science 253, 292–298 (1991).

192 P. Gaudreau, H. Paradis, Y. Langelier and P. Brazeau: J. Med. Chem. 33, 723–730 (1990).

193 H. Paradis, P. Gaudreau, P. Brazeau and Y. Langelier: J. Biol. Chem. 263, 16045–16050 (1988).

194 C.R. Brandt, R.L. Kintner, A.M. Pumfery, R.J. Visalli and D.R. Grau: J. Gen. Virol. 72, 2043–2049 (1991).

195 B.M. Dutia, M.C. Frame, J.H. Subak-Sharpe, W.N. Clarke and H.S. Marsden: Nature 321, 439–443 (1986).

196 D.J. Goldstein and S.K. Weller: Virology 166, 41–51 (1988).

197 A.D. Idowu, E.B. Fraser-Smith, K.L. Poffenberger and R.C. Herman: Antivir. Res. *17*, 145–156 (1992).

198 J.G. Jacobson, D.A. Leib, D.J. Goldstein, C.L. Bogard, P.A. Schaffer, S.K. Weller and D.M. Coen: Virology *173*, 276–283 (1989).

199 Y. Yamada, H. Kimura, T. Morishima, T. Daikoku, K. Maeno and Y. Nishiyama: J. Infect. Dis. *164*, 1091–1097 (1991).

200 J. Duan, M. Liuzzi, W. Paris, M. Lambert, C. Lawetz, N. Moss, J. Jaramillo, J. Gauthier, R. Deziel and M.G. Cordingley: Antimicrob. Agents Chemother. *42*, 1629–1635 (1998).

201 A.-M. Bonneau, P. Kibler, P. White, C. Bousquet, N. Dansereau and M.G. Cordingley: J. Virol. *70*, 787–793 (1996).

202 R.B. Pyles and R.L. Thompson: J. Virol. *68*, 4963–4972 (1994).

203 F. Focher, A. Verri, S. Spadari, R. Manservigi, J. Gambino and G.E. Wright: Biochem. J. *292*, 883–889 (1993).

204 R. Savva, K. McAuley-Hecht, T. Brown and L. Pearl: Nature *373*, 487–493 (1995).

205 H. Sun, C. Zhi, G.E. Wright, D. Ubiali, M. Pregnolato, A. Verri, F. Focher and S. Spadari: J. Med. Chem. *42*, 2344–2350 (1999).

206 M.A. Jacobson: AIDS Res. Hum. Retroviruses *10*, 917–923 (1994).

207 M.A. Polis, K.M. Spooner, B.F. Baird, J.F. Manischewitz, H.S. Jaffe, P.E. Fisher, J. Falloon, R.T. Davey Jr., J.A. Kovacs, R.E. Walker et al.: Antimicrob. Agents Chemother. *39*, 882–886 (1995).

208 L.B. Townsend, R.V. Devivar, S.R. Turk, M.R. Nassiri and J.C. Drach: J. Med. Chem. *38*, 4098–4105 (1995).

209 M.R. Underwood, R.J. Harvey, S.C. Stanat, M.L. Hemphill, T. Miller, J.C. Drach, L.B. Townsend and K.K. Biron: J. Virol. *72*, 717–725 (1998).

210 P.M. Krosky, M.R. Underwood, S.R. Turk, K. W.-H. Feng, R.K. Jain, R.G. Ptak, A.C. Westerman, K.K. Biron, L.B. Townsend and J.C. Drach: J. Virol. *72*, 4721–4728 (1998).

211 C. Addison, F.J. Rixon and V.G. Preston: J. Gen. Virol. *71*, 2377–2384 (1990).

212 G. Sherman and S.L. Bachenheimer: Virology *163*, 471–480 (1988).

213 G. Sherman and S.L. Bachenheimer: Virology *158*, 427–430 (1987).

214 S.K. Weller, E.P. Carmichael, D.P. Aschman, D.J. Goldstein and P.A. Schaffer: Virology *161*, 198–210 (1987).

215 L.B. Townsend, K.S. Gudmundsson, S.M. Daluge, J.J. Chen, Z. Zhu, G.W. Koszalka, L. Boyd, S.D. Chamberlain, G.A. Freeman, K.K. Biron et al.: Nucleosides & Nucleotides *18*, 509–519 (1999).

216 V.L. Zacny, E. Gershburg, M.G. Davis, K.K. Biron and J.S. Pagano: J. Virol. *73*, 7271–7277 (1999).

217 K. Takada: Int. J. Cancer *33*, 27–32 (1984).

218 K. Takada and Y. Ono: J. Virol. *63*, 445–449 (1989).

219 A.T. Jamieson, G.A. Gentry and J.H. Subak-Sharpe: J. Gen. Virol. *24*, 465–480 (1974).

220 R.B. Tenser: Intervirology *32*, 76–92 (1991).

221 F. Focher, C. Hildebrand, S. Freese, G. Ciarrocchi, T. Noonan, S. Sangalli, N. Brown, S. Spadari and G.E. Wright: J. Med. Chem. *31*, 1496–1500 (1988).

222 F. Focher, C. Hildebrand, S. Sangalli, D. Sandoli, G. Ciarrocchi, A. Rebuzzini, G. Pedrali-Noy, R. Manservigi, G.E. Wright, G. Brown et al.: Methods Findings Exptl. Clin. Pharmacol. *11*, 577–582 (1989).

223 C. Hildebrand, D. Sandoli, F. Focher, J. Gambino, G. Ciarrocchi, S. Spadari and G.E. Wright: J. Med. Chem. *33*, 203–206 (1990).

224   D.A. Leib, K.L. Ruffner, C. Hildebrand, P.A. Schaffer, G.E. Wright and D.M. Coen: Antimicrob. Agents Chemother. *34*, 1285–1286 (1990).

225   H. Xu, G. Maga, F. Focher, E.R. Smith, S. Spadari, J. Gambino and G.E. Wright: J. Med. Chem. *38*, 49–57 (1995).

226   I. Basnak, M. Sun, T.A. Hamor, F. Focher, A. Verri, S. Spadari, B. Wroblowski, P. Herdewijn and R.T. Walker: Nucleosides & Nucleotides *17*, 187–206 (1998).

227   J.L. Martin, C.E. Brown, N. Mathews-Davis and J.E, Reardon: Antimicrob. Agents Chemother. *38*, 2743–2749 (1994).

228   W.B. Parker and Y.C. Cheng: J. NIH Res. *6*, 57–61 (1994).

229   L.P. Kotra, Y. Xiang, M.G. Newton, R.F. Schinazi, Y.C. Cheng and C.K. Chu: J. Med. Chem. *40*, 3635–3644 (1997).

230   S. Spadari, G. Maga, F. Focher, G. Giarrocchi, R. Manservigi, F. Arcamone, M. Capobianco, A. Carcuro, F. Colonna, S. Iotti and A. Garbesi: J. Med. Chem. *35*, 4214–4220 (1992).

231   C.K. Chu, T.W. Ma, K. Shanmuganathan, C.G. Wang, Y.J. Xiang, S.B. Pai, G.Q. Yao, J.-P. Sommadossi and Y.-C. Cheng: Antimicrob. Agents Chemother. *39*, 979–981 (1995).

232   S.B. Pai, S.H. Liu, Y.L. Zhu, C.K. Chu, and Y.-C. Cheng: Antimicrob. Agents Chemother. *40*, 380–386 (1996).

233   J. Wang, M. Froeyen, C. Hendrix, G. Andrei, R. Snoeck, E. De Clercq and P. Herdewijn: J. Med. Chem. *43*, 736–745 (2000).

Antiviral Agents – Advances and Problems (E. Jucker, Ed.)
©2001 Birkhäuser Verlag, Basel (Switzerland)

Protease inhibitors as potential anti-viral agents for the treatment of picornaviral infections

Q. May Wang

Infectious Diseases Research
Lilly Research Laboratories
Eli Lilly and Company,
Indianapolis, IN 46285, USA

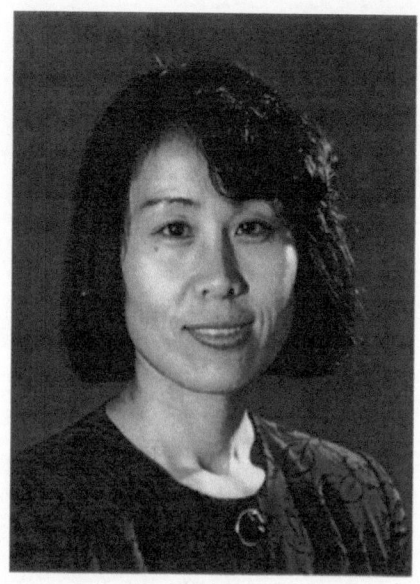

Q. May Wang

completed her B. S. in 1983 and M.S. degree in 1986, with a major of biology from Shandong University, China. She received her Ph.D. in biochemistry in 1991 from Purdue University, Indiana, and then conducted her postdoctoral training at Indiana University School of Medicine. She joined Lilly Research Laboratories as senior biochemist in 1995.

Summary

The picornavirus family contains several human pathogens including human rhinovirus (HRV) and hepatitis A virus (HAV). In the case of HRVs, these small single-stranded positive-sense RNA viruses translate their genetic information into a polyprotein precursor which is further processed mainly by two viral proteases designated 2A and 3C. The 2A protease (2Apro) makes the first cleavage between the structural and non-structural proteins, while 3C protease (3Cpro) catalyzes most of the remaining internal cleavages. It has been shown that both 2Apro and 3Cpro are cysteine proteases but their overall protein folding is more like trypsin-type serine proteases. Due to their unique protein structure and essential roles in viral replication, 2Apro and 3Cpro have been viewed as excellent targets for antiviral intervention. In recent years, considerable efforts have been made in the development of antiviral compounds targeting these proteases. This article summarizes the recent approaches in the design of novel 2A and 3C protease inhibitors as potential antiviral agents for the treatment of picornaviral infections.

Contents

Keywords

Picornavirus, human rhinovirus, hepatitis A virus, common cold, viral protease, 2A protease, 3C protease, viral protease inhibitors.

Glossary of abbreviations

2Apro, viral 2A protease; 3Cpro, viral 3C protease; EC50, 50% effective antiviral concentration, HAV, hepatitis A virus; HRV, human rhinovirus; PV, human poliovirus; IC50, 50% enzyme inhibition concentration; SAR, structure-activity relationship; MCPMK, Methoxysuccinyl-Ala-Ala-Pro-Val-chloromethylketone.

1 Introduction

Picornaviruses, a diverse group of small plus strand RNA viruses, are the major cause of numerous human diseases worldwide including poliomyelitis, acute hepatitis, myocarditis, and the common cold [1–4]. Family members include several well-known human pathogens such as polio viruses, hepatitis A virus (HAV), Coxsackie viruses, and over 100 serotypes of human rhinoviruses (HRVs) [1–4]. Despite the fact that some picornaviral infections are mild and self-limiting in healthy adults, serious sequelae of infection can occur in children or patients with pre-existing medical problems (see [3] and references therein). Therefore, development of effective vaccines and potent antiviral agents have been the major focus for the prevention or treatment of picornaviral infections.

231

Various effective prophylactic vaccines against the infections of poliovirus and HAV have been developed and are currently in use worldwide [2, 4]. In other cases, such as the common cold caused by Coxsackie viruses and HRVs, the development of prophylactic vaccines is particularly impractical due to the multiplicity of serotypes. For these picornaviral infections, extensive efforts have been devoted to searching for selective antiviral agents.

It has been proposed that interferon be used as primary mediator for control of picornaviral infections (see [3] for review). Interferon α demonstrated better effectiveness than interferon β for preventing HRV infections (see [3] and references therein]. However, potential use of interferon for therapy of established infection has been found to be ineffective even at very high doses [3].

Meanwhile, availability of the three-dimensional structure of rhinovirus has permitted the design of antiviral molecules interacting with the viral capsid proteins. Compounds acting through this mechanism include various isoxazole derivatives, flavinoids, and pyridazines [3, 5]. Recent clinical studies revealed that these inhibitors did not show significant relief of cold symptoms despite their antiviral efficacy (see [12] for review). In addition, antibodies or a soluble form of the intracellular adhesion molecule (ICAM-1), the receptor for the major group of HRVs, have been used to disrupt the viral attachment to the host cell surface and subsequent uncoating during cell entry [3, 6]. No clinical studies on these molecules have been reported [3].

Another approach under development is the selective inhibition of important viral enzymes or proteins by small molecules. Proteases encoded by viruses have long been viewed as attractive targets for antiviral intervention [11 for review]. The successful identification of HIV protease inhibitors and their use in therapy of AIDS has confirmed the validity of the viral proteases as antiviral targets [11]. In addition, proteases encoded by several other human pathogenic viruses including hepatitis C virus, cytomegolovirus, and herpes simplex viruses have also been actively used for development of antiviral agents (see [11] for review).

The picornaviral RNA genome encodes several nonstructural proteins which play important roles in the viral life cycle [1, 6–11]. Of these, a ~20 kDa cysteine protease termed 3C is one of the most extensively studied viral enzymes [7–9]. Another similar viral protease is designated 2A, encoded only by enteroviruses and HRVs, whose catalytic mechanism and roles in viral replication have also been defined [7–9]. With respect to the development of antipicornarviral agents, the 2A and 3C proteases have received much more attention than other viral enzymes [11, 12]. Compounds inhibiting 2A and 3C proteolytic activity have been identified through high throughput screening as well as rational design on the basis of their cleavage specificity and active site conformation. This article reviews the recent design and development of antiviral compounds targeting these proteases for the treatment of picornaviral infections in humans. A short introduction of the picornavirus infectious cycle, along with a brief summary of the biochemical characterization of the 2A and 3C enzymes are included to enhance understanding of these proteases. For more extensive analysis, excellent review articles are available [1–4, 6–10].

2   Picornaviruses

Picornaviruses are a group of small non-enveloped RNA viruses that possess a plus-strand RNA genome with a size of 7000–9000 nucleotides [1]. These viruses have been divided into five genera: aphthoviruses (foot-and-mouth-disease virus); cardioviruses (encephalomyocarditis virus and mengovirus); enteroviruses (polio virus and Coxsackie virus); hepatitis A virus; and rhinoviruses (for a detailed review see [1]). Many members of the picornavirus family are human and animal pathogens. For examples, the well-studied human polioviruses (PVs) are the major cause of poliomyelitis; hepatitis A virus (HAV) infects humans and causes type-A hepatitis; human rhinoviruses (HRVs) and Coxsackie viruses are associated with acute and chronic bronchitis and other respiratory tract illnesses; and the foot-and-mouth-disease viruses infect cloven-footed livestock animals [1–4]. In the case of HRVs, over a hundred HRV serotypes have been identified. It is believed that they may be responsible for over 50% of common colds in adults and children [3, 11].

In the past two decades, much attention has been focused on understanding the mechanisms of picornavirus replication and polyprotein processing [1–4, 7, 8, 13]. For most picornaviruses, the first step of the virus replication cycle is attachment of the virus to the host cell membrane followed by its penetration via endocytosis. Once entering the cell cytosol, the virus uncoats, releases its plus-strand RNA, and replicates its genomic information which is then translated into a single polyprotein with a size of ~250 kDa. This polyprotein precursor is subjected to proteolytic processing to generate mature viral structural proteins and functional viral enzymes. The capsid proteins subsequently assemble around newly made RNA genomes into progeny infectious virons which are finally released along with the host cell lysis [1, 3].

Picornaviruses share a common genomic organization and translational strategy. A generalized scheme of picornaviral genome organization and its polyprotein processing is illustrated in Figure 1 (also see figures in [1, 7–9]). The entire genome encodes 11–13 viral proteins, including four viral capsid structural proteins (VP1 through VP4) and 7–9 nonstructural proteins, depending on genus [1]. As the viruses translate their genomic information into a polyprotein precursor [1], the generation of mature viral proteins and enzymes from the polyprotein is essential to the viral replication and life cycle. The maturation cleavage process is mainly governed by a virally encoded 3C protease (3Cpro). All members of picornavirus family encode the 3Cpro, while only enteroviruses and HRVs contain an additional protease, designated 2A, which also participates in the maturation cleavage and regulation of host cell metabolism [7, 8, 13].

2.1 Viral 2A protease

As mentioned above, the 2A protease (2Apro) exists in only HRVs and enteroviruses including PVs and Coxsackie viruses [7, 8]. The 2Apro makes the first cleavage of the viral polyprotein as a cis or co-translational event [14–17]. This cleavage, taking place at the junction of the capsid protein VP1 and the N-terminus of 2A itself, separates the structural from the non-structural proteins (Fig. 1). In addition to its protease activity, the 2Apro has been found to participate in regulation of host cell metabolism. Unlike eukaryotic protein translation, viral protein translation occurs via a cap-independent mechanism. The cleavage of eukaryotic initiation factor eIF-4γ, also termed p220, has been found to be catalyzed by the 2Apro in the infected cells [16–21]. As eIF-4γ plays an important role in the initiation of cap-dependent protein synthesis, degradation of eIF-4γ may lead to an inhibition of cellular protein synthesis. Although it is not clear whether the cleavage of eIF-4γ is sufficient for a complete shut-off of host cell protein synthesis, expression of the 2Apro causes a significant reduction of cellular RNA polymerase II transcription [22, 23].

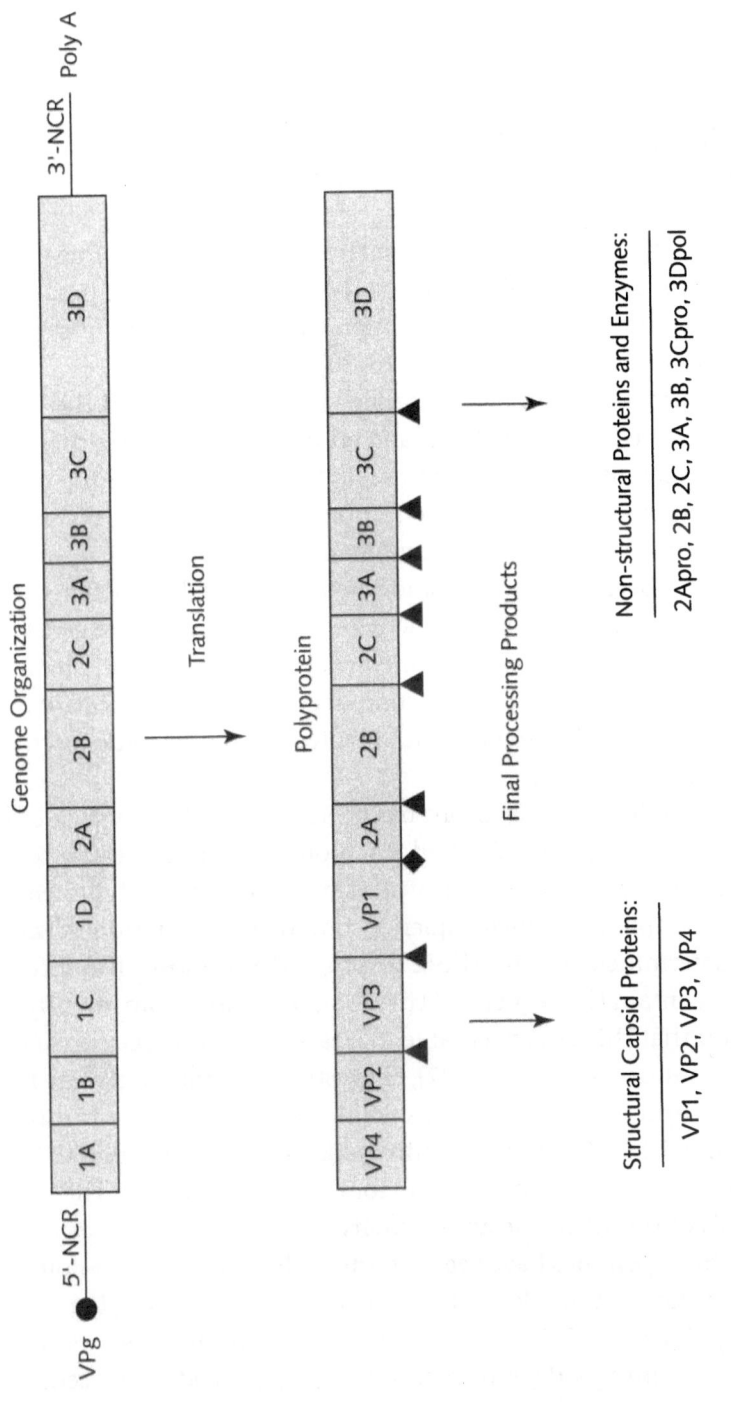

Fig. 1

Generalized schematic representation of picornavirus genome organization, polyprotein translation, and maturation cleavage. The cleavage sites for 2Apro and 3Cpro are indicated. Cleavage between the structural proteins VP4 and VP2 has been proposed to be an autocleavage event [8]. 3Dpol is the viral RNA-dependent RNA polymerase.

Viral 2Apro is classified as a cysteine protease [14, 17, 24]. This is supported by the observation that thiol alkalyting reagents can strongly inhibit the 2Apro catalytic activity [24, 25]. The catalytic triad of 2Apro has been defined as His-Asp-Cys through mutational analysis [14, 17, 19]. Although the 2Apro utilizes the thiol group of the cysteine residue as the nucleophile, both site-directed mutagenesis and amino acid sequence alignment data suggest that it is structurally more related to a group of small trypsin-like serine proteases than to a typical papain-like cysteine protease [17, 26–28]. Its unique protein structure and important roles in viral replication have made this protease an attractive target for antiviral intervention [26–30].

The active 2A proteases from PV, Coxsackie virus B4, HRV2, and HRV14 have been overexpressed in bacterial cells and purified by several groups [20, 25, 31–33]. The availability of large quantities of the recombinant 2Apro has greatly facilitated its biochemical characterization and efforts to identify specific inhibitors of this enzyme. The recombinant 2Apro's from HRV2 and Coxsackie virus have been purified to homogeneity from soluble fractions of the transformed bacterial cells [20], and active HRV14 2Apro can be generated through a refolding process [33]. Purified viral 2A has been found to be a zinc binding protein. Zn^{++} is a structural component required for formation or restoration of the active 2Apro but is not involved in the catalytic mechanism [29, 33, 34].

The cleavage specificity of the 2Apro has been extensively investigated using small synthetic peptides. Purified 2A proteases can process a 16-amino acid peptide derived from its cleavage site on the viral polyprotein [33, 35–38]. For example, a minimal sequence comprising nine residues (P8-P1') has been determined for the HRV2 2Apro and the most efficiently cleaved peptides contain the sequence –Thr–Xaa//Gly– [36]. More recently, it has been found that this enzyme is able to cleave the chromogenic peptides containing p-nitroanilide at P1 [37], suggesting that the P1 glycine is not essential for 2Apro recognition. Thus, all residues required for the 2A cleavage to occur exist within the N-terminal side of the scissile bond [37]. Similar substrate specificity has been found for the 2A protein from HRV14 [33]. On the basis of the 2Apro cleavage activity, several 2A protease assays using small synthetic peptides have been reported. These include end-point HPLC methods using peptides derived directly from the 2A processing site on its own viral polyprotein [35, 36] and continuous colorimetric assays utilizing peptides containing a P1' p-nitroanilide [33, 37]. In addition, sensitive 2Apro fluorometric assays, based on its cleavage of peptides that are modified with a fluorescence donor and quencher, have been reported recently [38].

2.2 Viral 3C protease

Unlike the 2A protease, 3C protein is encoded in all picornaviruses [1, 7, 8]. This ~20 kDa enzyme is responsible for the majority of the viral polyprotein maturation cleavages to generate functional viral proteins as shown in Figure 1. As a common feature, 3Cpro releases itself from the viral polyprotein through an autoproteolytic reaction [7, 8]. Processing reactions catalyzed by 3Cpro occur only at certain sites in the polyprotein and the enzyme mainly recognizes and cleaves the bonds formed between Gln-Gly, Gln-Ser, and Gln-Ala [7, 8]. Although the 3Cpro cleavage cascade order has not been clearly delineated, the activity of this protease in picornaviruses eventually results in the generation of mature viral proteins required for the completion of the viral replication cycle.

Similar to viral 2Apro, 3Cpro may significantly affect host cell metabolism. A number of important cellular proteins have been reported to be cleaved *in vivo* by this viral protease. These include cellular histone H3 protein, TATA-binding protein, a subunit of transcription factor IIIC, and the cAMP-responsible element binding protein [39–44]. As most of these proteins are cellular transcription factors, their degradation by 3Cpro causes inhibition of host cell transcription [39–44]. In addition to its proteolytic activity, it has been found that rhinovirus 3Cpro (in the form of its precursor, 3CD) can bind to the 5′-noncoding region of the viral genomic RNA and thus it may be involved in the formation of the viral replication complex [7, 45]. Amino acids involved in HRV 3Cpro RNA binding activity have been identified using site-directed mutagenesis and further confirmed by crystallographic studies [46–48].

The picornaviral 3C protein is also a cysteine protease. Interestingly, its overall architecture was originally predicted to be similar to the trypsin-type serine protease despite the existence of cysteine as the nucleophile in its active site center [26, 49, 50]. This hypothesis has been confirmed by the x-ray crystal structure of 3C proteins from both HRV14 and HAV [47, 51, 52]. The catalytic triad is composed of His-Glu-Cys and is positioned as seen in serine proteases [7, 26, 47, 51–53]. Viral 3Cpro has been widely considered as a target for the development of antiviral agents for several reasons. It is present in all members of the picornavirus family and all 3Cpro's studied to date share high degree of homology at amino acid level [9]. In addition, 3Cpro makes multiple cleavages on the viral polyprotein precursor, and thus controls the generation of the mature viral proteins. Inhibitors of this enzyme should be expected to have broad spectrum activity, block the viral replication process, and prevent new virion formation. Moreover, as a cysteine protease, 3Cpro has a serine protease folding pattern with no known cellular homologue [52]; this unique feature confers a potential high selectivity for 3C protease inhibitors.

The 3Cpro enzyme has been well studied with respect to its roles in viral replication and infection, biochemical characterization, and structure determination. Active 3C proteases from different members of the picornavirus family have been overproduced in bacterial expression systems [54–65]. Meanwhile, various assays based on the 3Cpro cleavage activity have been developed. These assays employ either viral polyprotein fragments or small peptides derived from the 3Cpro native cleavage sites as substrates [54, 64–74]. Some of these measurements can be used for large scale screening and thus have greatly facilitated identification and evaluation of 3C protease inhibitors [73, 74].

In addition, recent elucidation of the 3Cpro crystal structure together with substrate cleavage specificity studies have facilitated the rational design of inhibitors. X-ray crystallographic structure of both HAV and HRV14 3Cpro has been determined at 2.3 Å resolution [47, 51]. This cysteine protease folds into two six-stranded β-barrels with a long shallow substrate-binding groove located between the two domains [47, 51]. Both its overall protein structure and active site geometry are similar to mammalian trypsin-like serine proteases although it uses a cysteine residue as the nucleophile [47, 51].

With respect to the 3Cpro cleavage activity *in vitro*, purified recombinant 3C proteases can hydrolyze the peptides designed on the basis of the 3Cpro authentic cleavage sites in the viral polyprotein [64–83]. Primary amino acid sequence of the substrates plays an important role in the 3Cpro trans-cleavage activity [7, 8]. Early work on HRV14 3Cpro suggested that this enzyme could cleave peptide substrates containing at least six amino acids, that is, P4/P2′ [68]. It has a preference for a small nonpolar amino acid at P4 and Gly-

Pro at P1'-P2' downstream of the scissile bond [68]. More recent work reveals that all essential residues are located upstream of the scissile bond as the enzyme is able to cleave the peptides containing P1' p-nitroanilide [73]. This conclusion is supported by the model formed between the 3Cpro active site and the peptidyl p-nitroanilide [73]. Similar observations have been made for the 3Cpro from Coxsackie virus [82, 83].

3 Protease inhibitors against picornavirus infections

Success in developing small molecules as selective inhibitors of HIV protease has encouraged the effort to identify protease inhibitors against other viruses of clinical significance. Although the picornavirus family contains many human pathogens, the search for potent inhibitors against picornavirus infections has mainly focused on HRV, the major cause of common colds in humans. As discussed above, immunization of HRVs is precluded by its large number of serotypes, therefore, it has been suggested that selective inhibition of HRV by small molecules may be the most effective approach. Great energy has been directed at the design and synthesis of specific HRV inhibitors that target 2Apro and 3Cpro, and antipicornaviral compounds inhibiting 2Apro and 3Cpro have been described in the literature only recently. The most recent approaches in designing specific 2A and 3C protease inhibitors for treatment of HRV and picornavirus infections are summarized in the following sections.

3.1 Picornaviral 3C protease inhibitors

In recent years, structurally divergent molecules that inhibit picornaviral 3Cpro enzymes have been reported. Some of these 3Cpro inhibitors were developed through rational design based on the 3Cpro substrate specificity and active site folding; others have been identified through random screening using various 3Cpro enzymatic assays. Overall, the most potent 3Cpro inhibitors thus far described were generated through extensive SAR studies in combination with rational design. Inhibitors of viral 3Cpro enzyme can be classified into two groups: peptidic and nonpeptidic.

3.1.1 Peptidic 3C protease inhibitors

The use of peptide derivatives for inhibition of cellular and viral proteases has been widely described in the literature (see [11] and references therein). In general, typical peptidyl protease inhibitors consist of a few amino acids and an electrophilic anchoring warhead. These amino acids, mimicking the non-prime side sequence of the substrate, enhance the affinity of the inhibitor for the enzyme, and the warhead, pointing into the P1-P1′ pocket, interacts with the active site nucleophile and thus inhibits the protease cleavage activity. Some of the well known peptidic protease inhibitors include peptide aldehyde and Michael acceptor derivatives.

The design of potent peptidic protease inhibitors demands knowledge of the peptide substrate cleavage specificity of the target protease. In the case for HRV 3Cpro, most of its cleavages occur at the bond formed between P1 glutamine and P1′ glycine [7–9]. It has been found that cleavable peptide substrates for 3Cpro contain at least four amino acids upstream of the scissile bond [68]. It has a preference for a nonpolar amino acid with a small side chain at position P4 [68, 72–75]. Based on these studies, a group of tetrapeptide aldehydes, in which the P1glutamine is replaced with the corresponding aldehyde to function as an electrophilic anchoring group, has been synthesized and evaluated as potential inhibitors against HRV 3Cpro [76]. These molecules (compound 1 as a representative) inhibited purified HRV14 3C protease with an IC_{50} range of 0.6–10 μM and demonstrated a moderate antiviral activity in cell culture with EC_{50} values of 0.3–0.5 mM [76]. However, these aldehydes, carrying an unprotected glutamine side chain at P1, could form the thermodynamically more stable, yet inactive hemiaminal (1b) with diminished inhibitory activity against the enzyme [76].

To avoid the cyclization of P1 glutamine side chain, a dipeptide aldehyde (compound 2), containing a P1 methionine sulfone to mimic the glutamine residue, was described to be a competitive inhibitor of HRV14 3Cpro [77]. This compound displayed low cytotoxic activity and moderate antiviral efficacy with an EC_{50} of 3.4 μM in cell culture [77]. The efficient inhibition of HRV 3Cpro by this compound suggests that P1 methionine sulfone could replace the original glutamine present in the substrate [77].

In addition, a series of tripeptide aldehyde inhibitors of HRV 3Cpro was disclosed recently. They have been shown to reversibly inhibit 3Cpro with Ki values ranging from 5–640 nM [78]. Several of them displayed low micro-

1a

1b

2

3

4

molar antiviral activity in cell culture assays. For example, one of the most potent inhibitors (compound **3**) had a Ki of 6 nM against HRV14 3Cpro and an EC_{50} of 2.4 µM against HRV14 in cell culture [78]. This compound was also active against other serotypes of HRV [78]. A high-resolution structure of the 3Cpro co-crystalized with this compound was obtained. These studies suggest that a relatively large substituted alkyl and aryl amide can be tolerated at the S1 subsite of the 3Cpro [78].

A similar approach has been applied to the development of anti-HAV protease inhibitors. On the basis of the HAV 3Cpro preferred peptide substrates

[79–82], tetrapeptide aldehydes containing a side-chain protected P1 glutamine (dimethylamide of glutamine, compound 4) have been designed to inhibit the 3C protease from HAV [83]. These peptide aldehydes have been confirmed to be reversible slow-acting HAV 3Cpro inhibitors [83]. The most potent molecule (4) against HAV 3Cpro had a Ki of 42 nM; it also inhibited the 3Cpro from HRV14 with ~60-fold less potency, as the P2-P4 amino acids were not optimized for HRV 3Cpro [83]. Antiviral data and cytotoxicity information were not reported for these compounds.

In light of the relative low antiviral activity associated with the reversible aldehyde inhibitors for HRV 3C enzyme (76–78), an alternative approach of incorporating Michael acceptor moieties as the electron withdrawing group into 3Cpro peptide substrates has started thereafter. Hanzlik and co-workers have shown that peptidyl Michael acceptors containing an appropriate recognition peptide and a vinylogous amino acid ester can efficiently inhibit cysteine protease such as papain [84, 85]. Unlike peptidic aldehyde derivatives, Michael acceptors can form a very stable covalent complex with the viral protease and thus the inhibition is viewed as a largely irreversible reaction [84, 85]. Several groups have recently demonstrated inactivation of picornaviral 3Cpro using compounds of this type [86–89]. The first group of tetrapeptide Michael acceptors reported by Hanzlik and colleagues could inactivate HRV14 3C with IC_{50}s in submicromolar concentrations (compound 5 as representative), which were almost equal to one-half of the 3Cpro concentration used in the assay [86]. It has been found that Michael acceptors containing only one or two amino acids exhibited reduced enzyme inhibition and antiviral potency [86].

Independent to the above effort, a series of tripeptide Michael acceptors have been reported by scientists from Agouron Pharmaceuticals [87–93]. These compounds were synthesized with various Michael acceptor moieties as the electron-withdrawing group [87, 88]. In addition, to enhance the interaction between the inhibitor and the viral protease, compounds incorporated into the different sized peptides resembling the most preferred 3Cpro substrates were also prepared and evaluated [87, 88]. The resulting peptidyl inhibitors displayed 3Cpro inhibition with the k_{obs}/I as high as 800,000 $M^{-1}s^{-1}$ and antiviral activity with EC_{50} reaching 56 nM [87, 88]. Consistent with the previously established 3C cleavage specificity [68], Michael acceptors containing one or two amino acids displayed reduced 3Cpro inhibition and antiviral potency [87, 88]. In addition, incorporation of N-methyl amino acids into these tripeptidyl 3Cpro inhibitors has been explored [89]. The resulting compounds, containing an ethyl propenoate Michael acceptor moiety, demonstrated both 3Cpro inhibition and antiviral activity *in vitro* [89].

More recently, modifications have been introduced to the backbone amide moiety of the tripeptide Michael acceptors in order to improve their metabolic stability and bioavailability [90, 91]. In this regard, a group of P2-P3 ketomethylene-containing peptidomimetics were synthesized with an ethyl propenoate Michael acceptor moiety as the warhead [90, 91]. These backbone modified compounds demonstrated reduced 3Cpro inhibition but exhibited improved antiviral activity ($EC_{90} < 1$ µM) as compared to the corresponding peptide-derived molecules [90, 91]. As expected, the improved antiviral activity was accompanied with increased cell membrane permeability [90, 91].

Further modifications have been made on these ketomethylene-containing peptidomimetic compounds in order to improve enzyme inhibition potency. In particular, the P1-glutamine replacement by lactam moieties resulted in more potent 3Cpro inhibitors with improved antiviral properties as compared to the corresponding glutamine-derived peptidomimetic molecules [92]. The most potent inhibitors in this series, AG7088 (compound 6), exhibited broad antiviral spectrum with the mean antiviral activity of EC_{50} and EC_{90} values of 23 nM and 82 nM, respectively [91–93]. Examination of a panel of cellular serine proteases and cysteine proteases indicated that AG7088 was not active toward these cellular enzymes consistent with its low cytotoxicity data [91–93]. It has been claimed that AG7088 demonstrated antiviral activity when added late in the virus cycle [92]. Based on these attractive features, compound AG7088 has entered clinical trial in late of 1998 and currently it is in phase II clinical study. In parallel, attempts to use peptidic Michael acceptors as HAV 3C protease inhibitors have also been reported recently [94].

In addition to peptidyl aldehydes and Michael acceptors, another new generic group of peptidic 3Cpro inhibitors, azapeptides, have been reported most recently. For example, peptidyl bromomethylketonehydrazides containing a backbone modified glutamine irreversibly inactivated HRV 3Cpro with the second order inactivation rate constant up to $23,400 \ M^{-1}s^{-1}$ [95, 96]. This type of molecules inhibits cysteine proteases irreversibly by alkylating the thiol group of the active site cysteine [96]. Compound 7 in this class also displayed moderate antiviral activity against HRV1B in cell culture assay with an EC_{50} of 2.5 µg/ml [96]. In addition, azapeptide esters with a different reactive

5

6

leaving groups at P1 have been designed and examined as potential HRV14 3Cpro inhibitors [97]. Moderate 3Cpro inhibition by these molecules was observed, however, it was found that certain azapeptides are slow-turnover substrates for the viral protease, which might result in incomplete enzyme inhibition [97]. Similarly, a peptidyl monofluoromethylketone based on the preferred HAV 3Cpro peptide substrate was designed recently. This molecule (**8**) irreversibly inactivates HAV 3Cpro with a second order rate constant of 330 $M^{-1}s^{-1}$ by forming a stable complex with the enzyme [98]. At 5 µM this compound displayed antiviral activity [98].

3.1.2 Nonpeptidic viral 3C protease inhibitors

Work on peptidic protease inhibitors has provided important information for the further design and development of potent non-peptidic molecules. Based on these studies, it has been proposed that small molecules containing reactive carbonyl groups can specifically inhibit HRV 3Cpro via formation of a covalent hemithioacetal or Michael adducts with the active site thiol group [77, 83]. To date, several types of non-peptidic carbonyl compounds have been

7

8

synthesized and demonstrated to be viral 3C protease inhibitors. These include β-lactams [99], isatins [100], homophthalimides [101], and β-lactones [102].

A series of spiro indolinone β-lactams were first described in 1990 as potential mechanistic-based 3Cpro inhibitors [99]. Compound **9** was shown to have an IC_{50} of 20 µg/ml against HRV 3Cpro. However, this molecule was not selective as it inhibited human leukocyte elastase and cathepsin G with IC_{50} values of 0.4 and 4.0 µg/ml, respectively [99]. No antiviral data or cytotoxicity information is available for this compound.

Isatins (2,3-dioxindoles) have shown activity against HRV 3Cpro efficiently [100]. These HRV 3C protease inhibitors were designed through a combination of SAR studies, molecular modeling, and mechanical calculations. Inhibition of HRV 3Cpro by isatins was reversible with low nanomolar range K_i values (51 nM against HRV14 3C for compound **10**). Although several compounds in this group showed excellent selectivity against HRV 3Cpro with respect to several cellular proteases tested *in vitro*, antiviral data obtained from cell culture assay were found to be disappointing as most of the potent 3Cpro inhibitors displayed high cell toxicity [100].

Homophthalimides have also been identified as nonpeptidic HRV 3C protease inhibitors [101]. Based on the core structure identified through random screening against HRV 3Cpro, several potent compounds were identified in SAR studies. These compounds inhibit the HRV14 3C enzyme in the low micromolar range (IC_{50} value of 55.4 µM for compound 11). In addition, several homophthalimides displayed antiviral activity in cell culture assay which correlated well with the enzyme inhibition data [101].

More recently, β-lactones have been shown to be a new class of non-peptidic 3Cpro inhibitors that irreversibly inactivating HAV protease [102]. For example, compound 12 demonstrated a k_{inact}/K_I value of 3800 $M^{-1}s^{-1}$ against HAV 3Cpro [102]. It has be revealed that β-lactones inhibited HAV 3Cpro by alkylating the active site thiol group and thus covalent complex could be formed between the enzyme and these compounds [102]. Interestingly, it was stated that these β-lactones could also inhibit the counterpart enzyme from HRV14 [102]. No antiviral data were available for these compounds.

In addition to the above compounds generated through SAR studies, several other HRV 3Cpro inhibitors, identified from microbial fermentation extracts, have also been reported in literature [95–97]. These include naphthoquinone-lactol (13), a quinone-like citrinin (14), radicinin (15), and triterpene sulfates (16). Inhibition of HRV 3Cpro activity by these natural products was moderate with IC_{50} values in µg/ml or mM range [103–105]. Results regarding antiviral activity, cytotoxicity, and SAR studies are not available at the present time. With the exception of compound 16, all of these molecules appear to be capable of inactivating the 3Cpro active site nucleophile, as manifested by the presence of electrophilic groups, such as alkyl halides, aldehydes, ketones, α,β-unsaturated esters, quinones, or activated lactams. As this area of research receives more attention, a greater degree of chemical diversity is expected.

3.2 Viral 2A protease inhibitors

As discussed above, the viral 2Apro is another key enzyme involved in the replication and infection of both PV and HRVs. However, for several reasons much less attention has been given to the development of specific inhibitors against viral 2A protease as compared to the 3Cpro. First, unlike the 3Cpro which is present in all members of the picornavirus family, the 2Apro is encoded only in HRVs and enteroviruses [7, 8]. Secondly, the 2Apro makes only one cut at its own N-terminus as an intramolecular event [7, 8], making

9

10

11

12

13

14

15

16

the design of specific 2A protease inhibitor rather difficult. Finally, the lack of a crystal structure along with less developed biochemical understanding of the 2Apro, as compared to the 3Cpro, has hampered efforts to develop 2Apro inhibitors. Thus, it is not surprising that specific peptidic 2Apro inhibitors have not been reported to date.

As a cysteine protease, the 2Apro is sensitive to thiol alkylating reagents such as iodoacetamide and N-ethylmaleimide [25]. In addition, metal ions such as zinc have been described as a PV 2A enzyme inhibitor [25]. Inactivation of 2Apro by this thiophilic transition metal is probably through a direct binding of Zn^{++} to the active site thiol group of the protease [33]. Inhibition of the 2Apro cleavage activity by classic elastase-specific inhibitors has also been reported [24]. Methoxysuccinyl-Ala-Ala-Pro-Val-chloromethylketone (MCPMK) and elastatinal, both commercially available, could inhibit the 2Apro at low micromolar concentrations [24]. These classic serine protease inhibitors were also found to be active against viral replication in cell culture [24].

More recently, homophthalimides, originally designed to target the 3Cpro [94], have been found to inhibit HRV 2Apro activity at low micromolar concentration [98]. For example, compound 11 demonstrated an IC_{50} of 3.9 µM against HRV2 2Apro. Thus, the observed antiviral activity associated with homophthalimides might be explained as a dual inactivation of both 2Apro and 3Cpro *in vivo* [98]. Complexes formed between the 2Apro and the potent homophthalimides could be identified via mass spectrometry analysis [98], indicating that these molecules could directly interact with the enzyme. It is expected that potent compounds belonging to this group could be generated through extensive SAR studies on the basis of these initial 2Apro inhibition data [98].

4 Conclusions

The picornavirus family contains several human pathogens. These viruses are associated with human infectious diseases including acute hepatitis, common colds, and other upper respiratory tract infections. Despite the fact that effective prophylactic vaccines have been developed and used for prevention of HAV and PV infections, no satisfactory antiviral therapy or vaccine is available to date for treatment of the common cold caused by

HRVs and Coxsackie viruses, nor for the diseases caused by other viruses of the picornavirus family. The 2A and 3C proteases encoded by these viruses represent attractive targets for antiviral intervention [7, 8, 11]. The availability of purified active recombinant 2Apro and 3Cpro, success in development of convenient protease and antiviral cell culture assays, as well as our increasing understanding of their biochemical properties and structure conformation, have contributed greatly to the recent development of potent and selective protease inhibitors against picornavirus infections.

Meanwhile, since most of the picornaviral infections are generally mild [11, 107], the development of safe, inexpensive, and rapid-acting antivirals is particularly desirable. The search for clinically useful compounds against picornaviral infections has proved to be quite challenging. For example, clinical studies on the inhibitor blocking HRV attachment and uncoating process revealed that the compound displayed significant antiviral activity but no clinical benefit in treating established colds [108]. To warrant clinical development, the ideal antivirals should not only block viral replication but also diminish symptoms. It is noteworthy that the rapid progress made over the last three years is very encouraging and the first HRV protease inhibitors AG7088 has entered clinical trial. Therefore, one can remain optimistic about emergence of an effective protease inhibitor for treatment of picornavirus infections in the near future.

Acknowledgments

The author is grateful to Drs. Joe Colacino, Beverly Heinz, and Tony Zhang for helpful comments and critical reading of the manuscript.

References

1   Roeckert R.R., in: B.N. Fields et al. (eds.): Fields Virology. Raven Publishers, Philadelphia 1996, 609–654.

2   Melnick J.L., in: B.N. Fields et al. (eds.): Fields Virology. Raven Publishers, Philadelphia 1996, 655–712.

3   Couch R.B., in: B.N. Fields et al. (eds.): Fields Virology. Raven Publishers, Philadelphia 1996, 713–734.

4   Hollinger F.B. and Ticehurst J.R., in: B.N. Fields et al. (eds.): Fields Virology. Raven Publishers, Philadelphia 1996, 735–782.

5   Andries K., Dewindt B., Snoeks .J, Willebrords R., Stokbroekx R. and Lewi P.J.: Antiviral Res. 1, 213–225 (1991).

6   Rossmann M.G.: Protein Sci. 3, 1712–1725 (1994).

7   Porter A.G.: J. Virol. 67, 6917–6921 (1993).

8   Palmenberg A.C.: Annu. Rev. Microbiol. 44, 603–623 (1990).

9   Stanway G.: J. Gen. Virol. 71, 2483–2501 (1990).

10   Hellen C.U.T. and Wimmer E.: Virology 187, 391–397 (1992).

11   Mills J.S.: Antiviral Chem. Chemother. 7, 281–293 (1996).

12   Guiles J.W.: Exp. Opin. Ther. Patents 7, 123–128 (1997).

13   Krausslich H.G., Nicklin M.J., Lee C.K. and Wimmer E.: Biochimie 70, 119–130 (1988).

14   Toyoda H., Nicklin M.J., Murray M.G., Anderson C.W., Dunn J.J., Studier F.W. and Wimmer E.: Cell 45, 761–770 (1986).

15   Nicklin M.J., Krausslich H.G., Toyoda H., Dunn J.J. and Wimmer E.: Proc. Natl. Acad. Sci. USA 84, 4002–4006 (1987).

16   Krausslich H.G., Nicklin M.J., Toyoda H., Etchison D. and Wimmer E.: J. Virol. 61, 2711–2718 (1987).

17   Sommergruber W., Zorn M., Blaas D., Fessl F., Volkmann P., Maurer-Fogy I., Pallai P., Merluzzi V., Matteo M., Skern T. and Kuechler E.: Virology 169, 68–77 (1989).

18   Lloyd R.E., Grubman M.J. and Ehrenfeld E.: J. Virol. 62, 4216–4223 (1988).

19   Hellen C.U.T., Fäcke M., Kräusslich H.G., Lee C.K. and Wimmer E.: J. Virol. 65, 4226–4231 (1991).

20   Liebig H.D., Ziegler E., Yan R., Hartmuth K., Klump H., Kowalski H., Blaas D., Sommergruber W., Frasel L., Lamphear B., Rhoads R., Kuechler E. and Skern T.: Biochemistry 32, 7581–7588 (1993).

21   Sommergruber W., Ahorn H., Klump H., Seipelt J., Zoephel A., Fessl F., Krystek E., Blaas D., Kuechler E., Liebig HD. and Skern T.: Virology 198, 741–745 (1994).

22   Davies M.V., Pelletier J., Meerovitch K., Sonenberg N. and Kaufman R.J.: J. Biol. Chem. 266, 14714–14720 (1991).

23   Novoa I., Martinez-Abarca F., Fortes P., Ortin J. and Carrasco L.: Biochemistry 36, 7802–7809 (1997).

24   Molla A., Hellen C.U.T. and Wimmer E.: J. Virol. 67, 4688–4695 (1993).

25   König H. and Rosenwirth B.: J. Virol. 62, 1243–1250 (1988).

26   Bazan J.F. and Fletterick R.J.: Proc. Natl. Acad. Sci. USA 85, 7872–7876 (1988).

27   Cheah K.C., Leong L.E. and Porter A.G.: J. Biol. Chem. 265, 7180–7187 (1990).

28   Yu S.F. and Llyod R.E.: Virology 182, 615–625 (1991).

29   Sommergruber W., Seipelt J., Fessl F., Skern T., Liebig H.D. and Casari G.: Virology 234, 203–214 (1997).

30   Yu S.F., Benton P., Bovee M., Sessions J. and Lloyd R.E.: J. Virol. 69, 247–252 (1995).

31   Aldabe R., Feduchi E., Novoa I. and Carrasco L.: FEBS Lett. 377, 1–5 (1995).

32   Alvey J.C., Wyckoff E.E., Yu S.F., Lloyd R. and Ehrenfeld E.: J. Virol. 65, 6077–6083 (1991).

33   Wang Q.M., Johnson R.B., Cox G.A., Villarreal E.C., Churgay L.M. and Hale J.E.: J. Virol. 72, 1683–1687 (1998).

34   Voss T., Meyer R. and Sommergruber W.: Protein Sci. 4, 2526–2531 (1995).

35   Skern T., Sommergruber W., Auer H., Volkmann P., Zorn M., Liebig H.D., Fessl F., Blaas D. and Kuechler E.: Virology 181, 46–54 (1991).

36   Sommergruber W., Ahorn H., Zöphel A., Maurer-Fogy I., Fessl F., Schnorrenberg G., Liebig H.D., Blaas D., Kuechler E. and Skern T.:J. Biol. Chem. *267*, 22639–22644 (1992).

37   Wang Q.M., Sommergruber W. and Johnson R.B.: Biochem. Biophys. Res. Commun. *235*, 562–566 (1997).

38   Wang Q.M., Johnson R.B., Sommergruber W. and Shepherd T.A.: Arch. Biochem. Biophys. *356*, 12–18 (1998).

39   Falk M.M., Grigera P.R., Bergmann I.E., Zibert A., Multhaup G. and Beck E.: J. Virol. *64*, 748–756 (1990).

40   Clark M.E., Hämmerle T., Wimmer E. and Dasgupta A.: EMBO J. *10*, 2941–2947 (1991).

41   Clark M.E., Lieberman P.M., Berk A.J. and Dasgupta A.: Mol. Cell. Biol. 13, 1232–1237 (1993).

42   Joachims M., Harris K.S. and Etchison D.: Virology *211*, 451–461 (1995).

43   Yalamanchili P., Datta U. and Dasgupta A.: J. Virol. 71, 1220–1226 (1997).

44   Yalamanchili P., Weidman K. and Dasgupta A.: Virology *239*, 176–185 (1997).

45   Leong L.E.C., Walker P.A. and Porter A.G.: J. Biol. Chem. *268*, 25735–25739 (1993).

46   Walker P.A., Leong L.E.C. and Porter A.G.: J. Biol. Chem. *270*, 14510–14516 (1995).

47   Matthews D.A., Smith W.A., Ferre R.A., Codon B., Budahazi G., Sisson W., Villafranca J.E., Janson C.A., McElroy H.E., Gribskov C.L. and Worland S.: Cell *77*, 761–771 (1994).

48   Bergmann E.M., Mosimann S.C., Chernaia M.M., Malcolm B.A. and James M.N.: J. Virol. 71, 2436–2448 (1997).

49   Gorbalenya A.E., Blinov V.M. and Donchenko A.P.: FEBS Lett. *194*, 253–257 (1986).

50   Lawson M.A. and Semler B.L.: Proc. Natl. Acad. Sci. USA *88*, 9919–9923 (1991).

51   Allaire M., Chernaia M.M., Malcolm B.A. and James M.N.: Nature *369*, 72–76 (1994).

52   Malcolm B.A.: Protein Sci. *4*, 1439–1445 (1995).

53   Kean K.M., Teterina N.L., Marc D. and Girard M.: Virology *181*, 609–619 (1991).

54   Ivanoff L.A., Towatari T., Ray J., Korant B.D. and Petteway S.R. Jr.: Proc. Natl. Acad. Sci. USA *83*, 5392–5396 (1986).

55   Nicklin M.J., Harris K.S., Pallai P.V. and Wimmer E.: J. Virol. *62*, 4586–4593 (1988).

56   Libby R.T., Cosman D., Cooney M.K., Merriam J.E., March C.J. and Hopp T.P.: Biochemistry *27*, 6262–6268 (1988).

57   Takahara Y., Ando N., Kohara M., Hagino-Yamagishi K., Nomoto A., Itoh H., Numao N. and Kondo K.: Gene *79*, 249–258 (1989).

58   Knott J.A., Orr D.C., Montgomery D.S., Sullivan C.A. and Weston A.: Eur. J. Biochem. *182*, 547–555 (1989).

59   Aschauer B., Werner G., McCray J., Rosenwirth B. and Bachmayer H.: Virology *184*, 587–594 (1991).

60   Baum E.Z., Bebernitz G.A., Palant O., Mueller T. and Plotch S.J.: Virology *185*, 140–150 (1991).

61   Malcolm B.A., Chin S.M., Jewell D.A., Stratton-Thomas J.R., Thudium K.B., Ralston R. and Rosenberg S.: Biochemistry *31*, 3358–3363 (1992).

62   Miyashita K., Kusumi M., Utsumi R., Komano T. and Satoh N.: Biosci. Biotechnol. Biochem. *56*, 746–750 (1992).

63   Harmon S.A., Updike W., Jia X.Y., Summers D.F. and Ehrenfeld E.: J. Virol. *66*, 5242–5247 (1992).

64   Birch G.M., Black T., Malcolm S.K., Lai M.T., Zimmerman R.E. and Jaskunas S.R.: Protein Expr. Purif. *6*, 609–618 (1995).

65   Davis G.J., Wang Q.M., Cox G.A., Johnson R.B., Wakulchik M., Dotson C.A. and Villarreal E.C.: Arch. Biochem. Biophys. *346*, 125–130 (1997).

66   Cordingley M.G., Register R.B., Callahan P.L., Garsky V.M. and Colonno R.J.: J. Virol. *63*, 5037–5045 (1989).

67   Orr D.C., Long A.C., Kay J., Dunn B.M. and Cameron J.M.: J. Gen. Virol. *70*, 2931–2942 (1989).

68   Cordingley M.G., Callahan P.L., Sardana V.V., Garsky V.M. and Colonno R.J.: J. Biol. Chem. *265*, 9062–9065 (1990).

69   Hopkins J.L., Betageri R., Cohen K.A., Emmanuel M.J., Joseph C.R., Bax P.M., Pallai P.V. and Skoog M.T.: J. Biochem. Biophys. Methods *23*, 107–113 (1991).

70   McCall J.O., Kadam S. and Katz L.: BioTechnology *12*, 1012–1016 (1994).

71   Heinz B.A., Tang J., Iabus J.M., Chadwell F.W., Kaldor S.W. and Hammond M.: Antimicro. Agents & Chemother. *40*, 267–270 (1996).

72   Wang Q.M., Johnson R.B., Cox G.A., Villarreal E.C. and Loncharich R.J.: Anal. Biochem. *252*, 238–245 (1997).

73   Wang Q.M., Johnson R.B., Cohen J.D., Voy G.T., Richardson J.M. and Jungheim L.N.: Antiviral Chem. Chemother. *8*, 303–310 (1997).

74   Blair W.S. and Semler B.L.: J. Virol. *65*, 6111–6123 (1991).

75   Miyashita K., Okunishi J., Utsumi R., Komano T., Tamura T. and Satoh N.: Biosci. Biotechnol. Biochem. *60*, 705–707 (1996).

76   Kaldor S.W., Hammond M., Dressman B.A., Labus J.M., Chadwell F.W., Kline A.D. and Heinz B.A.: Bioorg. Med. Chem. Lett. *5*, 2021–2026 (1995).

77   Shepherd T.A., Cox G.A., McKinney E., Tang J., Wakulchik M., Zimmerman R.E. and Villarreal E.C.: Bioorg. Med. Chem. Lett. *6*, 2893–2896 (1996).

78   Webber S.E., Okano K., Little T.L., Reich S.H., Xin Y., Fuhrman S.A., Matthews D.A., Love R.A., Hendrickson T.F., Patick A.K. et al.: J Med. Chem. *41*, 2786–2805 (1998).

79   Jia X.Y., Ehrenfeld E. and Summers D.F.: J. Virol. *65*, 2595–2600 (1991).

80   Petithory J.R., Masiarz F.R., Kirsch J.F., Santi D.V. and Malcolm B.A.: Proc. Natl. Acad. Sci. USA *88*, 11510–11514 (1991).

81   Jewell D.A., Swietnicki W., Dunn B.M. and Malcolm B.A.: Biochemistry *31*, 7862–7869 (1992).

82   Schultheiss T., Sommergruber W., Kusov Y. and Gauss-Muller V.: J. Virol. *69*, 1727–1733 (1995).

83   Malcolm B.A., Lowe C., Shechosky S., McKay R.T., Yang C.C., Shah V.J., Simon R.J., Vederas J.C. and Santi D.V.: Biochemistry. *34*, 8172–8179 (1995).

84   Hanzlik R.P. and Thompson S.A.: J. Med. Chem. *27*, 711–712 (1984).

85   Liu S. and Hanzlik R.P.: J. Med. Chem. *35*, 1067–1075 (1992).

86   Kong J.S., Venkatraman S., Furness K., Nimkar S., Shepherd T.A., Wang Q.M., Aube J. and Hanzlik R.P.: J. Med. Chem. *41*, 2579–2587 (1998).

87   Dragovich P.S., Webber S.E., Babine R.E., Fuhrman S.A., Patick A.K., Matthews D.A., Lee C.A., Reich S.H., Prins T.J., Marakovits J.T. et al.: J. Med. Chem. *41*, 2806–2818 (1998).

88   Dragovich P.S., Webber S.E., Babine R.E., Fuhrman S.A., Patick A.K., Matthews D.A., Reich S.H., Marakovits J.T., Prins T.J., Zhou R et al.: J. Med. Chem. *41*, 2819–2834 (1998).

89   Dragovich P.S., Webber S.E., Prins T.J., Zhou R., Marakovits J.T., Tikhe J.G., Fuhrman S.A., Patick A.K., Matthews D.A., Ford C.E. et al.: Bioorg. Med. Chem. Lett. *9*, 2189– 2194 (1999).

90   Dragovich P.S., Prins T.J., Zhou R., Fuhrman S.A., Patick A.K., Matthews D.A., Ford C.E., Meador J.W. III, Ferre R.A. and Worland S.T.: J. Med. Chem. 42, 1203–1212 (1999).

91   Dragovich P.S., Prins T.J., Zhou R., Webber S.E., Marakovits J.T., Fuhrman S.A., Patick A.K., Matthews D.A., Lee C.A., Ford C.E.: J. Med. Chem. 42, 1213–1224 (1999).

92   Patick A.K., Binford S.L., Brothers M.A., Jackson R.L., Ford C.E., Diem M.D., Maldonodo F., Dragovich P.S., Zhou R., Prins T.J. et al.: Antimicrob. Agents Chemother. 43, 2444–2450 (1999).

93   Matthews D.A., Dragovich P.S., Webber S.E., Fuhrman S.A., Patick A.K., Zalman L.S., Hendrickson T.F., Love R.A., Prins T.J., Marakovits J.T. et al.: Proc. Natl. Acad. Sci. USA 96, 11000–11007 (1999).

94   Lall M.S., Malcolm B.A. and Vederas J.C.: Inhibitors of hepatitis A virus 3C proteinase. ACS annual meeting, A243 (1998).

95   Sham H.L., Rosenbrook W., Kati W., Betebenner D.A., Wideburg N.E., Saldivar A., Plattner J.J. and Norbeck D.W.: J. Chem. Soc. Perkin. Trans. I, 1081–1082 (1995).

96   Kati W.M., Sham H.L., McCall J.O., Montgomery D.A., Wang G.T., Rosenbrook W., Miesbauer L., Buke A., and Norbeck D.W.: Arch. Biochem. Biophys. 362, 363–375 (1999).

97   Venkatraman S., Kong J., NimKar S., Wang Q.M., Aube J. and Hanzlik R.P.: Bioorg. Med. Chem. Lett. 9, 577–580 (1999).

98   Morris T.S., Frormann S., Shechosky S., Lowe C., Lall M.S., Gauss-Muller V., Purcell R.H., Emerson S.U., Vederas J.C. and Malcolm B.A.: Bioorg. Med. Chem. 5, 797–807 (1997).

99   Skiles J.W. and McNeil D.: Tetrahedron Lett. 31, 7277–7280 (1990).

100   Webber S.E., Tikhe J., Worland S.T., Fuhrman S.A., Hendrickson T.F., Matthews D.A., Love R.A., Patick A.K., Meador J.W., Ferre R.A. et al.: J. Med. Chem. 39, 5072–5082 (1996).

101   Jungheim L.N., Cohen J.D., Johnson R.B., Villarreal E.C., Wakulchik M., Loncharich R.J. and Wang Q.M.: Bioorg. Med. Chem. Lett. 7, 1589–1594 (1997).

102   Lall M.S., Karvellas C. and Vederas J.C.: Organic Lett. 1, 803–806 (1999).

103   Singh S.B., Cordingley M.G., Ball R.G., Smith J.L., Dombrowski A.W. and Goetz M.A.: Tetrahedron Lett. 32, 5279–5282 (1991).

104   Kadam S., Podding J., Humphrey P.E., Karwowski J.P., Jackson M., Tennent S., Fung L., Hochlowski J., Rasmussen R. and McAlpine J.B.: J. Antibiotics. 46, 836–839 (1994).

105   Brill G.M., Kati W.M., Montgomery D., Karwowski J.P., Humphrey P.E., Jackson M., Clement J.J., Kadam S., Chen R.H. and McAlpine J.B.: J. Antibiotics. 49, 541–546 (1996).

106   Wang Q.M., Johnson R.B., Jungheim L.N., Cohen J.D. and Villarreal E.C.: Antimicrob. Agents Chemother. 42, 916–920 (1998).

107   Korant B.D., Towatari T., Ivanoff L., Patteway S., Brzin J., Lenarcic B. and Turk V.: J. Cell Biochem. 32, 91–95 (1996).

108   Hayden F.G., Hipskind G.J., Woerner D.H., Eisen G.F., Janssens M., Janssen P.A.J. and Andries K.: Antimicro. Agents Chemother. 39, 290–294 (1995).

Protease inhibitors as potential antiviral agents

Index